Recommended Dietary Allowances

10th Edition

Subcommittee on the Tenth Edition of the RDAs
Food and Nutrition Board
Commission on Life Sciences
National Research Council

NATIONAL ACADEMY PRESS
Washington, D.C.   1989

NATIONAL ACADEMY PRESS • 2101 CONSTITUTION AVE., NW • WASHINGTON, DC 20418

NOTICE: The project that is the subject of this report was approved by the Governing Board of the National Research Council, whose members are drawn from the councils of the National Academy of Sciences, the National Academy of Engineering, and the Institute of Medicine. The members of the committee responsible for the report were chosen for their special competences and with regard for appropriate balance. This report has been reviewed by a group other than the authors according to procedures approved by a Report Review Committee consisting of members of the National Academy of Sciences, the National Academy of Engineering, and the Institute of Medicine.

The study summarized in this report was supported by funds from the National Institutes of Health, United States Public Health Service, through Contract Nos. NO1-AM-0-2204 and NO1-DK-8-2236.

Library of Congress Cataloging-in-Publication

National Research Council (U.S.). Subcommittee on the Tenth Edition
of the RDAs.
    Recommended dietary allowances / Subcommittee on the Tenth Edition
of the RDAs, Food and Nutrition Board, Commission on Life Sciences,
National Research Council.—10th rev. ed.
        p.   cm.
    Rev. ed. of: Recommended dietary allowances / Committee on Dietary
Allowances, Food and Nutrition Board, Division of Biological
Sciences, Assembly of Life Sciences. National Research Council, 9th
rev. ed. 1980.
    Supported by funds from the National Institute of Health, United
States Public Health Service, contract no: NO1-DK-8-2236.
    Includes bibliographical references.
    ISBN 0-309-04041-8
    1. Nutrition.   2. Diet.   I. National Institutes of Health (U.S.)
II. National Research Council (U.S.). Committee on Dietary
Allowances. Recommended dietary allowances.   III. Title.
TX551.N393   1989
613.2'8—dc20
DNLM/DLC
for library of Congress   89-13176
                                                                       CIP

Printed in the United States of America

FOOD AND NUTRITION BOARD
SUBCOMMITTEE ON THE TENTH EDITION OF THE RDAS

RICHARD J. HAVEL *(Chairman)*, Cardiovascular Research Institute, University of California, San Francisco, California

DORIS H. CALLOWAY, Department of Nutritional Sciences, University of California, Berkeley, California

JOAN D. GUSSOW, Department of Nutrition Education, Teachers College, Columbia University, New York, New York

WALTER MERTZ, Human Nutrition Research Center, Agricultural Research Service, U.S. Department of Agriculture, Beltsville, Maryland

MALDEN C. NESHEIM, Provost, Cornell University, Ithaca, New York

Food and Nutrition Board Staff
SUSHMA PALMER, *Director*
PAUL R. THOMAS, *Program Officer*
FRANCES M. PETER, *Editor*
ALDON GRIFFIS, *Research Assistant*
MARIAN F. MILLSTONE, *Research Assistant*

The Food and Nutrition Board wishes to acknowledge the contributions of the Committee on Dietary Allowances that worked on the tenth edition from 1980 to 1985. The committee was chaired by the late Henry Kamin of Duke University Medical Center. Other members of the committee were Philip Farrell (University of Wisconsin, Madison), Helen A. Guthrie (Pennsylvania State University), Victor Herbert (Veterans Administration Medical Center, Bronx, New York), Robert Hodges (University of California, Irvine Medical Center), Max K. Horwitt (St. Louis University School of Medicine), Orville Levander (U.S. Department of Agriculture), Hellen Linkswiler (deceased; University of Wisconsin, Madison), James A. Olson (Iowa State University), and Peter L. Pellett (University of Massachusetts, Amherst). The Food and Nutrition Board staff included Myrtle L. Brown (executive secretary until August 1983), Sushma Palmer (director from July 1983), Linda D. Myers (project director), Frances M. Peter (editor), Marianne E. La Veille (research associate), and secretaries Susan Barron, Shirley E. Cole, Avis I. Harris, and Janie B. Marshall.

FOOD AND NUTRITION BOARD

iv

COMMISSION ON LIFE SCIENCES

The National Academy of Sciences is a private, nonprofit, self-perpetuating society of distinguished scholars engaged in scientific and engineering research, dedicated to the furtherance of science and technology and to their use for the general welfare. Upon the authority of the charter granted to it by the Congress in 1863, the Academy has a mandate that requires it to advise the federal government on scientific and technical matters. Dr. Frank Press is president of the National Academy of Sciences.

The National Academy of Engineering was established in 1964, under the charter of the National Academy of Sciences, as a parallel organization of outstanding engineers. It is autonomous in its administration and in the selection of its members, sharing with the National Academy of Sciences the responsibility for advising the federal government. The National Academy of Engineering also sponsors engineering programs aimed at meeting national needs, encourages education and research, and recognizes the superior achievements of engineers. Dr. Robert M. White is president of the National Academy of Engineering.

The Institute of Medicine was established in 1970 by the National Academy of Sciences to secure the services of eminent members of appropriate professions in the examination of policy matters pertaining to the health of the public. The Institute acts under the responsibility given to the National Academy of Sciences by its congressional charter to be an adviser to the federal government and, upon its own initiative, to identify issues of medical care, research, and education. Dr. Samuel O. Thier is president of the Institute of Medicine.

The National Research Council was organized by the National Academy of Sciences in 1916 to associate the broad community of science and technology with the Academy's purposes of furthering knowledge and advising the federal government. Functioning in accordance with general policies determined by the Academy, the Council has become the principal operating agency of both the National Academy of Sciences and the National Academy of Engineering in providing services to the government, the public, and the scientific and engineering communities. The Council is administered jointly by both Academies and the Institute of Medicine. Dr. Frank Press and Dr. Robert M. White are chairman and vice chairman, respectively, of the National Research Council.

Preface

This tenth edition of the *Recommended Dietary Allowances* (RDAs) reflects the work of two panels of the Food and Nutrition Board. The first, the Committee on Dietary Allowances, was appointed in 1980 and by 1985 had prepared a draft of this edition that, after an outside review overseen by the Report Review Committee of the National Research Council (NRC), was postponed for further consideration (Press, 1985). The second panel, a subcommittee of the Food and Nutrition Board (FNB) itself, was appointed in 1987 to complete this, the tenth edition of the RDAs.

The FNB subcommittee began work in June 1987 under sponsorship of the National Institute of Diabetes, Digestive, and Kidney Diseases. Throughout its efforts, the subcommittee was keenly aware of the breadth of expertise needed to address its charge. Accordingly, after establishing criteria for developing RDAs that would be applied across nutrients, the subcommittee held special meetings with invited experts on several nutrients and consulted widely on difficult-to-resolve issues and on the importance of new scientific data. Although the subcommittee sought the advice of others and considered the critiques of outside reviewers, it takes full responsibility for the recommendations and for any errors that may have escaped its attention.

This report has been approved by the Food and Nutrition Board and the NRC Report Review Committee. Both are satisfied that the tenth edition reflects a concurrence of scientific opinion and will be appropriate for use by governmental and private agencies as a basis for developing nutrition programs and policies pertaining to public health.

The subcommittee thanks the many consultants who provided advice and help in revising the draft report: Drs. John G. Bieri, Gladys Block, George M. Briggs (deceased), C. Wayne Callaway, Kenneth J. Carpenter, Frank Chytil, William E. Connor, Steven Cummings, Peter R. Dallman, Stanley N. Gershoff, DeWitt S. Goodman, J.-P. Habicht, Phillip Harvey, Michael N. Kazarinoff, Janet C. King, Orville A. Levander, Sheldon Margen, Velimir Matkovic, Donald B. McCormick, Dennis Miller, Curtis D. Morris, Suzanne Murphy, Susan M. Oace, Robert R. Recker, Floyd C. Rector, Jerry M. Rivers, Howerde E. Sauberlich, Ruth Schwartz, Barry Shane, E.L. Robert Stokstad, John W. Suttie, Barbara A. Underwood, Robert H. Wasserman, and Regina Ziegler. We also wish to thank the members of the Board's Committee on Nutritional Status During Pregnancy and Lactation and its three subcommittees, whose members reviewed and commented on this report.

The subcommittee is also grateful to Dr. Alvin G. Lazen of the Commission on Life Sciences and to the staff of the Food and Nutrition Board for their help during various phases of our work: Dr. Sushma Palmer, Frances Peter, Aldon Griffis, Marian Millstone, Marion Ramsey Roberts, Sandra Johnson, Molly McGlade, and especially Dr. Paul R. Thomas for his able support to the subcommittee throughout the study.

Richard J. Havel, *Chairman*
Food and Nutrition Board and
the Subcommittee on the Tenth
Edition of the RDAs

REFERENCE

Press, F. 1985. Postponement of the 10th edition of the RDAs. J. Am. Diet. Assoc. 85:1644–1645.

Contents

Recommended Dietary Allowances

10th Edition

1
Summary

Recommended Dietary Allowances (RDAs) have been prepared by the Food and Nutrition Board since 1941. The first edition was published in 1943 to provide "standards to serve as a goal for good nutrition." Because RDAs are intended to reflect the best scientific judgment on nutrient allowances for the maintenance of good health and to serve as the basis for evaluating the adequacy of diets of groups of people, the initial publication has been revised periodically to incorporate new scientific knowledge and interpretations. This is the tenth edition.

RDAs are defined in Chapter 2 as *the levels of intake of essential nutrients that, on the basis of scientific knowledge, are judged by the Food and Nutrition Board to be adequate to meet the known nutrient needs of practically all healthy persons*. This definition has remained essentially unchanged since 1974 (eighth edition). Individuals with special nutritional needs are not covered by the RDAs.

In principle, RDAs are based on various kinds of evidence: (1) studies of subjects maintained on diets containing low or deficient levels of a nutrient, followed by correction of the deficit with measured amounts of the nutrient; (2) nutrient balance studies that measure nutrient status in relation to intake; (3) biochemical measurements of tissue saturation or adequacy of molecular function in relation to nutrient intake; (4) nutrient intakes of fully breastfed infants and of apparently healthy people from their food supply; (5) epidemiological observations of nutrient status in populations in relation to intake; and (6) in some cases, extrapolation of data from animal experiments. In practice, there are only limited data on which estimates of nutrient requirements can be based.

1

In preparing this tenth edition of the RDAs, the subcommittee operated from the general assumption that modifications to the RDAs are justified mainly on the basis of substantive new information or where there were inconsistencies in the way evidence was evaluated in previous editions. The subcommittee reviewed the scientific literature published since the ninth edition as well as older studies on which the previous RDAs were based in cases where it was deemed important to reexamine the original data. For most nutrients, RDAs were established by first estimating the average physiological requirement for an absorbed nutrient. The subcommittee exercised judgment in adjusting this value by factors to compensate for incomplete utilization and to encompass the variation both in the requirements among individuals and in the bioavailability among the food sources of the nutrient. Therefore, the RDAs provide a safety factor appropriate to each nutrient and exceed the actual requirements of most individuals. The RDA for energy, however, reflects the mean population requirement for each group, since consumption of energy at a level intended to cover the variation in energy needs among individuals could lead to obesity in most persons.

MAJOR REVISIONS IN THE TENTH
EDITION AND THEIR BASES

The Summary Table in the back of this book summarizes the RDAs established by the subcommittee. It contains several changes that reflect advances in scientific knowledge in the past 9 years or new interpretations of data by the subcommittee. Changes include the following:

Age Groupings   Because peak bone mass is probably not attained before age 25 years, the age class of 19 to 22 years has been extended through age 24 for both sexes.

Reference Individuals   Heights and weights of reference adults in each age-sex class are the actual medians for the U.S. population of the designated age, as reported in the second National Health and Nutrition Examination Survey (NHANES II). In the previous edition, reference heights and weights were set at an arbitrary ideal. Therefore, differences from the ninth edition in allowances for nutrients based on body weight may simply reflect the difference in reference body weights.

Nutrients   RDAs for women during pregnancy and lactation are tabulated as absolute figures rather than as additions to the basic allowances. This is a convenience and reflects the subcommittee's judgment as to the precision with which the additional costs of reproduction and lactation are known. RDAs during lactation are now provided for the first and second 6-month periods to reflect the differences in the amount of milk produced (750 ml and 600 ml, respectively). In the ninth edition, a single allowance was provided throughout lactation based on secretion of 850 ml of milk. RDAs for infants who are not breastfed are based primarily on the amounts of nutrients provided by 750 ml (rather than 850 ml) of human milk plus an additional 25% (a result of adding 2 standard deviations) to allow for variance. In the ninth edition, allowances during the first 6 months of life did not include a consistent increment for individual variability.

Recommended Dietary Allowances

RDAs for some nutrients remain unchanged or were revised only slightly from the ninth edition. The following are major changes in this edition:

Energy Because reference weights are now actual medians rather than arbitrary ideals, the allowances are not directly comparable with values in the previous edition. Recommended allowances for adults were calculated by using empirically derived equations recently developed by the Food and Agriculture Organization for estimating resting energy expenditure and then multiplying the results by an activity factor representing light-to-moderate activity. Energy allowances range from 2,300 to 2,900 kcal/day for adult men and 1,900 to 2,200 kcal/day for adult women. Energy allowances in this edition and the previous one are similar, despite the different methods used to derive them.

Protein Protein allowances for adults are based on nitrogen balance studies, as recently recommended by the Food and Agriculture Organization, rather than on the factorial method used in the past. Despite this difference in the derivation of RDAs, the allowance for adult men and women remains at 0.8 g/kg of body weight per day. The increment estimated for pregnancy is reduced from 30 to 10 g/day; this revision is more heavily influenced by theory of nitrogen gain and efficiency with which dietary protein is converted to fetal, placental, and maternal tissues than by new evidence.

Vitamin K RDAs for vitamin K are established for the first time in this edition; they are based on recently published work. The RDA for adults and children is set at approximately 1 μg/kg of body weight. There is no recommended increment during pregnancy and lactation, because the effects of pregnancy on vitamin K requirements are unknown and lactation imposes little additional need for this nutrient.

Vitamin C   Allowances for vitamin C are largely unchanged from the ninth edition; for example, the RDA for adults of both sexes remains at 60 mg/day. An increment of 10 mg/day has been added for pregnant women to offset losses from the mother's body pool to the fetus; this is half the increment recommended in the previous edition. The subcommittee recommends that regular cigarette smokers ingest at least 100 mg of vitamin C per day, since smoking seems to increase metabolic turnover of the vitamin, leading to lower concentrations in the blood.

Vitamin B_6   An RDA of 0.016 mg of vitamin B_6 per gram of protein appears to ensure acceptable values for most indices of nutritional status in adults of both sexes; in the ninth edition, the RDA was 0.020 mg of vitamin B_6 per gram of protein. The RDA is established in relation to the upper boundary of acceptable levels of protein intake, i.e., twice the RDA for protein. The resulting vitamin B_6 allowances of 2.0 and 1.6 mg/day for adult men and women, respectively, are lower than those in the previous edition.

Folate   Folate allowances in this edition are much lower (often by 50% or more) than those in the ninth edition for all the age-sex groups. The basis for lowering the RDA is the recognition that diets containing about half the previous RDA maintain adequate folate status and liver stores. The folate allowance of approximately 3 μg/ kg body weight for adults and adolescents translates to 200 μg/day for the adult male and 180 μg/day for the adult female—an amount typically consumed in the United States and Canada by adults who show no evidence of poor folate status. During pregnancy, the RDA for folate is 400 μg/day—half the RDA in the ninth edition. The subcommittee considers this amount sufficient to build or maintain maternal folate stores and to support rapidly growing tissue.

Vitamin B_{12}   Vitamin B_{12} allowances in this edition are one-third to one-half lower than those in the ninth edition for all the age-sex groups. For example, the RDA for adults and adolescents of both sexes is now 2 rather than 3 μg/day and for children 1 to 10 years ranges from 0.7 to 1.4 rather than 2 to 3 μg/day. Reductions are based on recent data suggesting that the new allowances adequately sustain metabolic function and allow for biological variation, the maintenance of normal serum concentrations, and the build up or maintenance of substantial body stores; the latter is especially desirable in view of the increased prevalence of achlorhydria (which diminishes vitamin B_{12} absorption) and pernicious anemia beyond age 60.

Calcium In the ninth edition, the RDA for calcium for all adolescents was set at 1,200 mg/day to age 18, the approximate age at which longitudinal bone growth ceases. However, because peak bone mass is probably not attained before age 25, the subcommittee has extended this allowance through age 24 to promote full mineral deposition. For older ages, the allowance of 800 mg in the ninth edition is maintained. The subcommittee believes the most promising nutritional approach to reducing the risk of osteoporosis in later life is to ensure a calcium intake that allows the development of each individual's genetically programmed peak bone mass. It urges that special attention be paid to calcium intakes throughout childhood to age 25 years. The subcommittee emphasizes that the RDAs for calcium do not address the possible increased needs of persons who may have osteoporosis and should receive medical attention. RDAs for phosphorus parallel those for calcium except in infancy. In addition, the allowance for vitamin D, which promotes calcium absorption, is maintained at 10 μg/day throughout childhood to age 25 years.

Magnesium Increments of magnesium during pregnancy and lactation are far lower than in previous editions (reduced to $+20$ from $+150$ mg/day during pregnancy and to $+75$ and $+60$ from $+150$ mg/day during lactation); these amounts should be sufficient to meet the needs of the fetus and maternal tissue growth and to allow for individual variation. The allowance for children of both sexes between 1 and 15 years of age is 6.0 mg/kg, an amount above the levels that were found to be sufficient to support a positive magnesium balance in adolescent boys and girls. This allowance translates into RDAs for children that are considerably lower than the RDAs in the ninth edition, especially for preadolescent children.

Iron In setting RDAs for iron, it was the subcommittee's judgment that a dietary intake that achieves a target level of 300 mg of iron stores meets the nutritional needs of all healthy people, since, over several months, this level of stores provides for the iron needs of a person consuming a diet nearly devoid of iron. Using population-based data on iron intakes and status, turnover data, estimates of variability of iron losses among individuals, and distribution analysis, the subcommittee concluded that an RDA of 15 mg/day should meet the needs of essentially all healthy adolescent and adult women following usual dietary patterns and should provide a sufficient margin of safety. This allowance is a reduction from the 18 mg/day recommended in the ninth edition. The allowance for adult men and postmenopausal women remains at 10 mg/day.

A daily iron increment of 15 mg/day averaged over the entire pregnancy should be sufficient to meet maternal and fetal needs. Daily iron supplements are usually recommended, since the total need cannot be met by the iron content of habitual U.S. diets or by the iron stores of at least some women. No additional allowance of iron is recommended during lactation, since losses of iron in milk are less than menstrual loss, which is often absent during lactation. In contrast, the ninth edition recommended the continued use of the iron supplements prescribed during pregnancy for 2 to 3 months after birth to replenish iron stores.

The RDAs for iron are adequate for essentially all healthy people who daily consume diets containing 30 to 90 g of meat, poultry, or fish (containing highly absorbable heme iron) or foods containing 25 to 75 mg of ascorbate after preparation (to improve absorption of nonheme iron). People who eat little or no animal protein and whose diets are low in ascorbate may require higher amounts of food iron or vitamin C.

Zinc   In the ninth edition, the RDA for adults of both sexes was set at 15 mg/day. In the present edition, the allowance remains at 15 mg/day for adult men, but is reduced to 12 mg/day for adult women on the basis of their lower body weight.

Selenium   RDAs for selenium, established for the first time in this edition, are based on recent studies of Chinese men. The ninth edition provided a safe and adequate range for selenium intake, which for adults was 50 to 200 µg/day. In the present edition, the RDA for selenium in adults is set at 70 µg/day for men and 55 µg/day for women. RDAs for infants, children, and adolescents are extrapolated from adult values on the basis of body weight, and a factor is added for growth.

Estimated Safe and Adequate Daily Dietary Intakes

The ninth edition established a category of safe and adequate intakes for essential nutrients when data were sufficient to estimate a range of requirements, but insufficient for developing an RDA. This category, together with the caution that upper levels in the safe and adequate range should not be habitually exceeded because the toxic level for many trace elements may be only several times usual intakes, is maintained in the present edition. The table that includes this group of nutrients is similar to the corresponding table in the ninth edition, but incorporates several changes reflecting advances in scientific knowledge or new interpretations of data by the subcommittee.

Since vitamin K and selenium have been advanced to RDA status, they have been moved to the main Summary Table. Safe and adequate ranges are no longer provided for sodium, potassium, and chloride, since they are difficult to justify. Estimated minimum requirements for these electrolytes are provided for healthy persons at various ages (see Chapter 11). Minimum sodium requirements are estimated to range from 120 mg in the first 6 months of life to 500 mg/day in adulthood, and to increase during pregnancy and lactation; there is no known advantage in consuming large amounts of sodium and clear disadvantages for those susceptible to hypertension. Potassium requirements are estimated to range from 500 mg/day in early infancy to 2,000 mg/day in adulthood. Dietary recommendations for increased intake of fruits and vegetables, made in the recent Food and Nutrition Board report entitled *Diet and Health,* would yield a potassium intake of approximately 3,500 mg/day for adults—a level that could reduce the prevalence of hypertension and stroke.

Biotin In this edition, the estimated ranges of safe and adequate intakes for biotin are much lower for all age-sex groups than in the ninth edition (e.g., 30 to 100 µg/day for adolescents and adults compared to 100 to 200 µg/day). Improved analytical methods for biotin have reduced the estimates of daily intakes that are compatible with good health.

Copper Recent data on whole body surface losses of copper, along with data on urinary and fecal losses, indicate that a total dietary copper intake of approximately 1.6 mg/day is required to maintain balance in adult men. Therefore, 1.5 to 3 mg/day is recommended as a safe and adequate range of intake for adults and adolescents—a wider range than the 2 to 3 mg/day recommended in the ninth edition.

Manganese In this edition, a manganese intake of 2 to 5 mg/day is recommended for adolescents and adults of both sexes. This is a wider range of safe and adequate intakes compared to the range of 2.5 to 5 mg/day in the ninth edition. Since current dietary intakes of manganese appear to satisfy requirements, a recent survey showing the mean manganese intake of 2.7 and 2.2 mg for adult men and women, respectively, provides justification for the change.

Molybdenum   The estimated safe and adequate range of molybdenum intake for adults and adolescents of 75 to 250 µg/day is based on average reported intakes; the ranges for other age groups are derived from extrapolation on the basis of body weight. These provisional intakes are half the amounts recommended in the ninth edition, which were based on human balance studies; the present subcommittee believes these studies are inappropriate to use in estimating requirements for trace elements.

USES AND IMPLICATIONS OF THE RDAs

Over the years, RDAs have become widely known and applied. They are typically used for planning and procuring food supplies for population subgroups, for interpreting food consumption records of individuals and populations, for establishing standards for food assistance programs, for evaluating the adequacy of food supplies in meeting national nutritional needs, for designing nutrition education programs, and for developing new products in industry. The seventh edition of the RDAs (published in 1968) became the basis for establishing guidelines for the nutritional labeling of foods (known as the U.S. Recommended Daily Allowances, or USRDAs).

Because of the wide use of the RDAs, it is important to understand their appropriate applications and limitations. These are discussed in Chapter 2. Three points are of particular importance:

• The recommended allowances for nutrients are amounts intended to be consumed as part of a normal diet. If the RDAs are met through diets composed of a variety of foods derived from diverse food groups rather than by supplementation or fortification, such diets will likely be adequate in all other nutrients for which RDAs cannot currently be established.

• RDAs are neither minimal requirements nor necessarily optimal levels of intake. It is not possible at this time to establish optima. Rather, RDAs are safe and adequate levels (incorporating margins of safety intended to be sufficiently generous to encompass the presumed variability in requirement among people) reflecting the state of knowledge concerning a nutrient, its bioavailability, and variations among the U.S. population.

• Although RDAs are most appropriately applied to groups, a comparison of individual intakes, averaged over a sufficient length of time, to the RDA allows an estimate to be made about the probable risk of deficiency for that individual.

The subcommittee reemphasizes that RDAs can typically be met or closely approximated by diets that are based on the consumption of a variety of foods from diverse food groups that contain adequate energy. Such diets are entirely consistent with the type of dietary patterns advocated in the Food and Nutrition Board's report entitled *Diet and Health* to promote health and reduce risks of developing major chronic diseases. Together, the RDAs and the *Diet and Health* recommendations should be considered the appropriate basis for diet planning.

2

Definition and Applications

Recommended Dietary Allowances (RDAs) are the levels of intake of essential nutrients that, on the basis of scientific knowledge, are judged by the Food and Nutrition Board to be adequate to meet the known nutrient needs of practically all healthy persons.

The first edition of the *Recommended Dietary Allowances* (RDAs) was published in 1943 during World War II with the objective of "providing standards to serve as a goal for good nutrition." It defined, in "accordance with newer information, the recommended daily allowances for the various dietary essentials for people of different ages" (NRC, 1943). The origin of the RDAs[a] has been described in detail by the chairman of the first Committee on Recommended Dietary Allowances (Roberts, 1958). The initial publication has been revised at regular intervals; this is the tenth edition.

From their original application as a guide for advising "on nutrition problems in connection with national defense," RDAs have come to serve other purposes: for planning and procuring food supplies for population subgroups; for interpreting food consumption records of individuals and populations; for establishing standards for food assistance programs; for evaluating the adequacy of food supplies in

---

[a]Recommended Dietary Allowances (RDAs) should not be confused with U.S. Recommended Daily Allowances (USRDAs)—a set of values derived from the 1968 RDAs by the Food and Drug Administration as standards for nutritional labeling.

10

meeting national nutritional needs; for designing nutrition education programs; for developing new products in industry; and for establishing guidelines for nutrition labeling of foods. In most cases, there are only limited data on which estimates of nutrient requirements can be based.

ESTIMATION OF PHYSIOLOGICAL REQUIREMENTS

Where possible, the subcommittee established an RDA by first estimating the average physiological requirement for an *absorbed* nutrient. It then adjusted this value by factors to compensate for incomplete utilization and to encompass the variation both in requirements among individuals and in the bioavailability of the nutrient among the food sources. Thus, there is a safety factor in the RDAs for each nutrient, reflecting the state of knowledge concerning the nutrient, its bioavailability, and variations among the U.S. population. It is the intent of the subcommittee that the RDAs be both safe and adequate, but not necessarily the highest or lowest figures that the data might justify.

There is not always agreement among experts on the criteria for determining the physiological requirement for a nutrient. The requirement for infants and children may be equated with the amount that will maintain a satisfactory rate of growth and development; for an adult, it may be equated with an amount that will maintain body weight and prevent depletion of the nutrient from the body, as judged by balance studies and maintenance of acceptable blood and tissue concentrations. For certain nutrients, the requirement may be the amount that will prevent failure of a specific function or the development of specific deficiency signs—an amount that may differ greatly from that required to maintain body stores. Thus, designation of the requirement for a given nutrient varies with the criteria chosen.

Ideally, the first step in developing a nutrient allowance would be to determine the average physiological requirement of a healthy and representative segment of each age and sex group according to stipulated criteria. Knowledge of the variability among the individuals within each group would make it possible to calculate the amount by which the average requirement must be increased to meet the need of virtually all healthy people. Unfortunately, experiments in humans are costly and time-consuming, and even under the best of conditions, only small groups can be studied in a single experiment. Moreover, certain types of experiments are not possible for ethical reasons. Thus, estimates of requirements and their variability must often be derived from limited information.

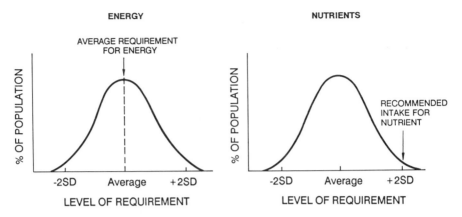

FIGURE 2-1 Distributions of requirements for energy and nutrients. SOURCE: Beaton, 1985, with permission.

If population requirements follow a normal, or Gaussian, distribution pattern (Figure 2-1), adding 2 standard deviations (SDs) to the observed mean requirement would cover the needs of most (i.e., 98%) individuals. With the possible exception of the protein requirement, however, there is little evidence that requirements for nutrients are normally distributed. The distribution of the iron requirements for women, for example, is skewed (NRC, 1986). In this report, therefore, each nutrient is treated individually to allow for variability within a population, as explained in the relevant chapters of this report.

Allowances for energy are established in a different manner than the allowances for specific nutrients. The RDA for energy reflects the mean population requirement for each age group. Energy needs vary from person to person; however, an additional allowance to cover this variation would be inappropriate because it could lead to obesity in the person with average requirements. Over the long term, a surplus of energy intake from any source is stored as fat, which may be detrimental to health.

ESTABLISHMENT OF DIETARY RECOMMENDATIONS

Recommended allowances for nutrients are amounts intended to be consumed as part of a normal diet. Therefore, it is necessary to take into account any factor that influences the absorption of food nutrients or the efficiency with which they are utilized. For some nutrients, a part of the requirement may be met by consumption of a substance that is subsequently converted within the body to the essential nutrient. For example, some carotenoids are precursors of vitamin A; since some or all of the vitamin A allowance can be met by dietary carotenoids, the efficiency with which these precursors are converted into vitamin A must be considered. The allowance for protein is expressed as if it were the RDA for a single dietary constituent. In fact, it is the sum of different requirements for several amino acids that occur in different proportions in various food proteins. For many nutrients, digestion, absorption, or both are incomplete and recommendations for dietary intake must make allowance for the portion of the ingested nutrient that is not absorbed. For example, the absorption of heme and nonheme iron differs; it is affected by other dietary components that are considered in establishing the RDA. The relative importance of such factors varies from nutrient to nutrient. Therefore, the degree to which the RDA, a *dietary* allowance, exceeds the *physiological* requirement also varies among nutrients. This is discussed in subsequent chapters.

Traditionally, RDAs have been established for essential nutrients only when data are sufficient to make reliable recommendations. The subcommittee that prepared the ninth edition of the RDAs created the category "Safe and Adequate Intakes" for nutrients with data bases insufficient for developing an RDA, but for which potentially toxic upper levels were known. In this category were three vitamins (vitamin K, biotin, and pantothenic acid), six trace elements (copper, chromium, fluoride, manganese, molybdenum, and selenium), and three electrolytes (sodium, potassium, and chloride). In this, the tenth edition, only minimal requirements are given for the electrolytes, and vitamin K and selenium have been advanced to RDA status.

HOW ARE RDAs TO BE MET?

Because there are uncertainties in the knowledge base, it is not possible to set RDAs for all the known nutrients. However, the RDAs can serve as a guide such that a varied diet meeting RDAs will probably be adequate in all other nutrients. Therefore, the subcommittee recommends that diets should be composed of a *variety* of foods that are derived from diverse food groups rather than by supplementation or fortification and that losses of nutrients during the processing and preparation of food should be taken into consideration in planning diets.

Diets of various types can be devised to meet recognized nutritional needs. However, RDAs should be provided from a selection of foods that are acceptable and palatable to ensure consumption. In addition to being a source of nutrients, food has psychological and social values that are important, although difficult to quantify.

RDAs relate to physiological requirements, where these are known. On the whole, the RDA committees tend to err on the side of generosity, since there is little evidence that small surpluses of nutrients are detrimental, whereas consistent uncompensated deficits, even small ones, over a long period can lead to deficiencies. Deficiency states in humans and animals have been reported for nutrients accorded RDA status. Such deficiencies are preventable or curable by the amounts of nutrients supplied by a well-selected diet. In the few cases where deficiency is commonly observed (e.g., iron deficiency in women), food fortification and individual supplementation are appropriate.

PHARMACOLOGIC AND TOXIC EFFECTS OF NUTRIENTS

In recent years, much attention and public interest have been focused on the possible effects of nutrients, often at high intakes, on conditions other than those associated with specific deficiencies. At higher levels of intake, both the toxicity and the pharmacological action of specific nutrients must be considered. All substances will cause harmful effects at some level of intake. For example, water or salt in excess can be lethal, large doses of vitamins A and D produce well-defined toxic syndromes, and even water-soluble vitamins (e.g., niacin and vitamin B_6) can cause adverse effects when taken in sufficiently large amounts. Several nutrients have specific therapeutic uses at high dosages (e.g., vitamin A and other retinoids are used in treating some types of skin disorders), but detrimental side effects after prolonged use. The pharmacological actions of nutrients differ in several ways from their physiological functions, namely:

• Doses greatly exceeding the amount of a nutrient present in foods are usually needed to obtain a therapeutic response.
• The specificity of the pharmacological action is often different from the physiological function.
• Chemical analogues of the nutrient that are often most effective pharmacologically may have little or no nutritional activity.

REFERENCE INDIVIDUALS

RDAs shown in the Summary Table at the end of this volume are expressed in terms of Reference Individuals in different age and sex

TABLE 2-1 Weights for Height of Adults in the United States[a]

Height cm	(in)	Weight, kg (lb)					
		Males, by percentile			Females, by percentile		
		15th	50th	85th	15th	50th	85th
147	(58)				45 (99)	55 (122)	72 (159)
152	(60)				49 (107)	60 (132)	75 (164)
157	(62)	57 (125)	64 (142)	76 (168)	51 (112)	60 (132)	77 (170)
163	(64)	58 (129)	67 (148)	79 (174)	54 (118)	63 (139)	79 (175)
168	(66)	61 (134)	71 (158)	83 (183)	55 (122)	64 (141)	81 (179)
173	(68)	65 (143)	76 (167)	88 (195)	59 (130)	67 (148)	83 (184)
178	(70)	67 (149)	79 (173)	93 (206)	61 (133)	69 (152)	78 (171)
183	(72)	73 (161)	83 (183)	99 (218)			
188	(74)	77 (171)	88 (194)	99 (217)			
193	(76)	85 (187)	103 (227)	106 (234)			

[a] Unpublished data from NHANES II (1976–1980) provided by the National Center for Health Statistics. Values rounded to nearest whole number. Subjects were ages 18 to 74 years. Height determined without shoes. Weight includes clothing weight, ranging from an estimated 0.09 to 0.28 kg (0.20 to 0.62 lb).

classes. The heights and weights of the Reference Individuals could have been set at some arbitrary ideal (e.g., 70 kg for adult men and 55 kg for adult women, as in the ninth edition). However, since weight is used as the basis for setting RDAs for many nutrients, the figures presented for adults in the Summary Table are the *actual* medians for the U.S. population of the designated age, as reported in the second National Health and Nutrition Examination Survey (NHANES II). Table 2-1 shows the actual weights for heights of adults in the United States. The use of these figures does not imply that the height-to-weight ratios for this population are ideal. The medians for those under 19 years of age were taken from Hamill et al. (1979) (Table 2-2). For groups or individuals with body mass substantially different from that of the Reference Individual, allowances can be adjusted using the median weight appropriate to the observed height.

The Summary Table in this report is similar to those in previous editions but features several changes. RDAs are now provided for the first and second 6 months of lactation to reflect the differences in the amount of milk produced. RDAs for women during pregnancy and lactation are now tabulated as absolute figures rather than as additions to the basic allowances. This is a convenience and reflects the subcommittee's judgment as to the precision with which the additional costs of reproduction and lactation are known. The RDAs displayed in the Summary Table are the sum of the RDAs for women

TABLE 2-2 Weight and Height of Males and Females Up to 18 Years in the United States[a]

Age	Males, by percentile						Females, by percentile					
	Weight, kg (lb)			Height, cm (in)			Weight, kg (lb)			Height, cm (in)		
	5th	50th	95th	5th	50th	95th	5th	50th	95th	5th	50th	95th
Months												
1	3.16	4.29 (9.4)	5.38	50.4	54.6 (21.5)	58.6	2.97	3.98 (8.8)	4.92	49.2	53.5 (21.1)	56.9
3	4.43	5.98 (13.2)	7.37	56.7	61.1 (24.1)	65.4	4.18	5.40 (11.9)	6.74	55.4	59.5 (23.4)	63.4
6	6.20	7.85 (17.3)	9.46	63.4	67.8 (26.7)	72.3	5.79	7.21 (15.9)	8.73	61.8	65.9 (25.9)	70.2
9	7.52	9.18 (20.2)	10.93	68.0	72.3 (28.5)	77.1	7.00	8.56 (18.8)	10.17	66.1	70.4 (27.7)	75.0
12	8.43	10.15 (22.3)	11.99	71.7	76.1 (30.0)	81.2	7.84	9.53 (21.0)	11.24	69.8	74.3 (29.3)	79.1
18	9.59	11.47 (25.2)	13.44	77.5	82.4 (32.4)	88.1	8.92	10.82 (23.8)	12.76	76.0	80.9 (31.9)	86.1
Years												
2	10.49	12.34 (27.1)	15.50	82.5	86.8 (34.2)	94.4	9.95	11.80 (26.0)	14.15	81.6	86.8 (34.2)	93.6
3	12.05	14.62 (32.2)	17.77	89.0	94.9 (37.4)	102.0	11.61	14.10 (31.0)	17.22	88.3	94.1 (37.0)	100.6
4	13.64	16.69 (36.7)	20.27	95.8	102.9 (40.5)	109.9	13.11	15.96 (35.1)	19.91	95.0	101.6 (40.0)	108.3
5	15.27	18.67 (41.1)	23.09	102.0	109.9 (43.3)	117.0	14.55	17.66 (38.9)	22.62	101.1	108.4 (42.7)	115.6
6	16.93	20.69 (45.5)	26.34	107.7	116.1 (45.7)	123.5	16.05	19.52 (42.9)	25.75	106.6	114.6 (45.1)	122.7
7	18.64	22.85 (50.3)	30.12	113.0	121.7 (47.9)	129.7	17.71	21.84 (48.0)	29.68	111.8	120.6 (47.5)	129.5
8	20.40	25.30 (55.7)	34.51	118.1	127.0 (50.0)	135.7	19.62	24.84 (54.6)	34.71	116.9	126.4 (49.8)	136.2
9	22.25	28.13 (61.9)	39.58	122.9	132.2 (52.0)	141.8	21.82	28.46 (62.6)	40.64	122.1	132.2 (52.0)	142.9

10	24.33	31.44 (69.2)	45.27	127.7	137.5 (54.1)	148.1	24.36	32.55 (71.6)	47.17	127.5	138.3 (54.4)	149.5		
11	26.80	35.30 (77.7)	51.47	132.6	143.3 (56.4)	154.9	27.24	36.95 (81.3)	54.00	133.5	144.8 (57.0)	156.2		
12	29.85	39.78 (87.5)	58.09	137.6	149.7 (58.9)	162.3	30.52	41.53 (91.4)	60.81	139.8	151.5 (59.6)	162.7		
13	33.64	44.95 (98.9)	65.02	142.9	156.5 (61.6)	169.8	34.14	46.10 (101.4)	67.30	145.2	157.1 (61.9)	168.1		
14	38.22	50.77 (111.7)	72.13	148.8	163.1 (64.2)	176.7	37.76	50.28 (110.6)	73.08	148.7	160.4 (63.1)	171.3		
15	43.11	56.71 (124.8)	79.12	155.2	169.0 (66.5)	181.9	40.99	53.68 (118.1)	77.78	150.5	161.8 (63.7)	172.8		
16	47.74	62.10 (136.6)	85.62	161.1	173.5 (68.3)	185.4	43.41	55.89 (123.0)	80.99	151.6	162.4 (63.9)	173.3		
17	51.50	66.31 (145.9)	91.31	164.9	176.2 (69.4)	187.3	44.74	56.69 (124.7)	82.46	152.7	163.1 (64.2)	173.5		
18	53.97	68.88 (151.5)	95.76	165.7	176.8 (69.6)	187.6	45.26	56.62 (124.6)	82.47	153.6	163.7 (64.4)	173.6		

SOURCE: Adapted from Hamill et al. (1979).

[a] Data in this table have been used to derive weight and height reference points in the present report. It is not intended that they necessarily be considered standards of normal growth and development. Data pertaining to infants 2 to 18 months of age are taken from longitudinal growth studies at Fels Research Institute. Ages are exact, and infants were measured in the recumbent position. The measurements were based on some 867 children followed longitudinally at the institute between 1929 and 1975. Data pertaining to children between 2 and 18 years of age were collected between 1962 and 1974 by the National Center for Health Statistics and involve some 20,000 individuals comprising nationally representative samples in three studies conducted between 1960 and 1974. In these studies, children were measured in the standing position with no upward pressure exerted on the mastoid processes. In the ninth edition of this report, data for children up to 6 years of age were taken from longitudinal growth studies in Iowa and Boston, where children were measured in the recumbent position. This explains the systematically smaller heights for 2- to 5-year-old children in this current table compared with those represented in previous editions. In this table, actual age is represented.

of reproductive age and increments as justified in the text. The 19- to 22-year age class in the ninth edition has been extended through 24 years for both sexes in consideration of the time required to attain peak bone mass. When extrapolating from Reference Individuals to specific population groups (e.g., military personnel), recommendations for nutrient intakes can be obtained by multiplying the number of people within the group by the RDAs for Reference Individuals, making allowances for the body sizes, age distribution, and physiological state (e.g., pregnant, lactating) of those in the group.

NUTRIENT ALLOWANCES FOR INFANTS

The starting point in estimating allowances for infants is usually the average amount of the nutrient consumed by thriving infants breastfed by healthy, well-nourished mothers. With a few exceptions, nutrients in a readily bioavailable form are present in human milk in proportions appropriate for adequate nutriture for the first 3 to 6 months of life. For this reason, RDAs for the very young infant are intended to serve as a guide for those who are not breastfed exclusively.

Since the previous edition, new data on breast milk production have emerged (e.g., Butte et al., 1984; Chandra, 1982; Hofvander et al., 1982; Neville et al., 1988). Average milk consumption for infants born at term is now accepted to be 750 ml for the first 6 months (with a coefficient of variation of approximately 12.5%), and 600 ml during the next 6 months when complementary foods are given. Maternal production is slightly higher than infant consumption, but it is subsumed within the variation. Therefore, the subcommittee accepts 750 ml and 600 ml as figures for both average milk production and consumption.

Recommendations for infants are subdivided into the first and second 6 months of life. Further subdivision of these age groups can be justified on physiological grounds, but the information base is not yet sufficient to establish nutrient allowances with such precision. RDAs for infants up to 6 months old are based primarily on the amounts of nutrients provided by 750 ml of human milk, plus an additional 25% (2 SDs) to allow for variance. RDAs during the second 6 months of life are consistent with infant feeding practices in the United States, i.e., increasing amounts of mixed solid foods are given to supplement milk or formula during that period.

NUTRIENT ALLOWANCES FOR THE ELDERLY

In this edition, as in previous editions of the RDAs, adults are divided into two age categories: 25 (or 23) to 50 years, and from 51 years upward. The subcommittee considered subdividing healthy older people into two groups, since increasing age may alter nutritional requirements due to changes in lean body mass, physical activity, and intestinal absorption. However, it concluded that data are insufficient to establish separate RDAs for people 70 years of age and older.

In applying the RDAs, one should remember that a given person may be physiologically younger or older than his or her chronological age would suggest and that it becomes increasingly difficult to define the term *healthy* with advancing age. There is some evidence that the elderly have altered requirements for some nutrients. For example, intestinal absorption, particularly of minerals, may be impaired. However, there is no evidence that an increased intake of nutrients above the RDAs is necessary, or that higher intakes will prevent the changes associated with aging.

CONDITIONS THAT MAY REQUIRE ADJUSTMENT IN APPLICATION OF RDAs

Climate

Ordinarily, adjustments made in clothing and housing protect the body against heat and cold. Therefore, adjustments in dietary allowances to compensate for environmental temperature changes rarely are necessary.

Prolonged exposure to high temperatures may reduce activity, energy expenditure, and therefore food intake. Except under extreme conditions, however, it is unlikely that this reduced food intake would greatly affect the nutriture of the individual. Sweat losses may need to be considered, as noted below.

Strenuous Physical Activity

Increased activity increases the need for energy and some nutrients. Such needs usually are met by the larger quantities of food consumed by active people, provided foods are sensibly selected.

In hot environments, activity increases water and salt losses through sweating and, if prolonged, can also lead to measurable losses of other essential nutrients. Special attention should be given to the immediate need for water under such conditions.

Clinical Considerations

RDAs apply to healthy persons. They do not cover special nutritional needs arising from metabolic disorders, chronic diseases, injuries, premature birth, other medical conditions, and drug therapies.

Data on the role of diet as a causal or contributing factor in chronic and degenerative disease lead to recommendations derived through approaches different from those used in developing RDAs for specific nutrients. Reference is made to relationships between dietary patterns and health in certain chapters; a detailed evaluation of relationships between dietary patterns and health can be found in the Food and Nutrition Board's publication *Diet and Health* (NRC, 1989) and *The Surgeon General's Report on Nutrition and Health* (DHHS, 1988).

APPLICATION OF RECOMMENDED DIETARY ALLOWANCES

Underlying all uses of the RDAs is the recognition that humans are highly adaptable. Throughout its existence, the human species has developed regulatory and storage mechanisms that permit it to survive in a variety of environments and to withstand periods of deprivation. These basic biological considerations, coupled with the fact that the RDAs include reasonable margins of safety, are the overriding considerations that should guide the user in applying the RDAs in specific situations. Experience with uses and misuses of the RDAs has indicated that certain areas require emphasis and clarification. These are discussed below.

In the Summary RDA Table at the end of this volume, nutrient intakes are expressed as quantities of a nutrient for a Reference Individual per day. However, the terms *per day* and *daily* should be interpreted as average intake over time. The length of time over which averaging should be achieved depends on the nutrient, the size of the body pool, and the rate of turnover of that nutrient. Some nutrients, such as vitamins A and B_{12}, can be stored in relatively large quantities and are degraded slowly. Others, such as thiamin, are turned over rapidly, and total deprivation in a person can lead to relatively rapid development of symptoms (i.e., in days or weeks, rather than in months). If the requirement for a nutrient is not met on a particular day, body stores or a surplus consumed shortly thereafter will compensate for the inadequacy. For most nutrients, RDAs are intended to be average intakes over at least 3 days; for others, (e.g., vitamins A and B_{12}), they may be averaged over several months.

Nutrient intake varies from day to day among individuals and for different nutrients. For example, the day-to-day variability in intake of some nutrients, such as protein and thiamin, is low, whereas vitamin A intake is highly variable. For this reason, dietary surveys that depend on single 24-hour recalls provide valid data only for the *population average* intake. A person who on one day may have consumed little of a given nutrient may on a subsequent day ingest considerably more. Only a time-averaged intake need approximate the RDA.

If a group average intake approximates that of the calculated group RDA, some persons within the group are consuming less than the RDA and others more. Except for energy, in which the average requirement of the population group is recommended, the RDAs are intended to be sufficiently generous to encompass the presumed (albeit unmeasured) variability in requirement among people. Thus, if a population's habitual intake approximates or exceeds the RDA, the probability of deficiency is quite low. Such comparisons between intake and RDA cannot, however, be used to conclude confidently that the requirements for a given person have or have not been met, because there is no assurance that the high (and low) consumers are the high (and low) requirers of the nutrient in question. Without knowing the distribution of intakes and requirements, there is no way to verify probable deficiency within a group. If individual intakes can be averaged over a sufficiently long period and compared with the RDA, the probable risk of deficiency for that individual can be estimated.

NUTRITIONAL ALLOWANCES AS GUIDELINES FOR FOOD SUPPLIES AND FOR HEALTH AND WELFARE PROGRAMS

The RDAs have been used by federal, state, and local health and welfare agencies as a starting point for determining the desirable nutrient content of foods and meals for school feeding programs, special food services, and various child-feeding programs, and as a basis for licensing and certification standards for such group facilities as day-care centers, nursing homes, and residential homes.

The attainment of RDAs should not be the only objective of food procurement or meal design for these programs. Since RDAs have not been set for all nutrients, meeting the RDAs from a wide variety of food classes is the best assurance that needs for non-RDA nutrients will be met. The foods selected must also be palatable and acceptable in other ways so they will be consumed over long periods in the required quantities. Although the subcommittee is aware that changes in the RDAs from the previous edition might have an impact on food assistance programs, it believes that modifications to these programs should be based on the recommendations in the Food and Nutrition Board's report *Diet and Health* (NRC, 1989) as well. Together, the RDAs and the *Diet and Health* recommendations should be considered the appropriate basis for diet planning.

In planning meals or food supplies, it is technically difficult and biologically unnecessary to design a single day's diet that contains all the RDAs for all the nutrients. Nor is there biological reason for expecting that each meal should contain a fixed percentage of an RDA for a nutrient. As stated previously, the RDAs are goals to be achieved over time—at least 3 days for nutrients that turn over rapidly, whereas one or several months might be adequate for more slowly metabolized nutrients. In practice, menus for congregate feeding should be designed so that the RDAs are met in a 5- to 10-day rotation.

REFERENCES

Beaton, G.H. 1985. Uses and limits of the use of the Recommended Dietary Allowances for evaluating dietary intake data. Am. J. Clin. Nutr. 41:155–164.

Butte, N.F., C. Garza, E.O. Smith, and B.L. Nichols. 1984. Human milk intake and growth in exclusively breast-fed infants. J. Pediatr. 104:187–195.

Chandra, R.K. 1982. Physical growth of exclusively breast-fed infants. Nutr. Res. 2:275–276.

DHHS (U.S. Department of Health and Human Services). 1988. The Surgeon General's Report on Nutrition and Health. Government Printing Office, Washington, D.C. 727 pp.

Hamill, P.V.V., T.A. Drizd, C.L. Johnson, R.B. Reed, A.F. Roche, and W.M. Moore. 1979. Physical growth: National Center for Health Statistics percentiles. Am. J. Clin. Nutr. 32:607–629.

Hofvander, Y., U. Hagman, C. Hillervik, and S. Sjolin. 1982. The amount of milk consumed by 1–3 months old breast- or bottle-fed infants. Acta Paediatr. Scand. 71:953–958.

Neville, M.C., R. Keller, J. Seacar, V. Lutes, M. Neifert, C. Casey, J. Allen, and P. Archer. 1988. Studies in human lactation: milk volumes in lactating women during the onset of lactation and full lactation. Am. J. Clin. Nutr. 48:1375–1386.

NRC (National Research Council). 1943. Recommended Dietary Allowances. Report of the Food and Nutrition Board, Reprint and Circular Series No. 115. National Research Council, Washington, D.C. 6 pp.

NRC (National Research Council). 1982. Diet, Nutrition, and Cancer. Report of the Committee on Diet, Nutrition, and Cancer, Assembly of Life Sciences. National Academy Press, Washington, D.C. 478 pp.

NRC (National Research Council). 1986. Nutrient Adequacy: Assessment Using Food Consumption Surveys. Report of the Subcommittee on Criteria for Dietary Evaluation, Food and Nutrition Board, Commission on Life Sciences. National Academy Press, Washington, D.C. 146 pp.

NRC (National Research Council). 1989. Diet and Health: Implications for Reducing Chronic Disease Risk. Report of the Committee on Diet and Health, Food and Nutrition Board, Commission on Life Sciences. National Academy Press, Washington, D.C. 750 pp.

Roberts, L.J. 1958. Beginnings of the Recommended Dietary Allowances. J. Am. Diet. Assoc. 34:903–908.

3
Energy

The energy requirement of an individual has been defined by a recent international working group as:

that level of energy intake from food which will balance energy expenditure when the individual has a body size and composition, and level of physical activity, consistent with long-term good health; and which will allow for the maintenance of economically necessary and socially desirable physical activity. In children and pregnant or lactating women the energy requirement includes the energy needs associated with the deposition of tissues or secretion of milk at rates consistent with good health (WHO, 1985).

For groups, recommended energy allowances represent the *average* needs of individuals. In contrast, recommended allowances for other nutrients are high enough to meet an upper level of requirement variability among individuals within the groups.

If energy intake is consistently above or below a person's requirement, a change in body energy stores can be expected. If the imbalance between intake and expenditure continues over long periods, changes in body weight or body composition will occur and may adversely affect health (see DHHS, 1988; NRC, 1989).

Recommended energy allowances are stipulated as kilocalories (kcal) per day[a] of physiologically available energy (i.e., the amount

---

[a] One kilocalorie is the amount of heat necessary to raise 1 kg of water from 15°C to 16°C. The accepted international unit of energy is the joule (J). To convert energy allowances from kilocalories to kilojoules (kJ), a factor of 4.2 may be used (1 kcal equals exactly 4.184 kJ). Because the energy content of diets is usually greater than 1,000 kJ, the preferred unit is the megajoule (MJ), which is 1,000 kJ.

24

of potential food energy that can be absorbed and utilized). Most food composition tables list physiologically available energy values based on digestibility trials of specific foods conducted by Atwater (Merrill and Watt, 1955). These *specific* energy values have been confirmed by others (Bernstein et al., 1955; Southgate and Durnin, 1970). The conventional *general* energy conversion factors of 4 kcal/g of food protein or food carbohydrate and 9 kcal/g of food fat (also derived by Atwater) are adequate for computation of the energy content of typical diets in the United States, but not of specific foods nor of diets based heavily on fibrous plant foods. Alcohol (ethanol) has a caloric value of 7 kcal/g, or 5.6 kcal/ml.

ESTIMATING ENERGY REQUIREMENTS

Total energy expenditure includes the energy expended at rest, in physical activity, and as a result of thermogenesis. These components, in turn, are affected by several variables, including age, sex, body size and composition, genetic factors, energy intake, physiologic state (e.g., growth, pregnancy, lactation), coexisting pathological conditions, and ambient temperature.

Resting Energy Expenditure

Unless levels of physical activity are very high, resting energy expenditure (REE) is the largest component of total energy expenditure. REE represents the energy expended by a person at rest under conditions of thermal neutrality. Basal metabolic rate (BMR) is more precisely defined as the REE measured soon after awakening in the morning, at least 12 hours after the last meal. REE is not usually measured under basal conditions. REE may include the residual thermic effect of a previous meal and may be lower than BMR during quiet sleep. In practice, BMR and REE differ by less than 10%, and the terms are used interchangeably.

REE is closely correlated with measures of lean body mass. In individuals of similar age, sex, height, and weight, differences in lean body mass account for approximately 80% of the variance in measured REE. Differences in lean body mass also account for most of the observed difference in REE between men and women, and between younger and older adults of similar heights and weights.

REE is commonly estimated by using any of several empirically derived equations. The values used in this volume were derived from

TABLE 3-1 Equations for Predicting Resting Energy Expenditure from Body Weight[a]

Sex and Age Range (years)	Equation to Derive REE in kcal/day	R^b	SD^b
Males			
0–3	$(60.9 \times wt^c) - 54$	0.97	53
3–10	$(22.7 \times wt) + 495$	0.86	62
10–18	$(17.5 \times wt) + 651$	0.90	100
18–30	$(15.3 \times wt) + 679$	0.65	151
30–60	$(11.6 \times wt) + 879$	0.60	164
> 60	$(13.5 \times wt) + 487$	0.79	148
Females			
0–3	$(61.0 \times wt) - 51$	0.97	61
3–10	$(22.5 \times wt) + 499$	0.85	63
10–18	$(12.2 \times wt) + 746$	0.75	117
18–30	$(14.7 \times wt) + 496$	0.72	121
30–60	$(8.7 \times wt) + 829$	0.70	108
> 60	$(10.5 \times wt) + 596$	0.74	108

[a] From WHO (1985). These equations were derived from BMR data.
[b] Correlation coefficient (R) of reported BMRs and predicted values, and standard deviation (SD) of the differences between actual and computed values.
[c] Weight of person in kilograms.

equations published by WHO (1985)[b] (Table 3-1). These calculated values are not completely accurate for individuals, but can serve as a guide for dietary planning. These equations take into account age, sex, and weight, but ignore height, which was found not to affect the precision of prediction appreciably.

Physical Activity

For most people, the second largest component of total energy expenditure is the energy expended in physical activity. In the past, estimates of energy requirements were based in part on the different physical activity levels associated with different occupations. With the introduction of labor-saving machinery, occupational energy expenditures and differences between occupations tended to decline. Renewed emphasis on physical fitness has led some people, but not

---

[b] In the United States, many investigators use the equations of Harris and Benedict (1919) to determine BMR. The values calculated from these equations do not differ significantly from those derived from the international equations used in this volume.

TABLE 3-2   Approximate Energy Expenditure for Various
Activities in Relation to Resting Needs for Males and Females of
Average Size[a]

Activity Category[b]	Representative Value for Activity Factor per Unit Time of Activity
Resting	REE × 1.0
Sleeping, reclining	
Very light	REE × 1.5
Seated and standing activities, painting trades, driving, laboratory work, typing, sewing, ironing, cooking, playing cards, playing a musical instrument	
Light	REE × 2.5
Walking on a level surface at 2.5 to 3 mph, garage work, electrical trades, carpentry, restaurant trades, house-cleaning, child care, golf, sailing, table tennis	
Moderate	REE × 5.0
Walking 3.5 to 4 mph, weeding and hoeing, carrying a load, cycling, skiing, tennis, dancing	
Heavy	REE × 7.0
Walking with load uphill, tree felling, heavy manual digging, basketball, climbing, football, soccer	

[a] Based on values reported by Durnin and Passmore (1967) and WHO (1985).
[b] When reported as multiples of basal needs, the expenditures of males and females are
similar.

all, to increase recreational activity, such as walking, jogging, and
sports, resulting in greater variability in the discretionary component
of energy expenditure. Thus, the traditional estimation of energy
needs according to occupation is no longer adequate.

For schoolchildren and people in sedentary occupations, long-term
well-being may depend on increasing physical activity during leisure
time. Indeed, for many Americans, increasing energy expenditure
through activity may be a more effective way of maintaining health,
including desirable body weight, than reduction in energy intake.
Increased activity promotes fitness and allows a more generous intake
of food, which makes for easier attainment of RDA levels of nutrients.

The energy costs of many different types of work and activity have
been measured (Durnin and Passmore, 1967; WHO, 1985[c]). Representative values are given in Table 3-2, expressed as multiples of
resting energy expenditure. Activities are aggregated according to

[c]The WHO (1985) report contains extensive references to the original investigations.
The reader is referred to that report for full documentation.

TABLE 3-3   Example of Calculation of Estimated Daily Energy
Allowances for Exceptionally Active and Inactive 23-Year-Old
Adults

STEP 1: DERIVATION OF ACTIVITY FACTOR[a]

Activity as Multiples of REE	Very Sedentary Day		Very Active Day	
	Duration (hr)	Weighted REE Factor	Duration (hr)	Weighted REE Factor
Resting 1.0	10	10.0	8	8.0
Very light 1.5	12	18.0	8	12.0
Light 2.5	2	5.0	4	10.0
Moderate 5.0	0	0	2	10.0
Heavy 7.0	0	0	2	14.0
TOTAL	24	33.0	24	54.0
MEAN		1.375		2.25

STEP 2: CALCULATION OF ENERGY REQUIREMENT, KCAL PER DAY

Gender	Resting Energy Expenditure[b]	Very Sedentary Day (REE × 1.375)	Very Active Day (REE × 2.25)
Male, 70 kg	1,750	2,406	3,938
Female, 58 kg	1,350	1,856	3,038

[a] Activity patterns are hypothetical. As an example of use of the ranges within a class of
   activity (Table 3-2), very light activity is divided between sitting and standing activities.
[b] From equations given in Table 3-1.

intensity of effort, such as resting, very light, light, moderate, and
heavy activity.

Energy requirement can be estimated, albeit imprecisely, if the
typical activity pattern is known. An average daily "activity factor"
can be calculated using the values in Table 3-2 for different activities,
weighted by the time engaged in such activities. The weighted activity
factor is multiplied by the REE (calculated from the equations in
Table 3-1, or measured) to derive energy requirement. An example
is shown in Table 3-3, in which energy expenditures of young adults
on unusually inactive and active days are compared. Estimated requirements for the inactive days are 1,500 and 1,200 kcal/day less
for males and females, respectively, than for the active days in the
example. A valid estimate of energy requirement would need to take
into account activity over a sufficiently long time (weekdays, week-
ends, season) to be representative.

A very sedentary person who habitually spends many hours a day
either lying or sitting is unlikely to expend the same amount of energy
at rest and for a given task as one who habitually undertakes more
strenuous activity several hours a day. A habitually sedentary person

TABLE 3-4 Factors for Estimating Daily Energy Allowances at Various Levels of Physical Activity for Men and Women (Ages 19 to 50)

Level of Activity	Activity Factor[a] (× REE)	Energy Expenditure[b] (kcal/kg per day)
Very light		
Men	1.3	31
Women	1.3	30
Light		
Men	1.6	38
Women	1.5	35
Moderate		
Men	1.7	41
Women	1.6	37
Heavy		
Men	2.1	50
Women	1.9	44
Exceptional		
Men	2.4	58
Women	2.2	51

[a] Based on examples presented by WHO (1985).

[b] REE was computed from formulas in Table 3-1 and is the average of values for median weights of persons ages 19 to 24 and 25 to 74 years: males, 24.0 kcal/kg; females, 23.2 kcal/kg.

would almost certainly have less muscle mass and might lack the physique to perform heavy physical work efficiently (Garrow and Blaza, 1982). Thus, differences in energy requirement are due both to pattern of activity and the body composition that results from that pattern of activity.

Activity factors associated with a range of activity patterns are listed in Table 3-4. These factors are similar to those specified by WHO (1985) and may be used as a rough guide to requirements if the proportion of time spent in different activities is unknown. Patterns typical of the U.S. population are in the categories light (1.5–1.6 × REE) or moderate (1.6–1.7 × REE). The activity factor of 1.3 × REE is a minimum value, reflecting 10 hours a day at rest and 14 hours of very light activity. This level may be lower than is compatible with desirable cardiovascular fitness (WHO, 1985).

Metabolic Response to Food

Metabolic rate increases after eating, reflecting the size and composition of the meal. It reaches a maximum approximately 1 hour after the meal is consumed and virtually disappears 4 hours afterward (Garrow, 1978). In relation to total energy expenditure, the thermic effect of meals is relatively small—on the order of 5 to 10% of energy ingested. Small differences in this component of energy expenditure could have significant cumulative long-term effects, but are generally undetectable, being lost in the day-to-day variation in energy metabolism.

Age

REE varies with the amount and composition of metabolically active tissue, which varies with age. The lean body mass of infants and young children contains a greater proportion of metabolically active organs than in adults. In adults, skeletal muscle, which has a lower rate of resting metabolism, is a major component of the lean body mass. Lean body mass declines beyond early adulthood at a rate of about 2 to 3% per decade, and the REE declines proportionately. Differences in body composition among age groups are reflected in the age-specific equations for calculating REE.

Activity patterns also vary with age. Unless constrained by the environment, children typically are active (1.7 to 2.0 × REE). Both physiological and social changes affect energy expenditure patterns of older adults. In the longitudinal study of aging conducted in Baltimore, Maryland, McGandy et al. (1966) found the activity component to be affected more than the REE over time and an especially sharp drop in activity after age 75. Elmstahl (1987) measured energy expenditure of very elderly institutionalized people (average age, 83 years) who had a variety of chronic conditions but were still able to participate in physical activity. The average energy expenditure of men and women was similar—1.45 to 1.50 × measured REE. Under laboratory conditions of controlled activity (sedentary, except for 0.5 hour cycling per day), the average expenditure of 68-year-old men was 1.58 × REE (Calloway and Zanni, 1980).

Sex

Differences in body composition of boys and girls occur as early as the first few months of life but are relatively small until children reach approximately 10 years of age. Thereafter, the differences in body composition become greater throughout adolescence. After maturity, men have proportionately greater muscle mass than do women, who have a greater proportion of body weight as fat. In adults, REE per unit of total body weight differs by approximately

10% between sexes. In the past, because of occupational differences, men and women often had markedly different energy expenditures, but their occupational activity requirements now are similar.

Growth

The cost of growth includes energy deposited as protein and fat plus the cost of their synthesis. The average energy cost is about 5 kcal/g of growth tissue gained (Roberts and Young, 1988). Except during the first year of life, growth is a very small (approximately 1%) component of total energy requirement.

Body Size

Persons with large (or small) bodies require proportionately more (or less) energy per unit of time for activities (e.g., walking) that involve moving mass over distance. Their total REE also will be higher (or lower) than the average for persons of the same sex and age. Energy allowances must be adjusted for the variation in requirements that result from these differences in body size. Adjustment will need to be greater for persons who are both large and active.

Weight may be used as a basis for adjusting energy allowances for different body sizes, provided the individuals are not appreciably over or under median weights for height within a given age and sex category (see Table 2-1 in Chapter 2). For obese or undernourished people, energy allowances should be adjusted according to the normal weight for their height.

Climate

In the United States, the ambient temperature of most living environments lies in the comfortable range of 20°C to 25°C (68°F to 77°F). Most people are protected against cold by warm clothes and heated environments. The effects of high temperatures are also minimized since many people also live and work in air-conditioned buildings. Not everyone is insulated from environmental exposure, however. When there is prolonged exposure to cold or heat, energy allowances may need adjustment.

The energy cost of work is slightly greater (approximately 5%) in a mean temperature below 14°C than in a warm environment (Johnson, 1963). A relatively small increase in energy expenditure (2% to 5%) is associated with carrying the extra weight of cold-weather clothing and footwear. Such clothing also increases energy expenditure by its so-called hobbling effect. If exposure to cold air or water leads to body cooling, energy needs will increase because of the increased metabolic rate associated with shivering and other muscle activity.

Energy requirements are also increased in people performing heavy work at a high temperature—37°C (99°F) or higher. Under such conditions, body temperature and metabolic rate increase, and extra energy is expended to maintain thermal balance (Johnson, 1963). Whereas little adjustment is necessary in environmental temperatures between 20°C and 30°C (68°F–86°F), energy allowances may need to be slightly increased wherever persons are required to be physically active in extreme heat.

With the above exceptions, no adjustment in energy allowance appears to be needed to compensate for change in climate, apart from climatic effects on physical activity patterns.

ESTIMATION OF ENERGY ALLOWANCES

Adults

In Table 3-5, recommended energy allowances for reference adults engaged in light to moderate activity are given for three age categories: 19 to 24 years, 25 to 50, and over age 50. Weights and heights of young adults between 19 and 24 years of age are close to those of mature adults; although some persons within this age group may still be growing, the very small energy need for growth is well within population variability. The recommended allowances should be adjusted to account for increased physical activity and for larger or smaller body size, but rarely for climate.

The recommended allowances for adults with a light-to-moderate activity level were calculated by using the WHO (1985) equations for the calculation of REE (Table 3-1) and multiplying the results by an activity factor. For men, the activity factor 1.67 × REE was used for the 19- to 24-year age group and 1.60 for those ages 25 to 50; for women, 1.60 and 1.55 were used for the respective age periods. These values are a blend of light and moderate classes of activity as suggested by WHO. For men of reference body size, the average allowance is 2,900 kcal/day; for women, it is 2,200 kcal. With light-to-moderate activity, the coefficient of variation in energy requirements of adults is approximately 20% (Garrow, 1978; McGandy et al., 1966; Todd et al., 1983). This range reflects variability in both the REE and the activity factor among the individuals in the group. This range does not cover the needs of persons with heavy activity patterns, for whom allowances should be adjusted to 2.0 × REE or higher.

TABLE 3-5   Median Heights and Weights and Recommended
Energy Intake

Category	Age (years) or Condition	Weight (kg)	Weight (lb)	Height (cm)	Height (in)	REE[a] (kcal/day)	Multiples of REE	Average Energy Allowance (kcal)[b] Per kg	Average Energy Allowance (kcal)[b] Per day[c]
Infants	0.0–0.5	6	13	60	24	320		108	650
	0.5–1.0	9	20	71	28	500		98	850
Children	1–3	13	29	90	35	740		102	1,300
	4–6	20	44	112	44	950		90	1,800
	7–10	28	62	132	52	1,130		70	2,000
Males	11–14	45	99	157	62	1,440	1.70	55	2,500
	15–18	66	145	176	69	1,760	1.67	45	3,000
	19–24	72	160	177	70	1,780	1.67	40	2,900
	25–50	79	174	176	70	1,800	1.60	37	2,900
	51+	77	170	173	68	1,530	1.50	30	2,300
Females	11–14	46	101	157	62	1,310	1.67	47	2,200
	15–18	55	120	163	64	1,370	1.60	40	2,200
	19–24	58	128	164	65	1,350	1.60	38	2,200
	25–50	63	138	163	64	1,380	1.55	36	2,200
	51+	65	143	160	63	1,280	1.50	30	1,900
Pregnant	1st trimester								+0
	2nd trimester								+300
	3rd trimester								+300
Lactating	1st 6 months								+500
	2nd 6 months								+500

[a] Calculation based on FAO equations (Table 3-1), then rounded.
[b] In the range of light to moderate activity, the coefficient of variation is ±20%.
[c] Figure is rounded.

The energy allowance for persons beyond age 50 is 1.5 × REE. This assumes continued light-to-moderate activity, which should be encouraged in the interest of maintaining muscle mass and well-being. It should not be assumed that the marked decline in activity often observed in the elderly is either inevitable or desirable. The average allowance for men of reference size (77 kg) is 2,300 kcal/day; for women, it is 1,900 kcal/day. A normal variation of ±20% is accepted as for younger adults. The requirements of persons beyond age 75 are likely to be somewhat less as a result of reduced body size, REE, and activity.

Pregnancy

Pregnancy imposes additional energy needs because of added maternal tissues and growth of the fetus and placenta. For a full-term pregnancy, during which the mother has gained 12.5 kg and has given birth to a 3.3-kg baby, total energy cost has been estimated to be 80,000 kcal (Hytten and Leitch, 1971). This estimate has been used in considering energy allowances for pregnancy (WHO, 1985). Alternative assumptions concerning the composition of tissue gained, observations of energy intake by pregnant women, and measurement of resting metabolism have led to estimates as low as 45,000 kcal (Durnin, 1986) and 68,000 kcal (van Raaij, 1989) to as high as 110,000 kcal (Forsum et al., 1988) as the cost of pregnancy in healthy, well-nourished women.

Epidemiological evidence suggests that adequate maternal weight gain, including some maternal fat storage, is needed to ensure that the size of the newborn is optimal for survival. Thus, storage of energy is included as part of the energy requirement of pregnancy.

Metabolic requirements and physical activity may change during pregnancy, but there are no well-documented studies providing the data from which to estimate changes in energy allowance for these two factors.

WHO (1985) estimated the energy allowance for pregnant women by dividing the gross energy cost (80,000 kcal) by the approximate duration of pregnancy (250 days following the first month), yielding an average value (after rounding) of 300 kcal/day for the entire pregnancy. The present subcommittee accepts this calculation with the caution that any diminution in activity with advancing pregnancy must be taken into account. Unless the woman begins pregnancy with depleted body reserves, additional energy intake is probably not required during the first trimester. An additional 300 kcal/day is recommended during the second and third trimesters.

Lactation

Energy requirements for lactation are proportional to the quantity of milk produced. The average energy content of human milk from well-nourished mothers is about 70 kcal/100 ml (WHO, 1985). The efficiency with which maternal energy is converted to milk energy is assumed to be approximately 80% (range, 76 to 94%) (Sadurkis et al., 1988; Thomson et al., 1970; WHO, 1985). Thus, approximately 85 kcal are required for every 100 ml of milk produced. Average milk secretion during the first 6 months of lactation is 750 ml/day; in the second 6 months, it is 600 ml/day. The coefficient of variation is 12.5%. Thus, the average woman would require an additional 640 kcal and 510 kcal/day in the first and second 6 months, respectively.

The upper boundary of requirements (+2 SD) would be 800 and 640 kcal.

Energy allowances during lactation may be partially met by extra fat stored during pregnancy. Such energy reserves, about 2 to 3 kg in women who gain 11 to 12 kg during pregnancy, normally are utilized during the first few months of breastfeeding. These fat stores can theoretically provide about 100 to 150 kcal/day during a 6-month lactation period. Accordingly, an additional average allowance of 500 kcal/day is recommended throughout lactation, which, assuming appropriate weight gain during pregnancy, may permit readjustment of maternal body fat stores upon termination of breastfeeding. The recommended allowance for women whose gestational weight gain is subnormal, or whose weight during lactation falls below the standard for their height and age, is an additional 650 kcal/day during the first 6 months.

Infants, Children, and Adolescents

For children less than 10 years of age, the energy requirement is estimated from intake associated with normal growth. Data on energy intakes recorded in studies of children in the United States, Canada, the United Kingdom, and Sweden have been compiled by WHO (1985). The international groups accepted the actual requirement to be 5% greater than these reported intakes, allowing for the likelihood that intake was underestimated.

The requirement figures of 108 kcal and 98 kcal/kg for infants from birth through 6 months and 6 months through 12 months, respectively, were estimated by WHO from intakes of healthy infants from developed countries. These figures are about 15% higher than recent estimates derived from energy expenditure measurements, using deuterium oxide methodology, with an allowance for the theoretical amount of energy deposited as tissue added in growth (Prentice et al., 1988). The new estimates, 95 kcal and 84 kcal/kg at the respective age periods, based on expenditure plus storage, can be taken as equal to dietary requirement if the metabolizable energy value of foods consumed (human milk, formula, beikost) is estimated correctly. Growth velocity is slower than the NCHS 50th centile in infants in these recent (1984–1988) studies and skinfold thickness is less than the Tanner standards developed in the 1950s (Tanner, 1984), indicating that infants are now leaner. There is, at present, insufficient evidence from which to judge whether or not this secular trend is desirable. Recognizing that infants self-regulate intake and that questions remain unanswered (including the question of metabolizable energy values), the subcommittee has elected to accept the WHO figures.

From birth through age 10 years, no distinction in energy requirement is made between sexes. Above age 10, separate allowances are recommended for boys and girls because of differences in the age of onset of puberty and evolving activity patterns. There is great variability in both the timing and magnitude of the adolescent growth spurt. Activity patterns are also quite variable. Thus, recommendations for these groups assume a wider range within which energy allowances can be adjusted individually to take account of body weight, activity, and rate of growth.

The recommended energy allowances from birth through age 10 years shown in Table 3-5 are those of the international agencies (WHO, 1985). Allowances for other age groups are adjusted to reflect typical activity patterns in the United States. Those for older girls and boys are based on a predicted activity factor of 1.7 at 11 years of age and a decrease to the adult light to moderate activity value of 1.6 by age 15 in girls and age 19 in boys.

COMPARISON OF RDA AND REPORTED INTAKES

Energy intakes of children as reported in both the 1977–1978 Nationwide Food Consumption Survey (USDA, 1984) and the 1976–1980 second National Health and Nutrition Examination Survey (NCHS, 1979) coincide with the allowances proposed for these age groups. From early adolescence onward in women and in men a few years later, reported average intakes are substantially below the RDA. Data from the 1986 Continuing Survey of Food Intakes by Individuals (USDA, 1988) indicate that mothers consume an average of 1,473 kcal/day, the same amount of energy as their children ages 1 to 5 years. It is commonly believed that adults underestimate food intake and that alcohol consumption in particular is underreported (NRC, 1986). If the underreported items are seasonings or adjuvants with low levels of essential nutrients (e.g., fats and oils, sweeteners) or alcoholic beverages, only energy intake will be affected seriously.

CHANGES IN ENERGY ALLOWANCES COMPARED TO NINTH EDITION

Reference weights in the present edition differ from those in the ninth. Thus, the allowances expressed as kcal/day are not directly comparable with values in the previous edition. Nevertheless, the changes made in adult allowances are generally small despite the different method used to derive the estimated allowances. The allowances for infants and children 7 to 10 years old are lower than in previous editions because of the new information on observed intakes of children in developed countries. For other ages, new allowances expressed per kilogram of body weight are trivially higher or lower than previously.

REFERENCES

Bernstein, L.M., M.I. Grossman, H. Kryzwicki, R. Harding, R.M. Berger, V.E. McGary, E. Francis, and L.M. Levy. 1955. Comparison of various methods for determination of metabolizable energy value of a mixed diet in humans. U.S. Army Med. Nutr. Lab. Rep. No. 168. Fitzsimons Army Hospital, Denver. 49 pp.

Calloway, D.H., and E. Zanni. 1980. Energy requirements and energy expenditure of elderly men. Am. J. Clin. Nutr. 33:2088–2092.

DHHS (U.S. Department of Health and Human Services). 1988. The Surgeon General's Report on Nutrition and Health. U.S. Government Printing Office, Washington, D.C. 727 pp.

Durnin, J.V.G.A. 1986. Energy requirements of pregnancy. An integration of the longitudinal data from the 5-country study. Pp. 147–154 in Nestlé Foundation Annual Report. Nestlé Foundation, Lausanne, Switzerland.

Durnin, J.V.G.A., and R. Passmore. 1967. Energy, Work, and Leisure. Heinemann Educational Books, London. 166 pp.

Elmstahl, S. 1987. Energy expenditure, energy intake and body composition in geriatric long-stay patients. Compr. Gerontol. A1:118–125.

Forsum, E., A. Sadurkis, and J. Wagner. 1988. Resting metabolic rate and body composition of healthy Swedish women during pregnancy. Am. J. Clin. Nutr. 47:942–947.

Garrow, J.S. 1978. Energy Balance and Obesity in Man, 2nd ed. Elsevier/North-Holland Biomedical Press, New York. 243 pp.

Garrow, J.S., and S. Blaza. 1982. Energy requirements in human beings. Pp. 1–21 in A. Neuberger and T.H. Jukes, eds. Human Nutrition. MTP Press, Lancaster, U.K.

Harris, J.A., and F.G. Benedict. 1919. A Biometric Study of Basal Metabolism in Man. Publication No. 279. Carnegie Institution, Washington, D.C.

Hytten, R.E., and I. Leitch. 1971. The Physiology of Human Pregnancy, 2nd ed. Blackwell Scientific Publications, Oxford. 599 pp.

Johnson, R.E. 1963. Caloric requirements under adverse environmental conditions. Fed. Proc. 22:1439–1446.

McGandy, R.B., C.H. Barrows, Jr., A. Spanias, A. Meredith, J.L. Stone, and A.H. Norris. 1966. Nutrient intakes and energy expenditure in men of different ages. J. Gerontol. 21:581–587.

Merrill, A.L., and B.K. Watt. 1955. Energy Value of Foods, Basis and Derivation. Agricultural Handbook No. 74. Human Nutrition Research Branch, Agricultural Research Service, U.S. Department of Agriculture. U.S. Government Printing Office, Washington, D.C. 105 pp.

NCHS (National Center for Health Statistics). 1979. Dietary Intake Source Data. DHEW Publ. No. 79-1221. NCHS, Hyattsville, Md.

NRC (National Research Council). 1986. Nutrient Adequacy: Assessment Using Food Consumption Surveys. Report of the Subcommittee on Criteria for Dietary Evaluation, Food and Nutrition Board, Commission on Life Sciences. National Academy Press, Washington, D.C. 146 pp.

NRC (National Research Council). 1989. Diet and Health: Implications for Reducing Chronic Disease Risk. Report of the Committee on Diet and Health, Food and Nutrition Board. National Academy Press, Washington, D.C. 750 pp.

Prentice, A.M., A. Lucas, L. Vasquez-Velasquez, P.S.W. Davies, and R.G. Whitehead. 1988. Are current dietary guidelines for young children a prescription for overfeeding? Lancet 2:1066–1069.

Roberts, S.B., and V.R. Young. 1988. Energy costs of fat and protein deposition in the human infant. Am. J. Clin. Nutr. 48:951–955.

Sadurkis, A., N. Kabir, J. Wagner, and E. Forsum. 1988. Energy metabolism, body composition, and milk production in healthy Swedish women during lactation. Am. J. Clin. Nutr. 48:44–49.

Southgate, D.A.T., and J.V.G.A. Durnin. 1970. Calorie conversion factors: an experimental reassessment of the factors used in calculation of the energy value of human diets. Br. J. Nutr. 24:517–535.

Tanner, J.M. 1984. Physical growth and development. Pp. 278–330 in J.O. Forfar and G.C. Arneil, eds. Textbook of Paediatrics, Vol. 1. Churchill Livingstone, Edinburgh.

Thomson, A.M., F.E. Hytten, and W.Z. Billewicz. 1970. The energy cost of human lactation. Br. J. Nutr. 24:565–572.

Todd, K.S., M. Hudes, and D.H. Calloway. 1983. Food intake measurement: problems and approaches. Am. J. Clin. Nutr. 37:139–146.

USDA (U.S. Department of Agriculture). 1984. Nationwide Food Consumption Survey. Nutrient Intakes: Individuals in 48 States, Year 1977–78. Report No. I-2. Consumer Nutrition Division, Human Nutrition Information Service. U.S. Department of Agriculture, Hyattsville, Md. 439 pp.

USDA (U.S. Department of Agriculture). 1988. Nationwide Food Consumption Survey. Continuing Survey of Food Intakes of Individuals. Women 19–50 Years and Their Children 1–5 Years, 4 Days, 1986. Report No. 86-3. Nutrition Monitoring Division, Human Nutrition Information Service. U.S. Department of Agriculture, Hyattsville, Md. 82 pp.

van Raaij, J.M.A., C.M. Schonk, S.H. Vermaat-Miedema, M.E.M. Peck, and J.G.A.J. Hautvast. 1989. Body fat mass and basal metabolic rate in Dutch women before, during, and after pregnancy: a reappraisal of energy cost of pregnancy. Am. J. Clin. Nutr. 49:765–772.

WHO (World Health Organization). 1985. Energy and Protein Requirements. Report of a Joint FAO/WHO/UNU Expert Consultation. Technical Report Series 724. World Health Organization, Geneva. 206 pp.

4

Carbohydrates and Fiber

Carbohydrates, along with fat and protein, are the macrocomponents of the diet—the principal dietary sources of energy. Alcohol (ethanol) is the only other important source of energy. The principal dietary carbohydrates are sugars and complex carbohydrates. The sugars include monosaccharides, such as glucose and fructose, and disaccharides, such as sucrose (table sugar), maltose, and lactose (milk sugar). Complex carbohydrates (polysaccharides) comprise starches and dietary fibers. Starches are polymers of glucose. Dietary fibers[a] are mainly indigestible complex carbohydrates in plant cell walls (cellulose, hemicellulose, and pectin) and a variety of gums, mucilages, and algal polysaccharides. Lignin is a noncarbohydrate component of dietary fiber in plant cell walls. Dietary fibers are converted to some extent into absorbable fatty acids by intestinal microorganisms. Pentoses and some carbohydrate-related compounds are present in the diet in smaller amounts. This category includes such substances as organic acids (e.g., citric and malic acids) and a number of polyols (e.g., sorbitol, xylitol), all of which have some energy value. Proximate analysis of foods commonly omits direct analysis of carbohydrate.

---

[a]Dietary fiber should not be confused with crude fiber, a nutritionally obsolete term that refers to the residue (primarily cellulose and lignin) remaining after food is treated with acid and alkali. Foods generally contain more dietary fiber than crude fiber, but no consistent quantitative relationship exists between the two. Some tables of food composition and some food labels present fiber content in terms of crude fiber. Little quantitative information is yet available on the individual components of dietary fiber in specific foods.

39

The value for carbohydrate content of foods given in compositional tables usually is "carbohydrate by difference," i.e., the residual weight after subtracting amounts of water, protein, fat, and ash found by analysis; this moiety includes sugars, starches, fiber, and small amounts of other organic compounds.

DIGESTIBLE CARBOHYDRATES

In the United States, the average intake of carbohydrates by adults was 287 g for males (USDA, 1986) and 177 g for females in 1985 (USDA, 1987). Of the carbohydrates in individual diets, an average of 41% comes from grain products and 23% comes from fruits and vegetables (Anderson, 1982; Wotecki et al., 1982). About half of the total digestible carbohydrate intake is made up of monosaccharides and disaccharides. These are found in fruits (sucrose, glucose, fructose, pentoses) and milk (lactose). Sugars in soft drinks, candies, jams, jellies, and sweet desserts are mainly sucrose and high-fructose corn syrup. Complex carbohydrates, which constitute the other half of digestible carbohydrate intake, are starches found predominantly in cereal grains and their products (flour, bread, rice, corn, oats, and barley), potatoes, legumes, and a few other vegetables.

Sugars and starches together are the major source of energy in the diet. In 1985, they provided an average of 45.3% of the energy in the diet of adult men in the United States (USDA, 1986). The corresponding figures for adult women and children 1 to 5 years of age were 46.4 and 52.0%, respectively (USDA, 1987). Eleven percent of the total energy intake, representing almost one-quarter of total carbohydrate intake, is provided by added sweeteners, mostly sucrose and high-fructose corn syrup (Glinsmann et al., 1986).

Fructose intake in the United States increased after the introduction of high-fructose corn syrup into the food supply in 1970. The product is formed by the enzymatic conversion of some of the glucose in cornstarch to fructose. Its fructose content ranges from 40% to almost 100%. In 1985, high-fructose corn syrup accounted for 30% of the total sweetener supply in the United States (Glinsmann et al., 1986; IFT, 1986). In soft drinks, for example, the use of sucrose has been almost completely abandoned in favor of a high-fructose corn syrup product containing 55% fructose, approximately 40% glucose, and about 5% other sugars (Bailey et al., 1988; GAO, 1984). It is unknown whether this increased intake of free fructose has any health consequences (Reiser and Hallfrisch, 1987).

Sugar alcohols, except for xylitol, occur naturally in fruits. Because these sweet substances are slowly and incompletely absorbed from the digestive tract and are less cariogenic than many other sugars, sugar alcohols such as sorbitol are useful in products intended for special diets and are often found in dietetic candies and chewing gum. In some people, however, sugar alcohols create a laxative effect due to their slow and incomplete absorption. Consumption of products containing an ounce or more of sorbitol, for example, may result in soft stools and diarrhea (IFT, 1986).

Pathophysiological Significance

Glucose absorbed in the intestine or produced by the liver is an important energy source for most tissues. Other dietary hexoses (fructose and the galactose moiety of the disaccharide lactose) are converted to glucose in the liver. Most amino acids, the glycerol component of fat, and some organic acids can be converted to glucose. Therefore, there is no absolute dietary requirement for carbohydrates, at least under most circumstances. In the absence of dietary carbohydrates, however, lipolysis of stored triglycerides and the oxidation of fatty acids increase and ketone bodies accumulate. A carbohydrate-free diet also is generally associated with an accelerated breakdown of dietary and tissue protein, loss of cations (especially sodium), and dehydration. These effects produced by low-carbohydrate diets or by fasting can be prevented by the daily ingestion of 50 to 100 g of carbohydrates (Calloway, 1971). Because of the desirability of limiting the intake of fat (see Chapter 5) and perhaps of protein (Chapter 6), the subcommittee recommends that more than half the energy requirement beyond infancy be provided by carbohydrates. One gram of carbohydrate yields 4 kcal. Thus, for people consuming as little as 2,000 kcal/day, the recommended intake would be at least 250 g. Similar recommendations, which emphasize an increased intake of complex carbohydrates rather than added sugars, have been made by other groups (see NRC, 1989).

Sugars, including sucrose in foods, provide the substrate for the microorganisms in the mouth that are responsible for tooth decay, particularly in children. Caries-producing potential depends on the ability of the carbohydrates to adhere to the tooth surface and the frequency of consumption, both of which affect the length of time carbohydrates are available as a bacterial substrate. Ingestion of other foods may inhibit the increase in oral hydrogen ion concentration associated with ingestion of sucrose and, hence, its cariogenicity. Thus, snacks of candies and other sweets may be more cariogenic than sugars consumed as part of a meal. An adequate intake of fluoride also inhibits tooth decay produced by dietary sugars.

DIETARY FIBER

Dietary fiber is the subject of considerable recent interest and extensive reviews (see, for example, LSRO, 1987; NRC, 1989; Vahouny and Kritchevsky, 1986). Because they are hygroscopic, dietary fibers soften the stool and, hence, promote normal elimination. Fiber-rich diets may also increase satiety. Some fiber components, including oat bran and pectin, also lower plasma cholesterol levels, either by binding bile acids or by other mechanisms.

The consumption of diets rich in plant foods (and therefore fiber) is inversely related to the incidence of cardiovascular disease, colon cancer, and diabetes (see NRC, 1989). Because an increase in dietary fiber consumption is almost invariably associated with a change in other dietary constituents, it is difficult to establish a clear relationship with dietary fiber alone. One plausible mechanism for an anticarcinogenic effect is the rapid passage of the digestive mass through the colon, thereby reducing the possibility that potential carcinogens have an opportunity to interact with the mucosal surface (NRC, 1982). In addition, the increased mass of the softer stool may dilute carcinogens.

Fibers may also bind to mineral elements. In this way, wheat bran may interfere with mineral absorption, but neither wheat bran nor other fibers, at the levels consumed in this country, appear to have an appreciable effect on the absorption of minerals (NRC, 1989).

In the United States, mean fiber intake is estimated to be approximately 12 g/day (Lanza et al., 1987). Over the last decade, many health organizations have recommended increasing the intake of complex carbohydrates in general or dietary fiber in particular (see, e.g., AHA, 1986; DHHS, 1986). The subcommittee recommends that a desirable fiber intake be achieved not by adding fiber concentrates to the diet, but by consumption of fruits, vegetables, legumes, and whole-grain cereals, which also provide minerals and vitamins (DHHS, 1986; NRC, 1982).

REFERENCES

AHA (American Heart Association). 1986. Dietary Guidelines for Healthy American Adults. Statement by the Nutrition Committee. AHA Publ. No. 71-003-C. American Heart Association, Dallas, Tex.

Anderson, T.A. 1982. Recent trends in carbohydrate consumption. Annu. Rev. Nutr. 2:113–132.

Bailey, L., L. Duewer, F. Gray, R. Hoskin, J. Putnam, and S. Short. 1988. Food consumption. Natl. Food Rev. 11:1–10.

Calloway, D.H. 1971. Dietary components that yield energy. Environ. Biol. Med. 1:175–186.

DHHS (U.S. Department of Health and Human Services). 1986. Diet, Nutrition & Cancer Prevention: The Good News. NIH Publ. No. 87-2878. U.S. Government Printing Office, Washington, D.C.

GAO (U.S. General Accounting Office). 1984. U.S. Sweetener/Sugar Issues and Concerns. Report No. GAO/RCED-85-19. U.S. General Accounting Office, Washington, D.C. 43 pp.

Glinsmann, W.H., H. Irausquin, and Y.K. Park. 1986. Evaluation of health aspects of sugars contained in carbohydrate sweeteners: report of Sugars Task Force, 1986. J. Nutr. 116:S1–S216.

IFT (Institute of Food Technologists). 1986. Sweeteners: Nutritive and non-nutritive. Food Technol. 40:195–206.

Lanza, E., D.Y. Jones, G. Block, and L. Kessler. 1987. Dietary fiber intake in the U.S. population. Am. J. Clin. Nutr. 46:790–797.

LSRO (Life Sciences Research Office). 1987. Physiological Effects and Health Consequences of Dietary Fiber. Federation of American Societies for Experimental Biology, Bethesda, Md. 236 pp.

NRC (National Research Council). 1982. Diet, Nutrition, and Cancer. A report of the Committee on Diet, Nutrition, and Cancer, Assembly of Life Sciences. National Academy Press, Washington, D.C. 478 pp.

NRC (National Research Council). 1989. Diet and Health: Implications for Reducing Chronic Disease Risk. Report of the Committee on Diet and Health, Food and Nutrition Board. National Academy Press, Washington, D.C. 750 pp.

Reiser, S., and J. Hallfrisch. 1987. Metabolic Effects of Dietary Fructose. CRC Press, Boca Raton, Fla.

USDA (U.S. Department of Agriculture). 1986. Nationwide Food Consumption Survey. Continuing Survey of Food Intakes by Individuals: Men 19–50 Years, 1 Day. 1985. Report No. 85-3. Nutrition Monitoring Division, Human Nutrition Information Service. U.S. Department of Agriculture, Hyattsville, Md. 94 pp.

USDA (U.S. Department of Agriculture). 1987. Nationwide Food Consumption Survey. Continuing Survey of Food Intakes by Individuals: Women 19–50 Years and Their Children 1–5 Years, 4 Days, 1985. Report No. 85-4. Nutrition Monitoring Division, Human Nutrition Information Service. U.S. Department of Agriculture, Hyattsville, Md. 182 pp.

Vahouny, G., and D. Kritchevsky, eds. 1986. Dietary Fiber, Basic and Clinical Aspects. Plenum Press, New York.

Wotecki, C.E., S.D. Welch, N. Raper, and R.M. Marston. 1982. Recent trends and levels of dietary sugars and other caloric sweeteners. Pp. 1–27 in S. Reiser, ed. Metabolic Effects of Utilizable Dietary Carbohydrates. Marcel Dekker, New York.

5
Lipids

Lipids are organic compounds with limited solubility in water. They are present in biologic systems mainly as energy stores within cells or as components of cell membranes. The *nonpolar* lipids occur mainly as esters of fatty acids that are virtually insoluble in water and enter metabolic pathways only after hydrolysis. The triacylglycerols (also called triglycerides or fats) are composed of three fatty acids esterified to glycerol. Cholesteryl esters are composed of a single fatty acid esterified to cholesterol. The *polar* or *amphipathic* lipids include fatty acids, in which the polar component is a negatively charged carboxyl ion; cholesterol, in which the polar component is an alcohol; sphingolipids, in which the polar group is phosphorylcholine (sphingomyelin) or a carbohydrate (glycosphingolipid); and glycerophosphatides (mainly lecithins), in which the polar component is a phosphate-containing aminoalcohol or polyalcohol. The term phospholipids encompasses glycerophosphatides and sphingomyelins.

The fatty acid components of lipids are classified as short-chain (less than 6 carbons), medium-chain (6 to 10 carbons), or long-chain (12 or more carbons). More than 90% of the fatty acids have an even number of carbon atoms. Fatty acids are also classified as saturated (lacking double bonds), monounsaturated (containing a single double bond), or polyunsaturated (containing more than one double bond). The polyunsaturated fatty acids are subdivided into those whose first double bond occurs either three carbon atoms from the methyl carbon (n-3 or ω-3) or six carbon atoms from the methyl carbon (n-6

44

or ω-6). The major saturated fatty acids in foods are palmitic acid (16 carbons) and stearic acid (18 carbons). The major monounsaturated fatty acid is oleic acid (18 carbons). The major polyunsaturated fatty acids in plant foods are linoleic acid, an n-6 fatty acid with 18 carbons and two double bonds, and linolenic acid, an n-3 fatty acid with 18 carbons and 3 double bonds. The major polyunsaturated fatty acids in fish are eicosapentaenoic acid (EPA), an n-3 fatty acid with 20 carbons and 5 double bonds, and docosahexaenoic acid (DHA), an n-3 fatty acid with 22 carbons and 6 double bonds.

Triglycerides are the principal lipid component of foods and the most concentrated source of energy among the macrocomponents of the diet (9 kcal/g). They can enhance palatability by absorbing and retaining flavors and by influencing the texture of foods. When fats are digested, emulsified, and absorbed, they facilitate the intestinal absorption (and perhaps also the transport) of the fat-soluble vitamins A, E, and D. Saturated and monounsaturated fatty acids and cholesterol can be readily synthesized from acetyl coenzyme A and thus are not essential dietary components. Small amounts of polyunsaturated fatty acids, which cannot be synthesized, are essential in the diet. They are precursors of important structural lipids (e.g., phospholipids in cell membranes) and of eicosanoids. Eicosanoids include prostaglandins (e.g., PGEs, PGFs, prostacyclin), thromboxanes, and leukotrienes.

Digestion of food fats and other lipids liberates free fatty acids, monoglycerides, and lesser amounts of monoacylphospholipids, which are then absorbed. The efficiency of fatty acid and monoglyceride absorption in healthy adults is high, ranging from 95 to 99%, whereas that of cholesterol ranges from 30 to 70%.

Fatty acids can be directly utilized as a source of energy by most body cells, with the exception of erythrocytes and cells of the central nervous system. Oxidative metabolism of long-chain fatty acids requires a carrier system (carnitine transferase) for mitochondrial transport. The central nervous system normally uses glucose as its major energy source, but the brain can utilize ketones that are produced during fatty acid catabolism when the supply of glucose is limited. Excess energy is stored principally as triglycerides within adipose tissue.

Cholesterol and phospholipids are major components of all cell membranes and of myelin. Cholesterol is also the precursor of the steroid hormones produced in the adrenal cortex and gonads, and of the bile acids produced in the liver.

DIETARY SOURCES AND USUAL INTAKES

More than one-third of the calories consumed by most people in the United States are provided by fat. Animal products in particular—red meats (beef, veal, pork, lamb), poultry, fish and shellfish, separated animal fats (such as tallow and lard), milk and milk products, and eggs—contribute more than half of the total fat to U.S. diets, three-fourths of the saturated fat, and all the cholesterol (NRC, 1988). In the U.S. Department of Agriculture (USDA) 1977-1978 Nationwide Food Consumption Survey, red meats were found to provide the major source of fat to Americans of all age groups other than infants (USDA, 1984). In the NHANES II survey, ground beef was found to be the single largest contributor of fat to the U.S. diet; mayonnaise, salad dressings, and margarine were the chief sources of linoleic acid; and eggs supplied the most cholesterol (Block et al., 1985).

Food supply disappearance data suggest that per capita consumption of fat in the United States has increased since the late 1970s. Although animal fats still predominate, the greater fat consumption can be attributed to vegetable products, reflecting increased use of margarines, vegetable shortenings, and edible oils (Bailey et al., 1988). Factors fostering the increased use of edible oils include the rapid growth of fast-food restaurants, in which many foods are cooked in oil, and the greater use of convenience foods that are fried or contain added oil (Raper and Marston, 1986).

Disappearance data, however, do not indicate the amount of fat actually consumed, because they are not adjusted for waste, spoilage, trimming, or cooking losses (NRC, 1988). Periodic surveys in which actual food consumption by individuals is measured indicate that people in the United States in fact have decreased the fat content of their diets. USDA surveys show that adults decreased their fat intake from 41% of total kcal in 1977 to 36.4% of total kcal in 1985–1986 (USDA, 1986, 1987). Although some of the decrease may reflect methodological differences, the results reflect changes in food selection as well. Since 1970, for example, consumption of red meat has declined, whereas consumption of poultry has increased and more low-fat milk than whole milk is being consumed (NRC, 1989).

ESSENTIAL FATTY ACIDS

Small amounts of linoleic acid must be present in the diet to maintain health. The inability of animals to produce linoleic acid is attributable to the lack of a δ-12 dehydrogenase to introduce a second double bond in its monounsaturated precursor (oleic acid). Once linoleic acid is available, however, it can be desaturated and elongated further to form arachidonic acid, a 20-carbon n-6 fatty acid with four double bonds. Thus, arachidonic acid is also considered an essential fatty acid, but only when linoleic acid deficiency exists. The third fatty acid traditionally classified as essential is the n-3 polyunsaturated fatty acid, α-linolenic acid. The role of linolenic acid in human nutrition is becoming clarified (Bivins et al., 1983; Neuringer and Connor, 1986). One possible case of deficiency has been described (Holman et al., 1982), and experiments in monkeys and rats have shown visual impairment and behavior differences after consumption of diets deficient in n-3 fatty acids (Neuringer and Connor, 1986). The retina and brain membranes are especially rich in docosahexaenoic acid. DHA and EPA can be synthesized from linolenic acid in the body or obtained directly in the diet from seafood. DHA and EPA are also synthesized by phytoplankton and algae and thus are abundant in fish and shellfish.

Linoleic and arachidonic acid, present in phospholipids, are important for maintaining the structure and function of cellular and subcellular membranes. In addition, n-6 and n-3 polyunsaturated fatty acids have been shown to be the precursors of eicosanoids (Glomset, 1985), which are important in the regulation of widely diverse physiological processes. A growing body of evidence indicates that nutritional status with respect to polyunsaturated fatty acids alters the production of eicosanoids. Consumption of fish rich in EPA can thereby modify platelet function and inflammatory responses.

Linoleic acid deficiency can be identified biochemically by analysis of plasma lipids. The characteristic abnormalities are low linoleic and arachidonic acid levels and elevated levels of 5,8,11-eicosatrienoic acid, a polyunsaturated, n-9 fatty acid produced from oleic acid. Studies in animals have shown that linoleic acid deficiency produces a variety of metabolic disturbances (Alfin-Slater and Aftergood, 1968). In infants fed formulas deficient in linoleic acid, drying and flaking of the skin have been observed (Wiese et al., 1958). Biochemical evidence of linoleic acid deficiency has also been found in premature infants whose fat intake is delayed (Friedman et al., 1976). Linoleic acid deficiency in adult humans was not reported until the early 1970s, when several investigators described such deficiency associated with scaly skin, hair loss, and impaired wound healing in hospitalized patients fed exclusively with intravenous fluids containing no fat (Collins et al., 1971; Paulsrud et al., 1972; Richardson and

Sgoutas, 1975). In addition, patients with malabsorption due to biliary atresia and cystic fibrosis may be deficient in linoleic acid (Farrell et al., 1985; Gourley et al., 1982).

Linoleic acid intake at levels from 1 to 2% of total dietary calories is sufficient to prevent both biochemical and clinical evidence of deficiency in several animal species and in humans (Holman, 1970). For infants consuming 100 kcal/kg body weight per day, this would correspond to a daily intake of approximately 0.2 g/kg. The American Academy of Pediatrics (AAP, 1985) has recommended that infant formulas provide at least 2.7% of energy as linoleic acid. For the average adult, a minimally adequate intake of linoleic acid is 3 to 6 g/day. This level is more than met by diets in the United States, since most vegetable oils are particularly rich sources of linoleic acid. In several studies, linoleic acid has been found to range from 5 to 10% of calories in diets providing 25 to 50% of energy as fat (Bieri and Evarts, 1973; Witting and Lee, 1975). As discussed in the section on vitamin E (see Chapter 7), large amounts of polyunsaturated fatty acids may increase the need for this fat-soluble, antioxidant nutrient. The Committee on Diet and Health of the Food and Nutrition Board recently recommended that the average population intake of n-6 polyunsaturated fatty acids remain at the current level of about 7% of calories and that individual intakes not exceed 10% of calories because of lack of information about the long-term consequences of a higher intake (NRC, 1989).

For many reasons, especially because essential fatty acid deficiency has been observed exclusively in patients with medical problems affecting fat intake or absorption, the subcommittee has not established an RDA for n-3 or n-6 polyunsaturated fatty acids. The rapid developments in the field of fat-soluble dietary factors, and their physiologic role in eicosanoid production, will require periodic reappraisal of their significance in nutrition and the regulation of metabolic functions. The possibility of establishing RDAs for these fatty acids should be considered in the near future. For example, Neuringer et al. (1988) proposed that the consumption of n-3 fatty acids in humans should be 10 to 25% that of linoleic acid, particularly during pregnancy, lactation, and infancy. Synthetic infant formulas generally contain only vegetable oils as their lipid sources and thus contain only 18-carbon polyunsaturates. Even when these formulas supply ample linolenic acid, DHA levels in the infants' erythrocyte membrane phospholipids are much lower than in those infants receiving either human milk or formulas supplemented with sources of longer-chain n-3 fatty acids (Carlson et al., 1986; Crawford et al., 1977). Also, the ratio of dietary linoleic acid to EPA and DHA can affect platelet function and inflammatory responses, and may thereby influence the development of certain chronic diseases, such as coronary heart disease and rheumatoid arthritis (Leaf and Weber, 1988).

OTHER CONSIDERATIONS

It has long been recognized that the amount and nature of fat ingested affects plasma cholesterol concentration, and that high blood cholesterol levels are strongly related to the incidence and risk of atherosclerotic vascular disease, especially coronary heart disease. Several types of evidence, including clinical dietary and drug trials, show that the cholesterol contained in the plasma's low-density lipoprotein (LDL) fraction is the principal detrimental component, whereas high levels of cholesterol in high-density lipoproteins (HDL) are associated with a reduced risk of coronary heart disease. Other factors, such as genetic background, cigarette smoking, hypertension, and obesity, also increase the risk of coronary artery disease (NRC, 1989). The strongest dietary determinant of blood cholesterol level is the saturated fatty acid content (NRC, 1989). The cholesterol content of the diet has an appreciable, but usually lesser influence. Increased intake of both these nutrients decreases LDL receptor activity in liver cells and increases LDL cholesterol levels in the blood (Spady and Dietschy, 1988).

In the past decade, considerable attention has been given to the potential role of dietary factors in the etiology and prevention of cancer. This subject has recently been reviewed in depth, and several organizations have proposed dietary guidelines toward lowering the risk of certain cancers. These guidelines have included the suggestion that total fat intake should be reduced (DHHS, 1988; NRC, 1982; NRC, 1989).

Additional research is needed to clarify the role of diet in carcinogenesis and to determine the proportion of energy that should be provided by dietary fats relative to other macrocomponents to reduce the risks of heart disease and cancer. However, a decrease in the average consumption of fat by Americans from its present level of approximately 36% of calories appears to be desirable. An additional benefit of reducing the fat content of the diet may be lower caloric intakes and hence a reduced prevalence of obesity and its adverse effects on health. After a comprehensive evaluation of the evidence, the Food and Nutrition Board's Committee on Diet and Health recommended that the fat content of the U.S. diet not exceed 30% of caloric intake, that less than 10% of calories should be provided from saturated fatty acids, and that dietary cholesterol should be less than 300 mg/day (NRC, 1989).

REFERENCES

AAP (American Academy of Pediatrics). 1985. Appendix K: Composition of human milk: normative data. Pp. 363–368 in G.B. Forbes, ed. Pediatric Nutrition Handbook. American Academy of Pediatrics, Elk Grove Village, Ill.

Alfin-Slater, R.B., and L. Aftergood. 1968. Essential fatty acids reinvestigated. Physiol. Rev. 48:758–784.

Bailey, L., L. Duewer, F. Gray, R. Hoskin, J. Putnam, and S. Short. 1988. Food consumption. Natl. Food Rev. 11:1–10.

Bieri, J.G., and R.P. Evarts. 1973. Tocopherols and fatty acids in American diets. The recommended allowance for vitamin E. J. Am. Diet. Assoc. 62:147–151.

Bivins, B.A., R.M. Bell, R.P. Rapp, and W.O. Griffen, Jr. 1983. Linoleic acid *versus* linolenic acid: what is essential? J. Parent. Ent. Nutr. 7:473–478.

Block, G., C.M. Dresser, A.M. Hartman, and M.D. Carroll. 1985. Nutrient sources in the American diet: quantitative data from the NHANES II survey. II. Macronutrients and fats. Am. J. Epidemiol. 122:27–40.

Carlson, S.E., P.G. Rhodes, and M.G. Ferguson. 1986. Docosahexaenoic acid status of preterm infants at birth and following feeding with human milk or formula. Am. J. Clin. Nutr. 44:798–804.

Collins, F.D., A.J. Sinclair, J.B. Royle, D.A. Coats, A.T. Maynard, and F.L. Leonard. 1971. Plasma lipids in human linoleic acid deficiency. Nutr. Metab. 13:150–167.

Crawford, M.A., A.G. Hassam, and B.M. Hall. 1977. Metabolism of essential fatty acids in the human fetus and neonate. Nutr. Metab. 21, Suppl. 1:187–188.

DHHS (U.S. Department of Health and Human Services). 1988. The Surgeon General's Report on Nutrition and Health. U.S. Government Printing Office, Washington, D.C. 727 pp.

Farrell, P.M., E.H. Mischler, M.J. Engle, D.J. Brown, and S.-M. Lau. 1985. Fatty acid abnormalities in cystic fibrosis. Pediatr. Res. 19:104–109.

Friedman, Z., A. Danon, M.T. Stahlman, and J.A. Oates. 1976. Rapid onset of essential fatty acid deficiency in the newborn. Pediatrics 58:640–649.

Glomset, J.A. 1985. Fish, fatty acids, and human health. N. Engl. J. Med. 312:1253–1254.

Gourley, G.R., P.M. Farrell, and G.B. Odell. 1982. Essential fatty acid deficiency after hepatic portoenterostomy for biliary atresia. Am. J. Clin. Nutr. 36:1194–1199.

Holman, R.T. 1970. Biological activities of and requirements for polyunsaturated acids. Pp. 607–682 in Progress in the Chemistry of Fats and Other Lipids, Vol. 9. Pergamon Press, New York.

Holman, R.T., S.B. Johnson, and T.F. Hatch. 1982. A case of human linolenic acid deficiency involving neurological abnormalities. Am. J. Clin. Nutr. 35:617–623.

Leaf, A., and P.C. Weber. 1988. Cardiovascular effects of n-3 fatty acids. N. Engl. J. Med. 318:549–557.

Neuringer, M.D., and W.E. Connor. 1986. N-3 fatty acids in the brain and retina: evidence for their essentiality. Nutr. Rev. 44:285–294.

Neuringer, M., G.J. Anderson, and W.E. Connor. 1988. The essentiality of N-3 fatty acids for the development and function of the retina and brain. Annu. Rev. Nutr. 8:517–541.

NRC (National Research Council). 1982. Diet, Nutrition, and Cancer. Report of the Committee on Diet, Nutrition, and Cancer, Assembly of Life Sciences. National Academy Press, Washington, D.C. 478 pp.

NRC (National Research Council). 1988. Designing Foods: Animal Product Options in the Marketplace. Report of the Committee on Technological Options to Improve the Nutritional Attributes of Animal Products, Board on Agriculture. National Academy Press, Washington, D.C. 367 pp.

NRC (National Research Council). 1989. Diet and Health: Implications for Reducing Chronic Disease Risk. Report of the Committee on Diet and Health, Food and Nutrition Board. National Academy Press, Washington, D.C. 750 pp.

Paulsrud, J.R., L. Pensler, C.F. Whitten, S. Stewart, and R.T. Holman. 1972. Essential fatty acid deficiency in infants induced by fat-free intravenous feeding. Am. J. Clin. Nutr. 25:897–904.

Raper, N.R., and R.M. Marston. 1986. Levels and sources of fat in the U.S. food supply. Pp. 127–152 in C. Ip, D.F. Birt, A.E. Rogers, and C. Mettlin, eds. Dietary Fat and Cancer. Alan R. Liss, New York.

Richardson, T.J., and D. Sgoutas. 1975. Essential fatty acid deficiency in four adult patients during total parenteral nutrition. Am. J. Clin. Nutr. 28:258–263.

Spady, D.K., and J.M. Dietschy. 1988. Interaction of dietary cholesterol and triglycerides in the regulation of hepatic low density lipoprotein transport in the hamster. J. Clin. Invest. 81:300–309.

USDA (U.S. Department of Agriculture). 1984. Nutrient Intakes: Individuals in 48 States, Year 1977–78. Nationwide Food Consumption Survey. Report No. I-2. Consumer Nutrition Division, Human Nutrition Information Service, Hyattsville, Md.

USDA (U.S. Department of Agriculture). 1986. Nationwide Food Consumption Survey. Continuing Survey of Food Intakes of Individuals: Men 19–50 Years, 1 Day, 1985. Report No. 85-3. Nutrition Monitoring Division, Human Nutrition Information Service. U.S. Department of Agriculture, Hyattsville, Md. 94 pp.

USDA (U.S. Department of Agriculture). 1987. Nationwide Food Consumption Survey. Continuing Survey of Food Intakes of Individuals: Women 19–50 Years and Their Children 1–5 Years, 4 Days, 1985. Report No. 85-4. Nutrition Monitoring Division, Human Nutrition Information Service. U.S. Department of Agriculture, Hyattsville, Md. 182 pp.

Wiese, H.F., A.E. Hansen, and D.J.D. Adam. 1958. Essential fatty acids in infant nutrition. J. Nutr. 58:345–360.

Witting, L.A., and L. Lee. 1975. Dietary levels of vitamin E and polyunsaturated fatty acids and plasma vitamin E. Am. J. Clin. Nutr. 28:571–576.

6
Protein and Amino Acids

Both animal and plant proteins are made up of about 20 common amino acids. The proportion of these amino acids varies as a characteristic of a given protein, but all food proteins—with the exception of gelatin—contain some of each. Amino nitrogen accounts for approximately 16% of the weight of proteins. Amino acids are required for the synthesis of body protein and other important nitrogen-containing compounds, such as creatine, peptide hormones, and some neurotransmitters. Although allowances are expressed as protein,[a] the biological requirement is for amino acids.

Proteins and other nitrogenous compounds are being degraded and resynthesized continuously. Several times more protein is turned over daily within the body than is ordinarily consumed, indicating that reutilization of amino acids is a major feature of the economy of protein metabolism. This process of recapture is not completely efficient, and some amino acids are lost by oxidative catabolism. Metabolic products of amino acids (urea, creatinine, uric acid, and other nitrogenous products) are excreted in the urine; nitrogen is also lost in feces, sweat, and other body secretions and in sloughed skin, hair, and nails. A continuous supply of dietary amino acids is required to replace these losses, even after growth has ceased.

---

[a]In this chapter, protein is equated with nitrogen × 6.25, i.e., crude protein containing 16% nitrogen. Specific food proteins have greater (cereals) or lesser (milk) percentages of nitrogen. See *USDA Agricultural Handbook Series 8* (1976–1989) for factors used in food composition tables.

Amino acids consumed in excess of the amounts needed for the synthesis of nitrogenous tissue constituents are not stored but are degraded; the nitrogen is excreted as urea, and the keto acids left after removal of the amino groups are either utilized directly as sources of energy or are converted to carbohydrate or fat.

Nine amino acids—histidine, isoleucine, leucine, lysine, methionine, phenylalanine, threonine, tryptophan, and valine—are not synthesized by mammals and are therefore dietarily essential or indispensable nutrients. These are commonly called the essential amino acids. Histidine is an essential amino acid for infants, but was not demonstrated to be required by adults until recently (Cho et al., 1984; Kopple and Swendseid, 1981). Under special circumstances (e.g., in premature infants or in people with liver damage), amino acids such as cystine and tyrosine, not normally essential, may become so because of impaired conversion from their precursors (Horowitz et al., 1981). Arginine is synthesized by mammals but not in amounts sufficient to meet the needs of the young of most species. Although it is not believed to be required by the human infant for normal growth, the need for arginine by the premature infant is unknown. When arginine is present in small amounts relative to other amino acids (such as in intravenous solutions or amino acid mixtures), or when liver function is compromised, arginine synthesis may be insufficient for adequate function of the urea cycle (Heird et al., 1972).

GENERAL SIGNS OF DEFICIENCY

Protein deficiency rarely occurs as an isolated condition. It usually accompanies a deficiency of dietary energy and other nutrients resulting from insufficient food intake. The symptoms are most commonly seen in deprived children in poor countries. Where protein intake is exceptionally low, there are physical signs—stunting, poor musculature, edema, thin and fragile hair, skin lesions—and biochemical changes that include low serum albumin and hormonal imbalances. Edema and loss of muscle mass and hair are the prominent signs in adults. Deficiency of this severity is very rare in the United States, except as a consequence of pathologic conditions and poor medical management of the acutely ill.

GENERAL PRINCIPLES FOR ESTIMATING PROTEIN REQUIREMENTS

At submaintenance levels of protein intake, a diminished turnover of tissue protein is accompanied by a reduced catabolic rate for the amino acids liberated by protein breakdown (Young and Scrimshaw, 1977). Similarly, turnover rate is increased with increased intake. In this way, the tissue protein pool can, within limits, enter a new steady state appropriate for the diminished or increased protein intake from food.

Under the experimental conditions of a protein-free diet, protein synthesis and breakdown continue by reutilizing amino acids. This process becomes very efficient, but some amino acids are still catabolized and the nitrogen is excreted. This lower limit, termed the *obligatory* nitrogen loss, has been extensively studied in adults fed protein-free diets. Values are remarkably uniform. In a series of 11 studies involving more than 200 adults ranging in age from 20 to 77 years, daily obligatory nitrogen losses averaged 53 mg (41–69 mg, range of study means) of nitrogen per kilogram daily (WHO, 1985).[b]

In the past, a factorial method was used as a basis for predicting the protein requirements of various age groups. For adults, the requirement for dietary protein was considered to be the amount needed to replace the obligatory nitrogen loss after adjustment for inefficiency in utilization of dietary protein and for the quality of the dietary protein consumed (i.e., its digestibility and amino acid composition). For children and pregnant and lactating women, an additional amount of protein for tissue growth or milk formation was incorporated into this factorial estimate of requirements. Because of the assumptions required, the validity of the factorial approach has been questioned.

WHO (1985) reviewed the evidence on protein requirements and concluded that adult protein allowances should be based on nitrogen balance studies. For older infants and children, data are sparse; thus, all lines of evidence were used by the subcommittee in estimating requirements—nitrogen balance and observed and theoretical needs for adequate growth. For pregnancy, nitrogen balance data were considered, but allowances continue to rely on theoretical deposition of protein in the fetus and adnexa. New information on human milk volume was used to estimate lactational requirements.

Protein synthesis and breakdown are energy-dependent and thus are sensitive to dietary energy deprivation. Consequently, the body's energy balance becomes an important factor in determining nitrogen balance and influences the apparent utilization of dietary protein.

---

[b]The WHO (1985) report contains extensive references to the original investigations. The reader is referred to that report for full documentation.

Protein requirements are determined and allowances established for conditions of adequate energy intake and balance.

Nitrogen Balance

Nitrogen balance is the difference between nitrogen intake and the amount excreted in urine, feces, and sweat, together with minor losses occurring by other routes. To estimate the protein requirement, levels of dietary protein below and near predicted adequate intake are fed and nitrogen balance is measured at each level. The requirement is estimated by interpolating or extrapolating the nitrogen balance data to the zero balance point (nitrogen equilibrium) for adults or to a defined level of positive balance (to allow for growth) for children.

Because of methodologic problems, it is difficult to attain exact measurement of intake and output of nitrogen (Hegsted, 1976), to determine the time required for adjustment at altered levels of protein intake (Rand et al., 1981), and to measure or otherwise account for nitrogen losses through routes other than urine and feces.

OTHER CRITERIA OF ADEQUACY

Most studies of protein requirements have been short. Because of the methodologic problems cited above, longer studies should provide a better basis for determining protein requirements[c]; they would permit the measurement of variables such as alterations in lean body mass or in growth rate of children, which respond more slowly to dietary inadequacy. In the few long-term studies that have been reported, investigators have explored the usefulness of various biochemical indices (e.g., serum aspartate and alanine amino transferase activities) (Garza et al., 1977), but no agreement on a sensitive and reliable marker has been reached (Solomons and Allen, 1983; WHO, 1985).

Because the human body can adapt to low and high intakes of nitrogen, there is a substantial difference between intakes barely sufficient to compensate for losses or to permit growth and intakes that may be associated with harmful effects. Since there are few criteria by which to evaluate the significance of the rate of protein turnover and pool size, value judgments must be made as to what is desirable

---

[c]The term protein requirement conventionally encompasses specific and nonspecific amino acid and amino nitrogen requirements.

in adults. For children, the protein required for growth is relatively small compared to that needed for maintenance. Nevertheless, satisfactory growth is a sensitive indicator of protein nutritional status.

The requirement for protein is reasonably well established for the very young child and the young male adult. For other age groups, much less information is available, and protein needs are estimated in part by interpolation or extrapolation based on reasonable biological principles.

THE REQUIREMENT FOR AMINO ACIDS

In determining the requirement for protein, the subcommittee first considered requirements for the essential amino acids. The required amounts of the nine essential amino acids must be provided in the diet, but because cystine can replace approximately 30% of the requirement for methionine, and tyrosine about 50% of the requirement for phenylalanine, these amino acids must also be considered. The essential amino acid requirements of infants, children, men, and women were studied extensively from 1950 to 1970. Except for infants, where the criterion was growth and nitrogen accretion, the requirement was accepted to be the amount of intake needed to achieve nitrogen equilibrium in short-term studies of adults or positive balance in children (see review by FAO/WHO, 1973; NRC, 1974; WHO, 1985). Estimates of amino acid requirements for various age groups are listed in Table 6-1.

In a novel approach to examining these requirements, the need for four amino acids was examined in children whose diets were strictly controlled because of inborn errors of metabolism and who were developing normally (Kindt and Halvorsen, 1980). Requirements determined in this way during the first 3 years of life are in good agreement with the values for isoleucine, leucine, phenylalanine plus tyrosine, and valine given in Table 6-1 for infants and 2-year-old children.

The requirement for histidine has not been quantified beyond infancy. Requirement values are difficult to establish because deficiency symptoms occur only after long periods of low intake. Kopple and Swendseid (1981) demonstrated that nitrogen balance diminished when histidine intake was less than 2 mg/kg per day, and increased when intake was increased to 4 mg/kg per day. WHO (1985) estimated the probable adult histidine requirement to be between 8 and 12 mg/kg per day by extrapolation from the infant requirement; this estimate is likely to be high, but safe.

TABLE 6-1 Estimates of Amino Acid Requirements[a]

	Requirements, mg/kg per day, by age group			
Amino Acid	Infants, Age 3–4 mo[b]	Children, Age ~2 yr[c]	Children, Age 10–12 yr[d]	Adults[e]
Histidine	28	?	?	8–12
Isoleucine	70	31	28	10
Leucine	161	73	42	14
Lysine	103	64	44	12
Methionine plus cystine	58	27	22	13
Phenylalanine plus tyrosine	125	69	22	14
Threonine	87	37	28	7
Tryptophan	17	12.5	3.3	3.5
Valine	93	38	25	10
Total without histidine	714	352	214	84

[a] From WHO (1985).

[b] Based on amounts of amino acids in human milk or cow's milk formulas fed at levels that supported good growth. Data from Fomon and Filer (1967).

[c] Based on achievement of nitrogen balance sufficient to support adequate lean tissue gain (16 mg N/kg per day). Data from Pineda et al. (1981).

[d] Based on upper range of requirement for positive nitrogen balance. Recalculated by Williams et al. (1974) from data of Nakagawa et al. (1964).

[e] Based on highest estimate of requirement to achieve nitrogen balance. Data from several investigators (reviewed in FAO/WHO, 1973).

The relatively low requirements estimated for adults have been confirmed by Inoue et al. (1988) using the nitrogen balance method. Studies of whole body lysine, leucine, valine, and threonine oxidation rates suggest that adult requirements for these essential amino acids have been underestimated. Approximations of average requirements according to the ^{13}C tracer studies are leucine, 40 mg/kg (Meguid et al., 1986a); lysine, 35 mg/kg (Meredith et al., 1986); threonine, 15 mg/kg (Zhao et al., 1986); and valine, 16 mg/kg (Meguid et al., 1986b). These new estimates have been challenged on methodologic and theoretical grounds (Millward and Rivers, 1986) and require further confirmation.

Studies on requirements for individual essential amino acids in the elderly are inconsistent. Some suggest that requirements are increased in the elderly; others indicate that they are decreased (Munro, 1983). In the one study in which the same methodology and design were applied to the elderly as in a study of young men, no differences in requirements between age groups were found (Watts et al., 1964).

The pattern of requirement for essential amino acids in the elderly is accepted to be the same as for younger adults.

There is no information on amino acid requirements of pregnant and lactating women.

The data demonstrate the unsatisfactory state of knowledge concerning amino acid requirements. The values in Table 6-1 are the best available and serve as the basis for calculation of amino acid requirement patterns at various ages and for procedures for the amino acid scoring of diets (see below).

RECOMMENDED ALLOWANCES FOR PROTEIN

In establishing an RDA for protein, three steps were followed: (1) The subcommittee first estimated the *average requirement* for *reference proteins* (i.e., highly digestible, high-quality protein such as egg, meat, milk, or fish) according to sex, age, and reproductive status of women. (2) The standard deviation of requirement was determined and average requirement values were increased accordingly to compute the recommended allowance of reference protein. (3) Amino acid scoring patterns were tabulated. These were based on requirements of various age groups for essential amino acids and for total protein. These patterns of requirement were reviewed in relation to U.S. food consumption patterns to determine if adjustment of the allowance for reference protein would be warranted in establishing the RDA for protein due to amino acid composition or protein digestibility of food proteins consumed.

The Requirement for Reference Protein and Its Variability

Adults   To determine the protein requirements of young male adults, WHO (1985) reviewed evidence from both short- and long-term nitrogen balance studies. On the basis of recalculated data from the short-term studies, the international group proposed a mean requirement of 0.61 g/kg per day for reference protein. Several relatively long-term studies (58 to 89 days) involving single levels of protein intake yielded similar estimates of requirement for subjects consuming egg-protein diets. By averaging the two sets of balance data (i.e., from the long- and short-term studies), a protein requirement of 0.6 g/kg per day (rounded) was obtained. This is accepted to be the average daily requirement for reference proteins. No data were available on the coefficient of variation for long-term studies, but for short-term studies, the mean coefficient of variation was estimated to be 12.5%. A value of 25% (2 SDs) above the average requirement would be expected to meet the needs of 97.5% of a normally distributed population. Thus, 0.75 g/kg per day (0.6 × 1.25) is the recommended allowance of reference protein for young male adults.

The international group examined the data from several short-term studies in which men were fed habitual mixed diets of ordinary food. The requirements were predicted to be 0.54 to 0.99 g/kg per day, the larger estimates deriving from diets of lower digestibility and quality. The adult requirement for absorbed protein appears not to differ between reference and practical diets.

There are fewer data for young adult women, but there is evidence (Calloway and Kurzer, 1982) that requirement values, when adjusted for body weight, are not substantially different from those for young adult men. Accordingly, the recommended allowance for reference protein is 0.75 g/kg per day for both sexes.

The Elderly The protein content of the adult body diminishes with age. More specifically, nonmuscle mass is little affected by age, whereas muscle diminishes extensively and is compensated for by an increase in body fat. These changes in muscle mass are related to whole-body protein turnover and changes in the rate of protein synthesis (Uauy et al., 1978a). Muscle protein turnover accounts for 30% of the total protein turnover in the young adult, but only 20% of that in the elderly (Munro, 1983). Serum albumin levels and daily albumin synthesis also decrease in elderly people who consume diets with adequate protein (Gersovitz et al., 1980).

Questions thus arise concerning the extent to which changes in protein metabolism affect protein requirements. Dietary protein needs might be expected to change during the aging process, i.e., to decrease due to lower rates of turnover, or to increase due to decreased efficiency of absorptive and metabolic processes and to decreased total food intake associated with reduced physical activity, or to become more variable due to disease and disability. There is surprisingly little information on which to base recommendations for protein intake in the elderly.

The early literature on this subject was reviewed by Irwin and Hegsted (1971). Only a few studies have been conducted in the more recent past, and their results are inconsistent. Zanni et al. (1979) concluded that 0.57 g of egg protein per kilogram of observed body weight (weights were above ideal for height) was adequate to sustain nitrogen equilibrium at a food energy intake of 30 kcal/kg, whereas Uauy et al. (1978b) found that 0.57 g/kg was insufficient for nearly all subjects and that needs were only barely met at 0.8 g/kg. According to Gersovitz et al. (1982), 0.8 g of egg protein per kilogram of body weight per day was insufficient to maintain nitrogen balance in the majority of elderly men and women studied over a 30-day period, but Cheng et al. (1978) found this level of protein to be adequate. In both of these studies, body weight was maintained; however, energy intake was lower in the study by Gersovitz and colleagues (1982), suggesting that activity patterns may have been different in the two groups or that nitrogen balance was improved by the higher food energy intake in the study by Cheng et al. (1978). Variations in activity level, disease prevalence, and use of therapeutic drugs are all potentially confounding variables.

The recommended allowance for reference protein (0.75 g/kg) is accepted to be the same for the elderly as for young adults. Because of the difference in body composition, this allowance is higher per unit of lean body mass and should allow for some decrement in utilization efficiency.

Pregnancy   Additional protein is required during pregnancy for the mother and the fetus (Hytten and Leitch, 1971). Maternal protein synthesis increases in order to support expansion of the blood volume, uterus, and breasts, and fetal and placental proteins are synthesized from amino acids supplied by the mother. The magnitude of the required increase in dietary intake remains uncertain, since different methods of estimation yield different figures.

The factorial method of estimating requirements for pregnancy is based on the amount of protein present in the fetus, placenta, and maternal tissues, including blood (Hytten and Leitch, 1971). It is calculated that 925 g of protein is deposited during a pregnancy involving 12.5 kg of maternal weight gain and an infant weighing 3.3 kg at term. The rate of nitrogen retention is not constant; for the first through third trimester, nitrogen deposition is estimated to be 0.11, 0.52, and 0.92 g/day, respectively (Table 6-2). Evidence from animal studies suggests, however, that relatively more protein may be stored during early gestation and mobilized at later stages of pregnancy (Naismith, 1977; Naismith and Morgan, 1976). Protein turnover is increased by the twelfth week of pregnancy (de Benoist et al., 1985); it remains high in the second trimester and the same (Jackson, 1987) or lower (Fitch and King, 1987) in the third trimester. Consequently, increased protein needs during pregnancy may be more uniform across time than the figures of Hytten and Leitch indicate.

Nitrogen balance data can also be used to estimate protein requirements during pregnancy. Almost all older balance studies have indicated that more nitrogen is retained during pregnancy than is

TABLE 6-2 Derivation of Reference Protein Allowance During Pregnancy

Trimester	Average Additional Storage of Nitrogen (g/day)[a]	Average Additional Storage +30%[b]	Corrected for Conversion Efficiency[c]	Additional Reference Protein (g/day)[d]
1	0.11	0.14	0.20	1.3
2	0.52	0.68	0.97	6.1
3	0.92	1.20	1.71	10.7
Average over entire pregnancy				6.0

[a] From WHO (1985). Assumes 3.3-kg infant birth weight.
[b] Coefficient of variation of birth weight assumed to be 15%.
[c] Assumes 70% conversion efficiency of dietary protein to tissue protein.
[d] Total nitrogen × 6.25.

predicted on the basis of fetal and placental growth and maternal tissue hypertrophy (Calloway, 1974). In more recent studies (Appel and King, 1979; Johnstone et al., 1981), nitrogen retentions have been found to be closer to the theoretical value if allowance is made for unmeasured losses. Nevertheless, data on changes in body weight and body potassium indicate that nitrogen retention under laboratory conditions is somewhat greater than can be accounted for only by the fetus and maternal supportive tissue (Appel and King, 1979; King et al., 1973). This suggests that protein might be retained at sites other than those now recognized, for example, in skeletal muscle. This possibility is supported in part by analyses of animal carcasses (King, 1975).

Dietary surveys in developed countries indicate that pregnant women eating self-selected diets generally consume somewhat larger amounts of protein than theoretical requirements. Moreover, satisfactory levels of protein intake tend to be associated with improved reproductive outcome (Higgins et al., 1973; Lechtig et al., 1975; Metcoff et al., 1981; Osofsky, 1975). However, such epidemiological data are confounded by the strong dietary correlation between protein and energy, as well as their metabolic interrelationships.

Despite these discrepancies between factorial and nitrogen balance estimates of nitrogen gain during pregnancy, the subcommittee concurs with WHO (1985) that the estimate of requirement should be based on the factorial method. The coefficient of variation in birth weight is 15%—a variance assigned to all components of pregnancy protein gain. The average storage value is thus increased by 30% to include the protein gains of virtually all healthy women during pregnancy. These values must be adjusted for the efficiency with which dietary protein is converted to fetal, placental, and maternal tissues; this is generally assumed to be 70%—the same as efficiency observed in infants. The additional allowance of reference protein needed to support the deposition of new tissue is calculated to be 1.3, 6.1, and 10.7 g/day during the first, second, and third trimesters of pregnancy, respectively (Table 6-2). There is also a maintenance requirement associated with the added lean tissue. To allow for this and because of the uncertainty about the rate of tissue deposition, the subcommittee recommends an additional allowance of 10 g of reference protein per day throughout pregnancy.

Lactation   The average protein (nitrogen $\times$ 6.25) content of mature human milk is approximately 1.1 g/100 ml, except during the first month when it is about 1.3 g/100 ml (WHO, 1985). Analyses of human milk composition in the United States, based on a study of 40 mothers in the first 4 months of lactation, show a fall in protein content from 1.36 g/100 ml to 1.12 g/100 ml during this period (Butte et al., 1984).

The average protein requirement for lactation is estimated from milk composition and the mean volume of milk produced, which is 750 ml/day, adjusted for 70% efficiency in the conversion of dietary protein to milk protein. The coefficient of variation is taken to be 12.5% (WHO, 1985); thus, the average requirement is increased by 25% to determine the recommended allowance of a reference protein. The allowance is calculated as follows:

$$\text{Additional protein required for lactation} = \frac{750 \text{ ml} \times 0.011 \text{ g protein per milliliter}}{0.70 \text{ efficiency}}$$
$$\times 1.25 \text{ for variance}$$
$$= 14.7 \text{ g/day.}$$

The volume of milk produced in the second 6 months of lactation is about 20% less than in the first 6 months, according to international data (WHO, 1985). No recent data from the United States have been published. If the international figure is accepted, then the additional allowance in this period is 11.8 g of reference protein per day. The recommended allowance of additional reference protein is 15 g/day during the first 6 months of lactation and 12 g/day thereafter.

Infants, Children, and Adolescents   During the first year of life, the protein content of the body increases from 11 to 15%, and body weight increases by approximately 7 kg. The average increase in body protein is about 3.5 g/day during the first 4 months of life and 3.1 g/day during the subsequent 8 months (Fomon, 1974). By 4 years of age, body protein content reaches the adult value of 18 to 19% of body weight (Widdowson and Dickerson, 1963). As the growth rate drops rapidly after the first year of life, the maintenance requirement represents a gradually increasing proportion of the total protein requirement.

For the first months of life, requirements are based on intake data because of the difficulty in accurately estimating allowances for growth and maturation of body composition. Infants breastfed by healthy, well-nourished mothers or fed human milk by bottle can grow at a satisfactory rate for about 4 months (Butte et al., 1984; Ferris et al., 1978; Fomon, 1986). Protein[d] intakes by breastfed infants range from 2.43 g/kg per day in the first month to 1.51 g/kg per day in the fourth month, averaging 2.04 g/kg per day in the first 3 months and 1.73 g/kg per day in the next 3 months (WHO, 1985). Breastfed infants in the United States grow satisfactorily at a mean protein intake of 1.68 g/kg per day (total nitrogen × 6.25) during the first 3 months (Butte et al., 1984). Probability assessment suggests that the true requirement appears to be less than mean intake; the figure proposed is 1.1 g/kg with a deviation of 0.1 to 0.2 g/kg (Beaton and Chery, 1988). The subcommittee has, however, accepted an average intake of 1.68 g/kg per day as the requirement between birth and 3 months of age, the reference being human milk protein. The protein needs of an infant up to 4 months of age will be met if the energy needs are met, provided the food is human milk or a formula that contains protein of a quality and quantity equivalent to that of human milk.

A modified factorial procedure for calculating the protein needs -of infants and children was examined by the WHO group. Values were assigned for a maintenance requirement, and an increment representing growth, the theoretical value for which was increased by 50% to allow for marked unevenness of daily growth rate and the inability of infants and children to store amino acids against intermittent needs. Efficiency of utilization was accepted to be 70%. These estimates were compared with data from the few studies of nitrogen balance in the age group 6 months to 9 years. Neither the factorial nor balance estimates were consistently higher or lower across age

---

[d]The figures given for protein are nitrogen × 6.25. Approximately 20% of the nitrogen in human milk is nonprotein nitrogen (e.g., amino acids, urea, nucleotides), much of which is assumed to be utilized by the infant, and by convention is calculated as if it were crude protein.

groups. Because there are large gaps in the experimental data, the modified factorial approach was used by the WHO group to estimate needs for all children. The international values are accepted by this subcommittee in establishing average requirements for reference protein beyond age 3 months. Table 6-3 provides examples of the steps involved in the calculations of daily allowances by the modified factorial approach. The coefficient of variation in requirements calculated in this manner is assumed to be 12.5%—the same as that established for maintenance requirements in adults. The factorially determined average requirement is accordingly increased by 25% to derive the recommended allowance for reference protein.

The tabulated values for reference protein allowances for the various age and sex groups are listed in Table 6-4. To convert these values to daily allowances of average U.S. dietary protein, one must examine these values in relation to the amino acid composition and digestibility of proteins consumed. Since the requirements of both amino acids and protein differ among age and sex groups, the quality of protein required to meet these needs will also vary.

Amino Acid Requirement Pattern According to Age

A pattern of requirements for amino acids in the total dietary protein is calculated by dividing each essential amino acid requirement by the recommended allowance of reference protein for the given age group (see Table 6-5).

The requirement pattern for infants is based on quantitative amino acid requirements (Table 6-1) divided by the reference protein allowance of infants 3 to 4 months of age (1.73 g/kg; Table 6-3)—the age at which the studies were made. WHO (1985) accepted for this age group a pattern based on the average composition of human milk protein. Both patterns are shown in Table 6-5. The variation in reported composition of human milk proteins is large, and a substantial portion of breast milk nitrogen is nonprotein. Given the difficulties in estimating the factors that affect the patterns, the values are in surprisingly good agreement. Only for tryptophan is the difference substantial. This subcommittee concludes that the composition of human milk should be used as a reference pattern for formulation of human milk substitutes for infants and as a guide to supplementary feeding of infants through 6 months of age.

The amino acid pattern shown for 2-year-old children should be applied to children ages 2 to 6, and that shown for children 10 to 12 years should be used for ages 6 to 13 years. The adult pattern is applicable to children above age 13 and adults. For children above

TABLE 6-3 Examples of the Derivation of Protein Allowances for Children and Adolescents by a Factorial Procedure[a]

Age	Growth Nitrogen Increment (mg/kg per day)[b]	Nitrogen Increment × 1.5 (mg/kg per day)[c]	Nitrogen Increment × 1.5, plus Correction for Efficiency at 70% (mg/kg per day)[d]	Nitrogen Maintenance Level (mg/kg per day)[e]	Total Nitrogen (mg/kg per day)	Allowance of Reference Protein (g/kg per day)[f] Mean	+2 SD[g]
Both sexes							
Months							
3–5.9	47	70	100	120	220	1.38	1.73
6–11.9	34	51	73	120	193	1.21	1.51
Years							
1	16	25	36	119	155	0.97	1.21
5	9	13	19	116	135	0.84	1.05
9	8	12	17	111	128	0.80	1.00
Males, years							
12	9	13	19	108	127	0.79	0.98
17	3	5	7	103	110	0.69	0.86
Females, years							
12	7	10	14	108	122	0.76	0.95
17	0	0	0	103	103	0.64	0.80

[a] From WHO (1985: Tables 32–34). These figures are examples of the derivation of requirements at various ages. For methodological details and a complete listing of ages, consult the WHO report.
[b] Increment for growth.
[c] 50% Additional nitrogen increment to allow for daily variation in growth rate and inability to store amino acids to be available when maximum growth occurs.
[d] Assuming a 70% efficiency of dietary protein utilization for growth.
[e] Data from WHO (1985).
[f] High-quality, highly digestible protein such as egg or milk. Protein is total nitrogen × 6.25.
[g] Individual variability. The coefficient of variation for both maintenance and growth was assumed to be 12.5%.

TABLE 6-4 Recommended Allowances of Reference Protein and U.S. Dietary Protein

Category	Age (years) or Condition	Weight (kg)	Derived Allowance of Reference Protein[a] (g/kg)	(g/day)	Recommended Dietary Allowance (g/kg)[b]	(g/day)
Both sexes	0–0.5	6	2.20[c]		2.2	13
	0.5–1	9	1.56		1.6	14
	1–3	13	1.14		1.2	16
	4–6	20	1.03		1.1	24
	7–10	28	1.00		1.0	28
Males	11–14	45	0.98		1.0	45
	15–18	66	0.86		0.9	59
	19–24	72	0.75		0.8	58
	25–50	79	0.75		0.8	63
	51+	77	0.75		0.8	63
Females	11–14	46	0.94		1.0	46
	15–18	55	0.81		0.8	44
	19–24	58	0.75		0.8	46
	25–50	63	0.75		0.8	50
	51+	65	0.75		0.8	50
Pregnancy	1st trimester			+1.3		+10
	2nd trimester			+6.1		+10
	3rd trimester			+10.7		+10
Lactation	1st 6 months			+14.7		+15
	2nd 6 months			+11.8		+12

[a] Data from WHO (1985).

[b] Amino acid score of typical U.S. diet is 100 for all age groups, except young infants. Digestibility is equal to reference proteins. Values have been rounded upward to 0.1 g/kg.

[c] For infants 0 to 3 months of age, breastfeeding that meets energy needs also meets protein needs. Formula substitutes should have the same amount and amino acid composition as human milk, corrected for digestibility if appropriate.

6 months and less than 2 years of age, a combination of the infant and preschool child figures should be used to evaluate a total diet. These values and recommendations are in general agreement with those of WHO (1985).

There are no established amino acid requirements and, hence, no amino acid patterns for pregnancy and lactation. The international group suggested that a pattern for the lactating woman's total diet could be developed by summing the adult protein and additional lactation allowances, calculating the proportion of each in the total, and applying the adult pattern to its fractional part (0.72) and the human milk pattern to the other (0.28). Values derived in this way are, in mg/g of protein: lysine, 31; methionine and cystine, 21; threonine, 19; and tryptophan, 9. A similar calculation is theoretically

TABLE 6-5   Amino Acid Requirement Patterns[a] Compared with the Composition of High-Quality Proteins[b] and the U.S. Diet[c]

Amino Acid	Amino Acid Requirement Pattern by Age Groups, mg/g protein				Reported Composition, mg/g protein				U.S. Diet, by age group	
	Infants	Children		Adults	Human Milk	Chicken Egg	Cow's Milk	Beef	1–3 years	All Ages
	3–4 months	~2 years	10–12 years							
Histidine	16	(19)[d]	(19)[d]	(11)[d]	26	22	27	34		
Isoleucine	40	28	28	13	46	54	47	48	54	52
Leucine	93	66	44	19	93	86	95	81	80	77
Lysine	60	58	44	16	66	70	78	89	70	68
Methionine plus cystine	33	25	22	17	42	57	33	40	35	35
Phenylalanine plus tyrosine	72	63	22	19	72	93	102	80	81	78
Threonine	50	34	28	9	43	47	44	46	40	39
Tryptophan	10	11	(9)[d]	5	17	17	14	12	12	12
Valine	54	35	25	13	55	66	64	50	57	54
Total without histidine	412	320	222	111	434	490	477	445	429	415

[a] Requirement pattern is calculated from amino acid requirements (Table 6-1) divided by the recommended allowance of reference protein. Protein allowance (in g/kg) is 1.73 for infants 3–4 months of age, 1.10 for children at 2 years of age, 0.99 for children 10–12 years of age, and 0.75 for adults (see Table 6-4). Except for infants, for whom the difference is trivial, and histidine for adults, patterns are identical with those reported by WHO (1985).

[b] From WHO (1985).

[c] From the 1977–1978 USDA Nationwide Food Consumption Survey (USDA, 1984).

[d] Values in parentheses are imputed.

possible for pregnancy, but more difficult because of the variety of tissues and proteins deposited.

Amino Acid Scoring of Dietary Protein Quality   To adjust for amino acid composition, a score is calculated according to the most limiting amino acid, i.e., the one in greatest deficit for the age group involved.

$$\text{Amino acid score} = \frac{\text{Content of individual essential amino acid in food protein (mg/g of protein)}}{\text{Content of same amino acid in reference pattern (mg/g of protein)}}$$

The amino acid score should be based on the appropriate pattern for age. Only four essential amino acids are likely to affect the protein quality of mixed human diets: lysine, the sulfur-containing amino acids (methionine plus cystine), threonine, and tryptophan. Scoring patterns for all the essential amino acids (presented in Table 6-5) are important for the formulation of special purpose diets in clinical practice.

CONSUMPTION AND AMINO ACID PATTERN OF PROTEINS IN THE U.S. DIET

Food consumption data from the U.S. Department of Agriculture's (USDA) 1977–1978 and 1985 surveys indicate that 14 to 18% of the total food energy intake is derived from protein (USDA, 1983, 1986, 1987). Despite wide variations in food energy intake, this proportion remains similar for both sexes and all age groups except infants. There is also little change as a function of household income, urbanization, or race. Food items likely to be underreported in surveys (e.g., alcoholic beverages, confections) would provide energy but little protein; hence, the percentage of energy from protein may be overestimated. Average consumption levels are, however, quite generous: about 50 g/day in preschool children; 70 to 85 g in older children; 90 to 110 g in male and 65 to 70 g in female adolescents and adults; and 75 to 80 g in men and 55 to 65 g in women over age 65.

Foods of animal origin contribute approximately 65% of the protein in the USDA survey, with the proportion from the meat and dairy groups varying somewhat with age (USDA, 1983). Similarly, the data from the second National Health and Nutrition Examination Survey (NHANES II) indicate that about 48% of the protein is derived from meat, fish, and poultry; 17% from dairy products; and 4% from eggs (Block et al., 1985). The importance of grain products as suppliers of protein is not always realized, particularly in populations ingesting diets rich in animal products. Cereal grains supply an average of 16 to 20% of the total protein intake in the United States.

The amino acid pattern in the diet consumed by children ages 1 to 3 years and all persons surveyed is given in Table 6-5. The pattern is uniform between the age groups and meets the requirement pattern levels for all age groups except infants. The U.S. consumption pattern also meets the provisional pattern for lactating women. Therefore, no adjustment to the recommended allowance for reference protein is required for people consuming a typical U.S. diet.

Digestibility The amino acid score alone may lead to an overestimation of the capacity of some proteins to meet physiological requirements unless digestibility is taken into account. When the amino acid score is multiplied by digestibility, it becomes analogous to the biologically determined net protein utilization (NPU). The NPU is the product of biological value (comparable to amino acid score) and true protein digestibility.

Differences in digestibility result from intrinsic differences in the nature of food protein and the nature of the cell wall, from the presence of other dietary factors that modify digestion (e.g., dietary fiber, polyphenols such as tannins, and enzyme inhibitors), and from chemical reactions (e.g., binding of the amino groups of lysine and cross-linkages), which may affect the release of amino acids by enzymatic processes. There are few data on the digestibility of specific amino acids in food proteins, and any differences are not captured in measurements of overall protein digestibility. Although it is known that there are differences between the pattern of amino acids in food protein, fecal matter, and portal blood, it is not now possible to provide finer adjustment than overall digestibility.

Representative data on the digestibility of some selected proteins are shown in Table 6-6. A more comprehensive listing of protein digestibility can be found in reports by Hopkins (1981) and FAO (1970). The true digestibility of reference proteins is assigned a value of 100 for translating requirements for reference proteins to recommended levels of intake for ordinary mixtures of dietary proteins. Since the mixed protein of a typical U.S. diet is shown to be as well digested as reference proteins, no adjustment for this factor is normally required.

Adjustment of Allowances for Dietary Quality Adjustment for exceptional dietary patterns can be made by deriving a weighted digestibility factor based on the digestibilities of the principal protein

TABLE 6-6   Values for the Digestibility of Protein in Humans[a]

Protein Source	True Digestibility (mean % + SD)	Digestibility Relative to Reference Proteins
Eggs	97 ± 3 ⎫	
Milk and cheese	95 ± 3 ⎬ 95	100
Meat and fish	94 ± 3 ⎭	
Maize	85 ± 6	89
Rice, polished	88 ± 4	93
Wheat, whole	86 ± 5	90
Wheat, refined	96 ± 4	101
Oatmeal	86 ± 7	90
Peanut butter	95	100
Soy flour	86 ± 7	90
Beans	78	82
Mixed U.S. diet	96[b]	101

[a] From WHO (1985). Apparent protein digestibility is the percentage of nitrogen intake that does not appear in the feces, i.e., $[(I - F) \times 100]/I$, where I = intake and F = fecal content. Estimates of true protein digestibility take into account the amount of nitrogen in feces when none is present in the diet plus the endogenous or obligatory loss, i.e., $[I - (F - F_o) \times 100]/I$, where F_o = obligatory fecal nitrogen. If F_o is not measured, 12 mg/kg body weight may be used for the calculation (WHO, 1985).

[b] Recalculated from apparent digestibility, using F_o = 12 mg of nitrogen per kilogram of body weight.

sources consumed and an amino acid score based on their contribution of essential amino acids. Such adjustment would rarely be warranted for the U.S. population. Shown in Table 6-7 is an example of calculations required to make an adjustment for an unusual diet—one in which the usual consumption pattern is reversed, i.e., only one-third of the protein from animal sources. A comparison of the amino acid pattern with the requirement patterns in Table 6-5 shows that lysine is low for the preschool age group and tryptophan is borderline. The limiting amino acid is lysine, which has a score of 51/58, or 88%. The amino acid pattern meets the requirement patterns of older children and adults, i.e., the score is 100. The weighted digestibility factor is 92%. Thus, the protein allowance for a 3-year-old child is $1.1 \times 100/88 \times 100/92$, or 1.4 g/kg. For older children and adults, an adjustment of the allowance would be made only for digestibility.

OTHER EFFECTS ON PROTEIN REQUIREMENTS

There is little evidence that muscular activity increases the need for protein, except for the small amount required for the develop-

TABLE 6-7   Example of Calculations Needed for Adjustment of
Protein Allowances for a Diet with 33% Animal- and 67%
Vegetable-Source Protein

Food	Portion of Total Dietary Protein	Contribution to Total Protein (mg)[a]				Digestibility Relative to Reference (%)
		Lysine	Sulfur-containing Amino Acids	Threonine	Tryptophan	
Milk	0.18	14	6	8	3	100
Chicken	0.15	12	6	6	2	100
Beans	0.10	7	2	4	1	82
Leaves	0.05	3	1	2	<1	86
Maize	0.42	11	15	15	3	89
Rice	0.10	4	4	3	1	93
TOTAL	1.0	51	34	38	<11	92[b]

[a] Amino acid contributed by the amount of protein from each source per gram of dietary
protein (total nitrogen × 6.25). For example, milk contains 487 mg of lysine per gram
of nitrogen or 78 mg per g protein (total nitrogen × 6.25), and 14 mg of lysine in 0.18
g of protein (total nitrogen × 6.25). Data from FAO (1970).

[b] Total diet average. Weighted for proportion of protein from each source, i.e., (0.18 ×
100) + (0.15 × 100) + (0.10 × 82) + (0.05 × 86) + (0.42 × 69) + (0.10 × 93) =
92%. Data from Table 6-6 and FAO (1970).

ment of muscles during physical conditioning (Torun et al., 1977).
Vigorous activity that leads to profuse sweating, such as in heavy
work and sports, and exposure to heat increases nitrogen loss from
the skin, but with acclimatization to a warm environment, the excessive skin loss is reduced and may be partially compensated by decreased renal excretion (WHO, 1985). In view of the margin of safety
in the RDA, no increment is added for work or training.

No added allowance is made here for the usual stresses encoun-
tered in daily living, which can give rise to transient increases in
urinary nitrogen output (Scrimshaw et al., 1966). It is assumed that
the subjects of experiments forming the basis for the requirement
estimates are usually exposed to the same stresses as the population
generally.

Extreme environmental or physiological stress increases nitrogen
loss (Cuthbertson, 1964). Infections, fevers, and surgical trauma can
result in substantial nitrogen loss through the urine and greatly increased energy expenditure. Therefore, severe infections and surgery should be treated as clinical conditions that require special dietary treatment. During convalescence from an illness that has led
to protein depletion, requirements for both protein and energy are
elevated because of the need to replace wasted tissues, just as they

are during periods of rapid growth. Premature infants also require special consideration with regard to amino acid composition of the formulas and level of protein intake.

COMPARISON OF CURRENT PROTEIN RECOMMENDATIONS TO THE 1980 RDAS

The RDAs for protein are summarized in Table 6-4. After rounding, allowances are (in g/kg per day): children 1 to 3 years old, 1.2; 4- to 6-year-old children, 1.1; 7- to 14-year-old children, 1.0; 15- to 18-year-old boys, 0.9; and all others (except infants), 0.8. The 1980 RDA for infants was 2.2 g/kg during the first 6 months and 2.0 g/kg for those between 6 and 12 months of age. The present RDA for the 6- to 12-month age group is somewhat lower, having been based on newer data on observed intakes of healthy children and theoretical growth requirements. Human milk or an equivalent substitute (i.e., formula containing as much protein and a similar amino acid pattern, corrected for digestibility if warranted) is recommended for infants from birth to 3 months of age. RDAs for other age and sex groups are essentially the same as the 1980 figures, but the derivation and justification are different, reflecting both new data and reexamination of older data. Present allowances for pregnancy and lactation are lower than in 1980: 10 g/day in contrast to 30 g/day in pregnancy, and 15 g/day rather than 20 g/day in lactation. The revised allowance for pregnancy is more heavily influenced by theory than by new evidence; the allowance for lactation is in accord with new information on breast milk production by women in the United States.

EXCESSIVE INTAKES AND TOXICITY

Because the system for disposal of excess nitrogen is efficient, protein intakes moderately above requirement are believed to be safe. Brenner et al. (1982) postulated that excess protein intake accelerates the processes that lead to renal glomerular sclerosis, a common phenomenon of aging. There is supportive evidence from studies in animals, but not in humans on this point. Urinary calcium excretion increases with increased protein intake if phosphorus intake is constant. If phosphorus intake increases with protein intake, as it does in U.S. diets, the effect of protein is minimized (Hegsted et al., 1981; Schuette and Linkswiler, 1982). It has been suggested, but not demonstrated, that a habitual high intake of protein might contribute to osteoporosis. This seems unlikely based on present evidence, at least for the range of intake by most people in the United States. Habitual intakes of protein in the United States are substantially above the requirement, and although there is no firm evidence that these intake levels are harmful, it has been deemed prudent to maintain an upper bound of no more than twice the RDA for protein (NRC, 1989).

REFERENCES

Appel, J., and J.C. King. 1979. Protein utilization in pregnant and nonpregnant women. Fed. Proc. 38:388.

Beaton, G.H., and A. Chery. 1988. Protein requirements of infants: a reexamination of concepts and approaches. Am. J. Clin. Nutr. 48:1403–1412.

Block, G., C.M. Dresser, A.M. Hartman, and M.D. Carroll. 1985. Nutrient sources in the American diet: quantitative data from the NHANES II survey. II. Macronutrients and fats. Am. J. Epidemiol. 122:27–40.

Brenner, B.M., T.W. Meyer, and T.H. Hostetter. 1982. Dietary protein intake and the progressive nature of kidney disease: the role of hemodynamically mediated glomerular injury in the pathogenesis of progressive glomerular sclerosis in aging, renal ablation, and intrinsic renal disease. N. Engl. J. Med. 307:652–659.

Butte, N.F., C. Garza, E.O. Smith, and B.L. Nichols. 1984. Human milk intake and growth in exclusively breast-fed infants. J. Pediatr. 104:187–195.

Calloway, D.H. 1974. Nitrogen balance during pregnancy. Pp. 79–94 in M. Winick, ed. Nutrition and Fetal Development. John Wiley & Sons, New York.

Calloway, D.H., and M.S. Kurzer. 1982. Menstrual cycle and protein requirements of women. J. Nutr. 112:356–366.

Cheng, A.H.R., A. Gomez, J.G. Bergan, T.C. Lee, F. Monckeberg, and C.O. Chichester. 1978. Comparative nitrogen balance study between young and aged adults using three levels of protein intake from a combination wheat-soy-milk mixture. Am. J. Clin. Nutr. 31:12–22.

Cho, E.S., H.L. Anderson, R.L. Wixom, K.C. Hanson, and G.F. Krause. 1984. Long-term effects of low histidine intake on men. J. Nutr. 114:369–384.

Cuthbertson, D.P. 1964. Physical injury and its effects on protein metabolism. Pp. 374–414 in H.N. Munro and J.B. Allison, eds. Mammalian Protein Metabolism, Vol II. Academic Press, New York.

de Benoist, B., A.A. Jackson, J.S. Hall, and C. Persaud. 1985. Whole-body protein turnover in Jamaican women during normal pregnancy. Human Nutr. Clin. Nutr. 39:167–179.

FAO (Food and Agriculture Organization). 1970. Amino-Acid Content of Foods and Biological Data on Proteins. Food Policy and Food Science Service, Nutrition Division. FAO Nutritional Studies No. 24. Food and Agriculture Organization, Rome. 285 pp.

FAO/WHO (Food and Agriculture Organization/World Health Organization). 1973. Energy and Protein Requirements. Report of a Joint FAO/WHO Ad Hoc Expert Committee. Technical Report Series No. 552; FAO Nutrition Meetings Report Series 52. World Health Organization, Rome. 118 pp.

Ferris, A.G., L.B. Vilhjalmsdottir, V.A. Beal, and P.L. Pellett. 1978. Diets in the first six months of infants in western Massachusetts. I. Energy-yielding nutrients. J. Am. Diet. Assoc. 72:155–160.

Fitch, W.L., and J.C. King. 1987. Protein turnover and 3-methylhistidine excretion in nonpregnant, pregnant and gestational diabetic women. Human Nutr. Clin. Nutr. 41C:327–339.

Fomon, S.J. 1974. Infant Nutrition, 2nd ed. W.B. Saunders, Philadelphia. 575 pp.

Fomon, S.J. 1986. Protein requirements of term infants. Pp. 55–68 in S.J. Fomon and W.C. Heiod, eds. Energy and Protein Needs During Infancy. Academic Press, New York.

Fomon, S.J., and L.J. Filer, Jr. 1967. Amino acid requirements for normal growth. Pp. 391–401 in W.L. Nyhan, ed. Amino Acid Metabolism and Genetic Variation. McGraw-Hill, New York.

Garza, C., N.S. Scrimshaw, and V.R. Young. 1977. Human protein requirements: a long-term metabolic nitrogen balance study in young men to evaluate the 1973 FAO/WHO safe level of egg protein intake. J. Nutr. 107:335–352.

Gersovitz, M., H.N. Munro, J. Udall, and V.R. Young. 1980. Albumin synthesis in young and elderly subjects using a new stable isotope methodology: response to level of protein intake. Metabolism 29:1075–1086.

Gersovitz, M., K. Motil, H.N. Munro, N.S. Scrimshaw, and V.R. Young. 1982. Human protein requirements: assessment of the adequacy of the current Recommended Dietary Allowance for dietary protein in elderly men and women. Am. J. Clin. Nutr. 35:6–14.

Hegsted, D.M. 1976. Balance studies. J. Nutr. 106:307–311.

Hegsted, D.M., S.A. Schuette, M.B. Zemel, and H.M. Linkswiler. 1981. Urinary calcium and calcium balance in young men as affected by level of protein and phosphorus intake. J. Nutr. 111:553–562.

Heird, W.C., J.F. Nicholson, J.M. Driscoll, Jr., N.J. Schullinger, and R.W. Winters. 1972. Hyperammonemia resulting from intravenous alimentation using a mixture of synthetic *L*-amino acids: a preliminary report. J. Pediatr. 81:162–165.

Higgins, A.C., E.W. Crampton, and J.E. Moxley. 1973. Nutrition and the outcome of pregnancy. Pp. 1071–1077 in R.O. Scow, ed. Endocrinology. Proceedings of the Fourth International Congress of Endocrinology, Washington, D.C., June 18–24, 1972. Excerpta Medica, Amsterdam.

Hopkins, D.T. 1981. Effects of variation in protein digestibility. Pp. 169–193 in C.E. Bodwell, J.S. Adkins, and D.T. Hopkins, eds. Protein Quality in Humans: Assessment and In Vitro Estimation. AVI Publishing, Westport, Conn.

Horowitz, J.H., E.B. Rypins, J.M. Henderson, S.B. Heymsfield, S.D. Moffitt, R.P. Bain, R.K. Chawla, J.C. Bleier, and D. Rudman. 1981. Evidence for impairment of transsulfuration pathway in cirrhosis. Gastroenterology 81:668–675.

Hytten, F.E., and I. Leitch. 1971. The Physiology of Human Pregnancy, 2nd ed. Blackwell Scientific Publications, Oxford. 599 pp.

Inoue, G., T. Komatsu, K. Kishi, and Y. Fujita. 1988. Amino acid requirements of Japanese young men. Pp. 55–62 in G.L. Blackburn, J.P. Grant, and V.R. Young, eds. Amino Acids: Metabolism and Medical Applications. John Wright, Boston.

Irwin, M.I., and D.M. Hegsted. 1971. A conspectus of research on protein requirements of man. J. Nutr. 101:387–429.

Jackson, A.A. 1987. Measurement of protein turnover during pregnancy. Human Nutr. Clin. Nutr. 41C:497–498.

Johnstone, F.D., D.M. Campbell, and I. MacGillivray. 1981. Nitrogen balance studies in human pregnacy. J. Nutr. 111:1884–1893.

Kindt, E., and S. Halvorsen. 1980. The need of essential amino acids in children. An evaluation based on the intake of phenylalanine, tyrosine, leucine, isoleucine, and valine in children with phenylketonuria, tyrosine amino transferase defect, and maple syrup urine disease. Am. J. Clin. Nutr. 33:279–286.

King, J.C. 1975. Protein metabolism in pregnancy. Clin. Perinatol. 2:243–254.

King, J.C., D.H. Calloway, and S. Margen. 1973. Nitrogen retention, total body [40]K and weight gain in teenage pregnant girls. J. Nutr. 103:772–785.

Kopple, J.D., and M.E. Swendseid. 1981. Effect of histidine intake on plasma and urine histidine levels, nitrogen balance and N[7]-methylhistidine excretion in normal and chronically uremic men. J. Nutr. 111:931–942.

Lechtig, A., J.P. Habicht, H. Delgado, R.E. Klein, C. Yarbrough, and R. Martorell. 1975. Effect of food supplementation during pregnancy on birthweight. Pediatrics 56:508–520.

Meguid, M.M., D.E. Matthews, D.M. Bier, C.N. Meredith, J.S. Soeldner, and V.R. Young. 1986a. Leucine kinetics at graded leucine intakes in young men. Am. J. Clin. Nutr. 43:770–780.

Meguid, M.M., D.E. Matthews, D.M. Bier, C.N. Meredith, and V.R. Young. 1986b. Valine kinetics at graded valine intakes in young men. Am. J. Clin. Nutr. 43:781–786.

Meredith, C.N., Z.M. Wen, D.M. Bier, D.E. Matthews, and V.R. Young. 1986. Lysine kinetics at graded lysine intakes in young men. Am. J. Clin. Nutr. 43:787–794.

Metcoff, J., E.R. Klein and B.L. Nichols, eds. 1981. Workshop on nutrition of the child: maternal nutritional status and fetal outcome. Am. J. Clin. Nutr. 34:653–817.

Millward, D.J., and J.P.W. Rivers. 1986. Protein and amino acid requirements in the adult human. J. Nutr. 116:2559–2561.

Munro, H.N. 1983. Protein nutriture and requirement in elderly people. Bibl. Nutr. Dieta 33:61–74.

Naismith, D.J. 1977. Protein metabolism during pregnancy. Pp. 503–511 in E.E. Philipp, J. Barnes, and M. Newton, eds. Scientific Foundations of Obstetrics and Gynaecology, 2nd ed. Year Book Medical Publishers, Chicago.

Naismith, D.J., and B.L. Morgan. 1976. The biphasic nature of protein metabolism during pregnancy in the rat. Br. J. Nutr. 36:563–566.

Nakagawa, I., T. Takahashi, T. Suzuki, and K. Kobayashi. 1964. Amino acid requirements of children: nitrogen balance at the minimum level of essential amino acids. J. Nutr. 83:115–118.

NRC (National Research Council). 1974. Improvement of Protein Nutriture. Report of the Committee on Amino Acids, Food and Nutrition Board. National Academy of Sciences, Washington, D.C. 201 pp.

NRC (National Research Council). 1989. Diet and Health: Implications for Reducing Chronic Disease Risk. Report of the Committee on Diet and Health, Food and Nutrition Board. National Academy Press, Washington, D.C. 750 pp.

Osofsky, H.J. 1975. Relationships between nutrition during pregnancy and subsequent infant and child development. Obstet. Gynecol. Surv. 30:227–241.

Pineda, O., B. Torun, F.E. Viteri, and G. Arroyave. 1981. Protein quality in relation to estimates of essential amino acids requirements. Pp. 29–42 in C.E. Bodwell, J.S. Adkins, and D.T. Hopkins, eds. Protein Quality in Humans: Assessment and In Vitro Estimation. AVI Publishing, Westport, Conn.

Rand, W.M., N.S. Scrimshaw, and V.R. Young. 1981. Conventional ("long-term") nitrogen balance studies for protein quality evaluation in adults: rationale and limitations. Pp. 61–94 in C.E. Bodwell, J.S. Adkins, and D.T. Hopkins, eds. Protein Quality in Humans: Assessment and In Vitro Estimation. AVI Publishing, Westport, Conn.

Schuette, S.A., and H.M. Linkswiler. 1982. Effects on Ca and P metabolism in humans by adding meat, meat plus milk, or purified proteins plus Ca and P to a low protein diet. J. Nutr. 112:338–349.

Scrimshaw, N.S., J.-P. Habicht, M.L. Piche, B. Cholakos, and G. Arroyave. 1966. Protein metabolism of young men during university examinations. Am. J. Clin. Nutr. 18:321–324.

Solomons, N.W., and L.H. Allen. 1983. The functional assessment of nutritional status: principles, practice and potential. Nutr. Rev. 41:33–50.

Torun, B., N.S. Scrimshaw, and V.R. Young. 1977. Effect of isometric exercises on body potassium and dietary protein requirements of young men. Am. J. Clin. Nutr. 30:1983–1993.

Uauy, R., J.C. Winterer, C. Bilmazes, L.N. Haverberg, N.S. Scrimshaw, H.N. Munro, and V.R. Young. 1978a. The changing pattern of whole body protein metabolism in aging humans. J. Gerontol. 33:663–671.

Uauy, R., N.S. Scrimshaw, and V.R Young. 1978b. Human protein requirements: nitrogen balance response to graded levels of egg protein in elderly men and women. Am. J. Clin. Nutr. 31:779–785.

USDA (U.S. Department of Agriculture). 1976–1989. USDA Agricultural Handbook Series 8. Foods—Raw, Processed, Prepared. Comparison of Nutrient Data Research. Human Nutrition Information Service. U.S. Department of Agriculture, Washington, D.C. (various pagings)

USDA (U.S. Department of Agriculture). 1983. Nationwide Food Consumption Survey 1977–1978. Food Intakes: Individuals in 48 States, Year 1977–78. Report No. I-1. Consumer Nutrition Division, Human Nutrition Information Service. U.S. Department of Agriculture, Hyattsville, Md. 617 pp.

USDA (U.S. Department of Agriculture). 1984. Nationwide Food Consumption Survey. Nutrient Intakes: Individuals in 48 States, Year 1977–78. Report No. I-2. Consumer Nutrition Division, Human Nutrition Information Service. U.S. Department of Agriculture, Hyattsville, Md. 439 pp.

USDA (U.S. Department of Agriculture). 1986. Nationwide Food Consumption Survey. Continuing Survey of Food Intakes by Individuals. Men 19–50 Years, 1 Day, 1985. Report No. 85-3. Nutrition Monitoring Division, Human Nutrition Information Service. U.S. Department of Agriculture, Hyattsville, Md. 94 pp.

USDA (U.S. Department of Agriculture). 1987. Nationwide Food Consumption Survey. Continuing Survey of Food Intakes by Individuals: Women 19–50 Years and Their Children 1–5 Years, 4 Days, 1985. Report No. 85-4. Nutrition Monitoring Division, Human Nutrition Information Service, Hyattsville, Md. 182 pp.

Watts, J.H., A.N. Mann, L. Bradley, and D.J. Thompson. 1964. Nitrogen balances of men over 65 fed the FAO and milk patterns of essential amino acids. J. Gerontol. 19:370–374.

WHO (World Health Organization). 1985. Energy and Protein Requirements. Report of a Joint FAO/WHO/UNU Expert Consultation. Technical Report Series 724. World Health Organization, Geneva. 206 pp.

Widdowson, E.M., and J.W.T. Dickerson. 1963. Chemical composition of the body. Pp. 1–247 in C.L. Comar and F. Bronner, eds. Mineral Metabolism: An Advanced Treatise, Vol II. The Elements, Part A. Academic Press, New York.

Williams, H.H., A.E. Harper, D.M. Hegsted, G. Arroyave, and L.E. Holt, Jr. 1974. Nitrogen and amino acid requirements. Pp. 23–63 in Improvement of Protein Nutriture. Report of the Committee on Amino Acids, Food and Nutrition Board. National Academy of Sciences, Washington, D.C.

Young, V.R., and N.S. Scrimshaw. 1977. Human protein and amino acid metabolism and requirements in relation to protein quality. Pp. 11–54 in C.E. Bodwell, ed. Evaluation of Proteins for Humans. AVI Publishing, Westport, Conn.

Zanni, E., D.H. Calloway, and A.Y. Zezulka. 1979. Protein requirements of elderly men. J. Nutr. 109:513–524.

Zhao, X.H., Z.M. Wen, C.N. Meredith, D.E. Matthews, D.M. Bier, and V.R. Young. 1986. Threonine kinetics at graded threonine intakes in young men. Am. J. Clin. Nutr. 43:795–802.

7
Fat-Soluble Vitamins

VITAMIN A

Vitamin A designates a group of compounds essential for vision, growth, cellular differentiation and proliferation, reproduction, and the integrity of the immune system (Goodman, 1984b; Moore, 1957; Olson, 1984; Sporn et al., 1984). Retinol, retinaldehyde, and retinoic acid, naturally occurring compounds with some vitamin A activity, and a large number of synthetic analogs with or without vitamin A activity are collectively termed retinoids. Retinoids vary qualitatively as well as quantitatively in vitamin A activity. Dietary retinoic acid, for example, does not fulfill all the metabolic needs for vitamin A, since it does not protect against night blindness or reproductive dysfunction. The body's need for vitamin A can be met by dietary intake of preformed retinoids with vitamin A activity (usually in animal products) or by consumption of carotenoid precursors of vitamin A such as β-carotene, α-carotene, and cryptoxanthin formed by plants and present in some animal fats.

The structural requirements for vitamin A biological activity are very strict and apply both to retinoids and to carotenoids (Wolf and Johnson, 1960). Of more than 500 carotenoids found naturally, only about 50 are precursors of retinol (i.e., have provitamin A activity) (Isler, 1971; Olson, 1983, 1984). All-*trans* β-carotene is the most active on a weight basis and makes the most important quantitative contribution to human nutrition (Bauernfeind, 1972; Moore, 1957; Underwood, 1984)

Preformed vitamin A is present in foods of animal origin mainly as retinyl ester (Goodman and Blaner, 1984). In the small intestine,

78

retinyl esters are hydrolyzed; the products are associated first with lipid globules and then with bile salt-containing mixed micelles in the upper part of the small intestine. These mixed micelles contain carotenoids as well as retinol. However, absorption of retinol and carotenoids, especially β-carotene, differs in several ways. For example, in physiological amounts, retinol is more efficiently absorbed than are most carotenoids, e.g., 70 to 90% compared to 20 to 50% (Bauernfeind, 1972; Reddy and Sivakumar, 1972). However, carotenoids present in oils are well absorbed (Rao and Rao, 1970). As the amount ingested increases, the efficiency of retinol absorption usually remains high (60 to 80%), whereas carotenoid absorption falls markedly to levels as low as 10% or less (Bauernfeind, 1972; Olson, 1972).

Absorbed retinol is largely esterified in intestinal mucosal cells and incorporated into chylomicrons, as is the portion of absorbed β-carotene and other biologically active carotenoids that is not cleaved in intestinal cells. Most absorbed β-carotene normally is converted to retinol (and then to retinyl esters) in mucosal cells. The retinyl esters and carotenoids are taken up from the blood with chylomicron remnants, mainly in the liver by hepatocytes (Blomhoff et al., 1982; Goodman and Blaner, 1984). Studies in animals have shown that when liver reserves of vitamin A are adequate, much of the newly absorbed retinol is transferred from hepatocytes to stellate cells of the liver and stored as retinyl esters (Blomhoff et al., 1982, 1985). In well-nourished individuals, the storage efficiency of ingested vitamin A in the liver is more than 50% (Sauberlich et al., 1974), and the liver contains ≥90% of the total body stores of the vitamin (Underwood, 1984). In vitamin A-depleted rats, liver stores are reduced and the kidneys and other tissues contain an appreciable percentage (10 to 50%) of the small amount of total body reserve. In humans, carotenoids are deposited more widely, including localization in adipose tissues and adrenals; relatively small amounts are found in the liver (Raica et al., 1972).

Retinol circulates in the blood as a 1:1:1 trimolecular complex with retinol-binding protein (RBP) and transthyretin (TTR) (Goodman, 1984a). RBP is released from the liver in combination with retinol, and the holo-RBP complex combines with TTR in the blood. Subsequently, retinol is slowly metabolized in the liver to numerous products, some of which are conjugated with glucuronic acid or taurine, and eliminated in the bile (Sporn et al., 1984). Of the total retinol metabolized, approximately 70% of the metabolic products appear in the feces and 30% are excreted in the urine. Almost all these excreted products are biologically inactive metabolites. For a more detailed review of retinol metabolism, see Goodman and Blaner (1984).

General Signs of Deficiency

Vitamin A deficiency is found most commonly in children under 5 years of age and is usually due to an insufficient dietary intake. Deficiency also occurs as a result of chronic fat malabsorption. Prominent clinical signs are ocular, and range—in increasing severity—from night blindness and conjunctival xerosis to corneal xerosis, ulceration, and sometimes liquefaction. Collectively, these symptoms and signs are referred to as xerophthalmia (Sommer, 1982). Irreversible corneal lesions associated with partial or total blindness are termed keratomalacia. Other less specific deficiency signs may include loss of appetite, hyperkeratosis, increased susceptibility to infections, and metaplasia and keratinization of epithelial cells of the respiratory tract and other organs. Although rare in the United States, vitamin A deficiency is a major nutritional problem in some parts of the nonindustrialized world, causing a number of the more than 500,000 new cases of active corneal lesions that occur annually in children (FAO, 1988).

The Nutritional Relationship Between Preformed Vitamin A, Biologically Active Retinoids, and Carotenoids

Vitamin A activity is often expressed as international units (IU), derived both from preformed vitamin A and from carotenoids. This has led to confusion, since the term IU was based on studies that did not take into account the poor absorption and bioavailability of carotenoids. Solely on the basis of growth-promoting action in rats under controlled conditions, 1 IU of vitamin A activity has been defined as equal either to 0.30 μg of all-*trans* retinol or to 0.60 μg of all-*trans* β-carotene. In studies in humans, the same relationship held when small oral doses of synthetic all-*trans* retinyl acetate and of synthetic all-*trans* β-carotene were used to cure vitamin A deficiency (i.e., 1 μg of retinol was equivalent to about 2 μg of β-carotene) (Sauberlich et al., 1974).

The bioavailability of carotenoids in many foods is not as great as that of retinol or of pure carotenoid supplements. As noted above, pure carotenoids are absorbed from the intestine less well than retinol. Furthermore, provitamin A carotenoids other than β-carotene yield only half the vitamin A activity of β-carotene. On the basis of all these considerations, the assumed relationship between the biological effectiveness of β-carotene and retinol was changed, so that 6 μg of dietary β-carotene was assumed to be nutritionally equivalent to 1 μg of retinol (FAO/WHO, 1967; NRC, 1980). The vitamin A activity in foods is thus currently expressed as *retinol equivalents* (RE): 1 RE is defined as 1 μg of all-*trans* retinol, 6 μg of all-*trans* β-carotene, or 12 μg of other provitamin A carotenoids. This definition of retinol equivalent is now generally accepted throughout the world (Bieri and McKenna, 1981) and has been included, together with IU, in the recent revision of *Agriculture Handbook Series 8* of the U.S. Department of Agriculture (USDA, 1976–1989).

Dietary Sources and Usual Intakes

The richest sources of preformed retinol are liver and fish liver oils, and appreciable quantities are also present in whole and fortified milk and in eggs. Biologically active carotenoids are found in abundance in carrots and in dark-green leafy vegetables such as spinach (USDA, 1976–1989). Because only a few carotenoids serve as provitamin A compounds and because many other yellow and orange carotenoid and other pigments are present in plants, the color intensity of a fruit or vegetable is not a reliable indicator of its content of provitamin A. Data from the second (1976–1980) National Health and Nutrition Examination Survey (NHANES II) indicate that the major contributors of vitamin A or provitamin A in the U.S. diet are liver, carrots, eggs, vegetable-based soups, and whole-milk products (Block et al., 1985). Fortified food products also contribute substantially to the dietary intake of vitamin A in the United States. In addition, recent surveys indicate that approximately one-third of the U.S. adult population consumes vitamin supplements regularly, including vitamin A in doses often meeting or exceeding the 1980 RDAs (McDonald, 1986; Stewart et al., 1985).

In view of the incomplete data on the carotenoid content of foods, it is not possible to state precisely what percentage of vitamin A activity in the diet is contributed by carotenoids. With improved methodology, current studies of the carotenoid content of vegetables should yield more reliable figures (Khachik et al., 1986).

Using available food composition data, the USDA found the average vitamin A intake of adult men to be 1,419 RE (USDA, 1986). The corresponding intakes for adult women and children 1 to 5 years of age were 1,170 RE and 1,049 RE, respectively (USDA, 1987). Less than one-third of total vitamin A activity in the diets of these groups came from carotenoids.

Recommended Allowances

Adults Estimates of vitamin A intakes have been based on the amounts needed (1) to correct impaired dark adaptation, abnormal electroretinograms, and follicular hyperkeratosis among vitamin A-depleted subjects; (2) to increase the concentration of retinol in the plasma of depleted subjects to the normal range; and (3) to maintain a normal plasma concentration of retinol in well-nourished subjects (Rodriguez and Irwin, 1972). Some studies in humans suggest that at liver storage concentrations above 20 μg/g, an adequate supply of retinol is available to maintain normal plasma levels and to meet tissue needs (Amedee-Manesme et al., 1984, 1987, 1988). By contrast, average liver concentrations were 149 μg/g in specimens obtained from humans at autopsy (Raica et al., 1972). In a human vitamin A depletion-repletion study, initial body pools of vitamin A were estimated to range from 315 to 877 mg. At the time vitamin A deficiency signs appeared, the body vitamin A pool was reduced by approximately one-half (Sauberlich et al., 1974).

Induced vitamin A depletion and repletion have been conducted only in a few adult males in two studies. During World War II, Hume and Krebs (1949) in Sheffield, England, investigated the human requirements for vitamin A. Vitamin A deficiency symptoms included dryness of skin, impaired dark adaptation, eye discomfort, and low plasma retinol levels (<15 μg/dl). Of the 16 subjects studied, only three had changes in dark adaptation of sufficient magnitude to serve as a criterion to investigate the curative ability of varying amounts of retinol or β-carotene. One subject was given 390 μg of retinol per day—an amount sufficient to improve his dark adaptation but to improve his low plasma retinol levels only transiently. Supplementation with 780 μg of retinol per day for 45 days had little further effect on the subject's plasma retinol level (an initial level of 17 μg/dl was increased to 21 μg/dl). However, daily retinol supplements of 7,200 μg returned his plasma retinol level to his initial level of 33 μg/dl and higher.

Two other subjects were repleted with two different levels of β-carotene. One received 768 μg daily but did not improve until the dose was increased to 1,500 μg of β-carotene daily. The other subject, who had a milder vitamin A deficiency, promptly improved with daily β-carotene supplements of 1,500 μg. From the results of the one subject, Hume and Krebs (1949) concluded that a daily retinol intake of 390 μg represented the minimum protective dose. They recommended, however, that a daily intake of 750 μg of retinol be considered as the vitamin A requirement of the adult human. This figure should be raised by 20% to 900 μg to correct for an error in the conversion factor used in the analytical measurements of Hume and Krebs (Leitner et al., 1960).

In the study by Sauberlich et al. (1974), eight volunteer adult males were depleted of vitamin A. There was considerable variation among them in the time of occurrence of vitamin A deficiency signs. Abnormal electroretinograms occurred at plasma retinol levels of 4 to 11 μg/dl and impaired dark adaptation was observed at plasma retinol levels of 3 to 25 μg/dl, whereas follicular hyperkeratosis was found at plasma retinol levels of 7 to 37 μg/dl. Plasma levels below 30 μg/dl were associated with a mild degree of anemia that responded only to vitamin A supplementation (Hodges et al., 1978).

Daily retinol supplements of 300 μg partially corrected the abnormal electroretinograms, whereas supplements of 600 μg/day corrected the condition completely in one subject and to a great extent in two others. This suggests that 600 μg/day is the minimum physiological need for retinol to prevent eye changes in adult men. However, the skin lesions failed to clear promptly with this level of intake. The skin lesions were among the earliest manifestations of vitamin A deficiency, occurring in some subjects with plasma retinol levels higher than 30 μg/dl. Hence, maintenance of a plasma retinol level above 30 μg/dl in adult men appears desirable to prevent vitamin A deficiency manifestations and to ensure modest body stores of the vitamin.

After 103 days of vitamin A depletion, the plasma vitamin A levels ranged from 29 to 34 μg/dl. Radioisotopic labeling of the body pool of vitamin A indicated that the average rate of utilization at this state of depletion was 910 μg of vitamin A per day (range, 570 to 1,250 μg). This suggests that a daily retinol intake of 900 μg would maintain a plasma retinol level of 30 μg/dl and provide a modest body pool of vitamin A in most adult men. For women, the requirement would be reduced in proportion to body weight.

The amount of β-carotene necessary to meet the vitamin A requirement of adult men was approximately twice that of retinol, although in some instances the amount required appeared to be less than double. A β-carotene intake of 1,200 μg/day was comparable to a retinol intake of 600 μg/day. The β-carotene was provided to the subjects under optimal conditions for absorption (dissolved in corn oil); under normal dietary states, the bioavailability of β-carotene (in vegetables and fruits) would be considerably less.

An international committee (FAO, 1988) analyzed the data obtained in this study of Sauberlich et al. (1974) and interpreted these results differently. They calculated the mean dietary intake of retinol required to maintain a minimal reserve in adult males to be 526 μg/day. Given the limited number of subjects in the Sauberlich study, the large observed variation in the depletion rate of body stores, and the assumptions required for the calculation, it is difficult to accept 526 μg/day as a basis for establishing the allowance for vitamin A. Furthermore, none of the data provide a valid basis for estimating the population variance of the requirement of adults or children.

Other earlier studies suggest that the daily vitamin A requirement for adult men ranges from 750 to 1,200 μg of retinol. For instance, Jeghers (1937) reported a minimal retinol intake of 1,200 μg/day; Basu and De (1941) concluded that 900 μg of retinol per day was needed to prevent impaired dark adaptation in adults; and Wagner (1940) reported that 750 μg of retinol per day was required to produce visual normality. In a recent population-based study of Gambian women whose vitamin A intake came almost entirely from provitamin A carotenoids, Villard and Bates (1987a) found that vitamin A adequacy was achieved with daily intakes as low as 500 RE. However, the actual provitamin A activity of dietary carotenoids and the applicability of this study to women in the U.S. population are uncertain.

Clinical observations, radiometric findings on body pools of vitamin A, and vitamin A utilization rates suggest that the maintenance of a plasma retinol level above 20 μg/dl appears to be essential, while a plasma level above 30 μg/dl would be desirable to ensure modest body stores of the vitamin. These plasma levels would be associated with utilization rates of vitamin A of 570 to 1,250 μg/day found for the eight adult men in the study of Sauberlich et al. (1974). Hence, 600 μg of retinol per day represents a minimal intake that would not necessarily support optimal levels of liver stores of retinol or plasma retinol levels.

Since the data are limited, and the study of Sauberlich et al. (1974) suggests that the individual requirement for adult men varies considerably, it is the judgment of the subcommittee that there is no reason to alter the RDA for adult men from the value of 1,000 RE recommended in the ninth edition of the RDAs. The RDA for adult women is set at 800 RE on the basis of their lower body weight.

Healthy elderly Americans (65 years of age and older) ingest the same average amounts of vitamin A as do other adults (DHEW, 1979; USDA, 1984) and have normal plasma vitamin A levels (DHEW, 1974; Garry et al., 1987). Although diseases that adversely affect vitamin A absorption, storage, and transport may be more common among the elderly than among other age groups, the vitamin A status of otherwise healthy elderly people does not appear to require special attention.

Pregnancy and Lactation   Vitamin A is required for growth, for cellular differentiation, and for the normal development of fetuses. Most, if not all, vitamin A transferred to the fetus is derived from holo-RBP in maternal plasma. The median retinol concentration in fetal liver is low (<25 μg/g) and does not increase appreciably, even when the mother is given vitamin A supplements (Wallingford and Underwood, 1986). During the last trimester, the total body pool of vitamin A in the fetus increases only by approximately 1.3 mg (Montreewasuwat and Olson, 1979). In contrast, the total body pool would be 209 mg in a 63-kg woman whose liver contains a vitamin A concentration of 100 μg/g (Mitchell et al., 1973; Raica et al., 1972). If the mean fetal utilization of vitamin A for the last 13 weeks (91 days) were 200 μg/day, 18 mg of vitamin A, or only 9% of the total mean maternal stores, would be required. For most women in our society, therefore, no increment of vitamin A intake is necessary during pregnancy.

The range of vitamin A in human milk from well-nourished women in the United States and Europe is about 0.4 to 0.7 μg of retinol per milliliter (Wallingford and Underwood, 1986). If the mean daily milk volume is 750 ml, the daily secretion of vitamin A in the milk would be 300 to 525 μg. Over a 6-month period, 54 to 95 mg of vitamin A would be secreted, i.e., 26 to 45% of the total mean maternal reserve of 209 mg. To maintain maternal liver reserves, account for normal variation in milk volume, and provide a margin of safety, therefore, a daily increment of 500 RE is recommended during the first 6 months of lactation. Inasmuch as the mean daily human milk volume falls to 600 ml after 6 months, a daily increment of 400 RE should suffice during this later period. The efficiency with which vitamin A ingested by a well-nourished mother is transferred to the milk is not readily defined. In vitamin A-depleted lactating women and those chronically ingesting low intakes, however, dietary supplements increase the concentration of vitamin A in the milk (Venkatachalam et al., 1962; Villard and Bates, 1987b).

Infants and Children   As noted above, the milk of well-nourished U.S. and European women contains 40 to 70 μg/dl retinol and 20 to 40 μg/dl of carotenoids (mainly as β-carotene). In terms of retinol equivalents, carotenoids contribute approximately 10% of the vitamin A value of milk. If a retinol concentration of 40 μg/dl and a milk consumption of 750 ml/day are accepted as adequate, the intake of vitamin A for an infant would be 300 μg of retinol per day. The coefficient of variation in the vitamin A content of human milk is

48% (Gebre-Medhin et al., 1976). The relevance of this variance to the actual requirement of the infant is unclear, primarily because signs of vitamin A deficiency and reduced growth rate are not generally apparent in children receiving as little as 100 to 200 μg of retinol a day (Batista, 1969; Patwardhan, 1969; Reddy, 1971) and because infants who are breastfed by well-nourished women in the United States do not show signs of vitamin A deficiency. Thus, a daily intake of 375 μg of retinol (300 μg + 2 SDs) seems sufficient to meet the needs of essentially all healthy infants.

Because the need for vitamin A during rapid growth greatly exceeds that for the maintenance of adequate reserves in adults (Underwood, 1984), the RDA remains relatively constant as the growth rate falls but the body weight increases. In the absence of specific data on the needs of children, the retinol allowance of 375 μg seems adequate from birth to about 1 year of age. Thereafter, RDA values are extrapolated to the adult level on the basis of body weight. Allowances of 400, 500, and 700 RE daily are recommended for the age groups of 1 to 3, 4 to 6, and 7 to 10 years, respectively, with no distinction between males and females.

The 11- to 14-year group and older age groups are considered separately by sex because of differences in lean body mass that occur during this period of development and the different hormonal influences on blood values of the vitamin independent of vitamin A status (Pilch, 1987). Recommended intakes during the adolescent years are similar to those for adults.

Other Factors Affecting Recommended Allowances

The absorption and utilization of carotenoids and vitamin A are enhanced by dietary fat, protein, and vitamin E, and are depressed by the presence of peroxidized fat and other oxidizing agents in the food. The absorption of carotenoids and vitamin A is markedly reduced when diets contain very little (≤ 5 g/day) fat. At low carotenoid intakes, conversion of β-carotene to retinol may, however, be more efficient. Deficiencies of a variety of other nutrients, including protein, α-tocopherol, iron, and zinc, also adversely affect vitamin A transport, storage, and utilization. (For review and references, see Underwood, 1984.)

The ability of retinoids to prevent, suppress, or retard some experimentally produced cancers at sites such as the skin, bladder, and breast in animal models is well established. However, neither intake of foods rich in preformed vitamin A nor concentration of retinol in plasma appears to be associated with the risk of any type of cancer in humans (NRC, 1989). On the other hand, most carotenoids, unlike vitamin A, trap free radicals (Burton and Ingold, 1984) and quench singlet oxygen, which can cause neoplastic changes in cells. Because only about 10% of carotenoids in nature show provitamin A activity, any anticancer effects that carotenoids possess might be related more to their rather unique antioxidant or other properties than to their conversion into vitamin A (Bendich and Shapiro, 1986; Olson, 1986; NRC, 1989). This possibility is supported by a report that the ingestion of carrots and squash was *not* associated with any protection against neoplasia, whereas the intake of tomatoes, containing some β-carotene but mainly lycopene with no provitamin A activity, was protective (Colditz et al., 1985). In addition, a recent epidemiological study correlated the dietary intake of carotenoid-rich vegetables with a lowered risk of lung cancer among white men in New Jersey (Ziegler et al., 1986). This subject has been reviewed in the National Research Council reports on *Diet, Nutrition, and Cancer* (NRC, 1982) and *Diet and Health* (NRC, 1989). At this time, it is not possible to draw any conclusions about how this information relates to setting RDAs for vitamin A, but it does suggest that a generous intake of carotenoid-rich foods may be of benefit.

Excessive Intakes and Toxicity

When ingested in very high doses, either acutely or chronically, preformed vitamin A causes many toxic manifestations, including headache, vomiting, diplopia, alopecia, dryness of the mucous membranes, desquamation, bone abnormalities, and liver damage (Bauernfeind, 1980). Signs of toxicity usually appear only with sustained daily intakes, including both foods and supplements, exceeding 15,000 μg of retinol (50,000 IU) in adults and 6,000 μg of retinol (20,000 IU) in infants and young children (Bauernfeind, 1980). These doses are more than 10 times higher than the RDA and usually cannot be obtained from foods, except by the sustained ingestion of large amounts of liver or fish liver oils, which are particularly rich in vitamin A.

A high incidence (≥ 20%) of spontaneous abortions and of birth defects, including malformations of the cranium, face, heart, thymus, and central nervous system, has been observed in the fetuses of women ingesting therapeutic doses (0.5 to 1.5 mg/kg) of 13-*cis* retinoic acid (isotretinoin) during the first trimester of pregnancy (Lammer et al., 1985). Large daily doses of retinyl esters or retinol (≥ 6,000 RE or 20,000 IU) may cause similar abnormalities (Costas et al., 1987; Miller et al., 1987; Stange et al., 1978).

A single oral dose of 60 mg of retinol in oil (60,000 RE or 200,000 IU) is well tolerated by children and has been successfully used prophylactically in preschool Asian children (Bauernfeind, 1980). Transient symptoms of acute toxicity with no lasting effects have, however, occurred in 1 to 3% of children given the high dose supplement (WHO, 1982). Single doses of vitamin A up to 300 mg (300,000 RE or 1 million IU) administered to adults have resulted in only minor, transient toxic signs (Olson, 1983)

Carotenoids, even when ingested in very large amounts for weeks to years, are not known to be toxic (Bauernfeind, 1980; Miller et al., 1987; Olson, 1983). The main reasons for their lack of toxicity are their markedly reduced efficiency of absorption at high doses and relatively limited conversion to vitamin A in the intestine, liver, and other organs (Brubacher and Weiser, 1985). On the other hand, carotenoids taken in large doses for several weeks are absorbed well enough to color the adipose tissue stores, including the subcutaneous fat. Thus, the skin, especially the palms of the hands and the soles of the feet, appears yellow. This coloration gradually disappears when the high intake is discontinued. For food products containing large quantities of carotenoids, it would be advisable in nutritional labeling to distinguish between retinol, which in large amounts is toxic, and carotenoids, which are not.

References

Amedee-Manesme, O., D. Anderson, and J.A. Olson. 1984. Relation of the relative dose response to liver concentration of vitamin A in generally well-nourished surgical patients. Am. J. Clin. Nutr. 39:898–902.

Amedee-Manesme, O., M.S. Mourey, A. Hanck, and J. Thearasse. 1987. Vitamin A relative dose response test: validation by intravenous injection in children with liver disease. Am. J. Clin. Nutr. 46:286–289.

Amedee-Manesme, O., R. Luzeau, J.R. Wittepen, A. Hanck, and A. Sommer. 1988. Impression cytology detects subclinical vitamin A deficiency. Am. J. Clin. Nutr. 47:875–878.

Basu, N.M., and N.K. De. 1941. Assessment of vitamin A deficiency amongst Bengalees and determination of the minimal and optimal requirements of vitamin A by a simplified method for measuring visual adaptation in the dark. Indian J. Med. Res. 29:591.

Batista, M. 1969. Consideracoes—sobre o problema da Vitamina A no Nordeste Brasileiro. Hospital (Rio de Janeiro) 75:817–832.

Bauernfeind, J.C. 1972. Carotenoid vitamin A precursors and analogs in foods and feeds. J. Agric. Food Chem. 20:456–473.

Bauernfeind, J.C. 1980. The Safe Use of Vitamin A. International Vitamin A Consultative Group. The Nutrition Foundation, Washington, D.C.

Bendich, A., and S.S. Shapiro. 1986. Effect of β-carotene and canthaxanthin on the immune responses of the rat. J. Nutr. 116:2254–2262.

Bieri, J.G., and M.C. McKenna. 1981. Expressing dietary values for fat-soluble vitamins: changes in concepts and terminology. Am. J. Clin. Nutr. 34:289–295.

Block, G., C.M. Dresser, A.M. Hartman, and M.D. Carroll. 1985. Nutrient sources in the American diet: quantitative data from the NHANES II Survey. I. Vitamins and minerals. Am. J. Epidemiol. 122:13–26.

Blomhoff, R., P. Helgerud, M. Rasmussen, T. Berg, and K.R. Norum. 1982. In vivo uptake of chylomicron [3H] retinyl ester by rat liver: evidence for retinol transfer from parenchymal to nonparenchymal cells. Proc. Natl. Acad. Sci. U.S.A. 79:7326–7330.

Blomhoff, R., M. Rasmussen, A. Nilsson, K.R. Norum, T. Berg, W.S. Blaner, M. Kato, J.R. Mertz, D.S. Goodman, U. Eriksson, and P.A. Peterson. 1985. Hepatic retinol metabolism: distribution of retinoids, enzymes and binding proteins in isolated rat liver cells. J. Biol. Chem. 250:13660–13665.

Brubacher. G.B., and H. Weiser. 1985. The vitamin A activity of β-carotene. Int. J. Vit. Nutr. Res. 55:5–15.

Burton, G.W., and K.U. Ingold. 1984. β-carotene: an unusual type of lipid antioxidant. Science 224:569–573.

Colditz, G.A., L.G. Branch, R.J. Lipnick, W.C. Willett, B. Rosner, B.M. Posner, and C.H. Hennekens. 1985. Increased green and yellow vegetable intake and lowered cancer deaths in an elderly population. Am. J. Clin. Nutr. 41:32–36.

Costas, K., R. Davis, N. Kim, A.S. Stark, S. Thompson, H.L. Vallet, and D.L. Morse. 1987. Use of supplements containing high-dose vitamin A—New York State, 1983–1984. J. Am. Med. Assoc. 257:1292–1297.

DHEW (U.S. Department of Health, Education, and Welfare). 1974. First Health and Nutrition Examination Survey, United States, 1970–72. Health Resources Administration. U.S. Department of Health, Education, and Welfare, Rockville, Md.

DHEW (U.S. Department of Health, Education, and Welfare). 1979. Dietary Intake Source Data: United States, 1971–74. Vital and Health Statistics, DHEW Publ. No. (PHS) 79-1221. National Center for Health Statistics, Public Health Service, U.S. Department of Health, Education, and Welfare, Hyattsville, Md. 421 pp.

FAO (Food and Agriculture Organization). 1988. Requirements of Vitamin A, Iron, Folate, and Vitamin B12. Report of a Joint FAO/WHO Expert Consultation. FAO Food and Nutrition Series No. 23. Food and Agriculture Organization, Rome. 107 pp.

FAO/WHO (Food and Agriculture Organization/World Health Organization). 1967. Requirements of Vitamin A, Thiamine, Riboflavin, and Niacin. Report of a Joint Food and Agriculture Organization/World Health Organization Expert Committee. FAO Nutrition Meetings Report Series No. 41. WHO Technical Report Series No. 362. World Health Organization, Geneva.

Garry, P.J., W.C. Hunt, J.L. Bandrofchak, D. VanderJagt, and J.S. Goodwin. 1987. Vitamin A intake and plasma retinol levels in healthy elderly men and women. Am. J. Clin. Nutr. 46:989–994.

Gebre-Medhin, M., A. Vahlquist, Y.U. Hofvander, and B. Vahlquist. 1976. Breast milk composition in Ethiopian and Swedish mothers. 1. Vitamin A and β-carotene. Am. J. Clin. Nutr. 29:441–451.

Goodman, D.S. 1984a. Plasma retinol-binding protein. Pp. 41–88 in M.B. Sporn, A.B. Roberts, and D.S. Goodman, eds. The Retinoids, Vol. 2. Academic Press, Orlando, Fla.

Goodman, D.S. 1984b. Vitamin A and retinoids in health and disease. N. Engl. J. Med. 310:1023–1031.

Goodman, D.S., and W.S. Blaner. 1984. Biosynthesis, absorption, and hepatic metabolism of retinol. Pp. 1–39 in M.B. Sporn, A.B. Roberts, and D.S. Goodman, eds. The Retinoids, Vol. 2. Academic Press, Orlando, Fla.

Hodges, R.E., H.E. Sauberlich, J.E. Canham, D.L. Wallace, R.B. Rucker, L.A. Mejia, and M. Mohanram. 1978. Hematopoietic studies in vitamin A deficiency. Am. J. Clin. Nutr. 31:876–885.

Hume, E.M., and H.A. Krebs. 1949. Vitamin A Requirement of Human Adults. Report of the Vitamin A Subcommittee, Accessory Food Factors Committee, Medical Research Council. Special Report Series No. 264. Her Majesty's Stationery Office, London. 145 pp.

Isler, O., ed. 1971. Carotenoids. Birkhauser, Basel.

Jeghers, J. 1937. The degree and prevalence of vitamin A deficiency in adults. J. Am. Med. Assoc. 109:756.

Khachik, F., G.R. Beecher, and N.F. Whittaker. 1986. Separation, identification, and quantification of the major carotenoids and chlorophyll constituents of green vegetables by liquid chromatography. J. Agric. Food Chem. 34:603–616.

Lammer, E.J., D.T. Chen, R.M. Hoar, N.D. Agnish, P.O. Benke, J.T. Braun, C.J. Curry, P.M. Fernhoff, A.W. Grix, I.T. Lott, J.M. Richard, and S.C. Sun. 1985. Retinoic acid embryopathy. N. Engl. J. Med. 313:837–841.

Leitner, Z.A., T. Moore, and I.M. Sharman. 1960. Vitamin A and vitamin E in human blood—levels of vitamin A and carotenoids in British men and women, 1948–57. Br. J. Nutr. 14:157–169.

McDonald, J.T. 1986. Vitamin and mineral supplement use in the United States. Clin. Nutr. 5:27–33.

Miller, R.K., K. Brown, J. Cordero, D. Dayton, B. Hardin, M. Greene, C. Grabowski, A. Hendricks, E. Hook, R. Jensh, G. Kimmel, J. Manson, K.O. Shea, J. Schardein, and R. Staples. 1987. Position paper by the Teratology Society: vitamin A during pregnancy. Teratology 35:267–275.

Mitchell, G.V., M. Young, and C.R. Seward. 1973. Vitamin A and carotene levels of a selected population in metropolitan Washington, D.C. Am. J. Clin. Nutr. 26:992–997.

Montreewasuwat, N., and J.A. Olson. 1979. Serum and liver concentrations of vitamin A in Thai fetuses as a function of gestational age. Am. J. Clin. Nutr. 32:601–606.

Moore, T. 1957. Vitamin A. Elsevier, Amsterdam.

NRC (National Research Council). 1980. Recommended Dietary Allowances, 9th revised ed. Report of the Committee on Dietary Allowances, Food and Nutrition Board, Division of Biological Sciences, Assembly of Life Sciences. National Academy of Sciences, Washington, D.C. 185 pp.

NRC (National Research Council). 1982. Diet, Nutrition, and Cancer. Report of the Committee on Diet, Nutrition, and Cancer, Assembly of Life Sciences. National Academy Press, Washington, D.C. 496 pp.

NRC (National Research Council). 1989. Diet and Health: Implications for Reducing Chronic Disease Risk. Report of the Committee on Diet and Health, Food and Nutrition Board. National Academy Press, Washington, D.C. 750 pp.

Olson, J.A. 1972. The prevention of childhood blindness by the administration of massive doses of vitamin A. Isr. J. Med. Sci. 8:1199–1206.

Olson, J.A. 1983. Formation and function of vitamin A. Pp. 371–412 in J.W. Porter, ed. Polyisoprenoid Synthesis, Vol. II. John Wiley & Sons, New York.

Olson, J.A. 1984. Vitamin A. Pp. 1–43 in L. Machlin, ed. The Handbook of Vitamins. Marcel Dekker, New York.

Olson, J.A. 1986. Carotenoids, vitamin A and cancer. J. Nutr. 116:1127–1130.

Patwardhan, V.N. 1969. Hypovitaminosis A and epidemiology of xerophthalmia. Am. J. Clin. Nutr. 22:1106–1118.

Pilch, S.A. 1987. Analysis of vitamin A data from the Health and Nutrition Examination Surveys. J. Nutr. 117:636–640.

Raica, N., Jr., J. Scott, L. Lowry, and H.E. Sauberlich. 1972. Vitamin A concentration in human tissues collected from five areas in the United States. Am. J. Clin. Nutr. 25:291–296.

Rao, C.N., and B.S.N. Rao. 1970. Absorption of dietary carotenes in human subjects. Am. J. Clin. Nutr. 23:105–109.

Reddy, V. 1971. Observations on vitamin-A requirement. Indian J. Med. Res. 59:34–37.

Reddy, V., and B. Sivakumar. 1972. Studies on vitamin A absorption. Indian Pediatr. 9:307–310.

Rodriguez, M.S., and M.I. Irwin. 1972. A conspectus of research on vitamin A requirements of man. J. Nutr. 102:909–968.

Sauberlich, H.E., H.E. Hodges, D.L. Wallace, H. Kolder, J.E. Canham, J. Hood, N. Raica, Jr., and L.K. Lowry. 1974. Vitamin A metabolism and requirements in the human studied with the use of labelled retinol. Vitam. Horm. 32:251–275.

Sommer, A. 1982. Nutritional Blindness: Xerophthalmia and Keratomalacia. Oxford University Press, Oxford.

Sporn, M.B., A.B. Roberts, and D.S. Goodman, eds. 1984. The Retinoids, Vols. 1 and 2. Academic Press, Orlando, Fla.

Stange, L., K. Carlstrom, and M. Erickson. 1978. Hypervitaminosis A in early human pregnancy and malformations of the central nervous system. Acta Obstet. Gynecol. Scand. 57:289–291.

Stewart, M.L., J.T. McDonald, A.S. Levy, R.E. Schucker, and D.P. Henderson. 1985. Vitamin/mineral supplement use: a telephone survey of adults in the United States. Am. J. Diet. Assoc. 85:1585–1590.

Underwood, B.A. 1984. Vitamin A in animal and human nutrition. Pp. 281–392 in M.B. Sporn, A.B. Roberts, and D.S. Goodman, eds. The Retinoids, Vol. 1. Academic Press, Orlando, Fla.

USDA (U.S. Department of Agriculture). 1976–1989. USDA Agricultural Handbook Series 8. Comparison of Foods—Raw, Processed, Prepared. Nutrient Data Research, Human Nutrition Information Service. U.S. Department of Agriculture, Washington, D.C. (various pagings)

USDA (U.S. Department of Agriculture). 1984. Table 2A-1. Nutritive value of food intake. Average per individual per day, 1/1977–78. Pp. 154–155 in Nationwide Food Consumption Survey. Nutrient Intakes: Individuals in 48 States, Year 1977–78. Report No. I-2. Consumer Nutrition Division, Human Nutrition Information Service. U.S. Department of Agriculture, Hyattsville, Md.

USDA (U.S. Department of Agriculture). 1986. Nationwide Food Consumption Survey. Continuing Survey of Food Intakes of Individuals: Men 19–50 Years, 1 Day, 1985. Report No. 85-3. Nutrition Monitoring Division, Human Nutrition Information Service. U.S. Department of Agriculture, Hyattsville, Md. 94 pp.

USDA (U.S. Department of Agriculture). 1987. Nationwide Food Consumption Survey. Continuing Survey of Food Intakes by Individuals: Women 19–50 Years and Their Children 1–5 Years, 4 Days, 1985. Report No. 85-4. Nutrition Monitoring Division, Human Nutrition Information Service. U.S. Department of Agriculture, Hyattsville, Md. 182 pp.

Venkatachalam, P.S., B. Belavady, and C. Gopalan. 1962. Studies on vitamin A nu-
    tritional status of mothers and infants in poor communities of India. J. Pediatr.
    61:262–268.
Villard, L., and C.J. Bates. 1987a. Dietary intakes of vitamin A precursors by rural
    Gambian pregnant and lactating women. Hum. Nutr. Appl. Nutr. 41A:135–145.
Villard, L., and C.J. Bates. 1987b. Effects of vitamin A supplementation on plasma
    and breast milk vitamin A levels in poorly nourished Gambian women. Hum.
    Nutr. Clin. Nutr. 41C:47–58.
Wagner, K.H. 1940. Die experimentelle Avitaminose A beim Menschen. Seyler's Z.
    Physiol. Chem. 264:153.
Wallingford, J.C., and B.A. Underwood. 1986. Vitamin A deficiency in pregnancy,
    lactation, and the nursing child. Pp. 101–152 in J.C. Bauernfeind, ed. Vitamin
    A Deficiency and its Control. Academic Press, New York.
WHO (World Health Organization). 1982. Control of Vitamin A Deficiency of Xe-
    rophthalmia. A Report of a Joint WHO/UNICEF/USAID/Helen Keller Inter-
    national/IVACG Meeting. Technical Report Series No. 672. World Health Or-
    ganization, Geneva. 70 pp.
Wolf, G., and B.C. Johnson. 1960. Metabolic transformations of vitamin A. Vitam.
    Horm. 18:403–415.
Ziegler, R.G., T.J. Mason, A. Stemhagen, R. Hoover, J.B. Schoenberg, G. Gridley,
    P.W. Virgo, and J.F. Fraumeni, Jr. 1986. Carotenoid intake, vegetables, and the
    risk of lung cancer among white men in New Jersey. Am. J. Epidemiol. 123:1080–
    1093.

VITAMIN D

Vitamin D (calciferol) is essential for the proper formation of the skeleton and for mineral homeostasis. Exposure of the skin to ultraviolet light catalyzes the synthesis of vitamin D_3 (cholecalciferol) from 7-dehydrocholesterol. The other major form of the vitamin, D_2 (ergocalciferol), is the product of the ultraviolet light-induced conversion of ergosterol in plants. The effectiveness of exposure to sunlight or ultraviolet light in curing or preventing rickets was shown early in the twentieth century (Chick et al., 1923).

General Signs of Deficiency

Vitamin D deficiency is characterized by inadequate mineralization of the bone. In children, severe deficiency results in deformation of the skeleton (rickets). In the adult, vitamin D deficiency leads to undermineralization of the bone matrix osteoid; the resulting hypocalcemia is accompanied by secondary hyperthyroidism that can lead to excessive bone loss and, in the extreme, bone fractures (osteomalacia) (Nordin, 1973). The prolonged periods required to produce vitamin D deficiency in animals and humans is attributed to the slow release of vitamin D-related steroids from fat depots and skin.

Because milk and other foods are fortified with vitamin D, rickets is very rare in many countries. However, vitamin D deficiency occurs in some infants who are breastfed without supplemental vitamin D or exposure to sunlight (Edidin et al., 1980; Hayward et al., 1987), in the elderly (Egmose et al., 1987; Omdahl et al., 1982; Reid et al., 1986), and in people with vitamin D malabsorption (Rosen and Chesney, 1983). Abnormalities in calcium homeostasis and bone metabolism can also occur when the conversion of vitamin D to biologically active forms is compromised due to disease states. For example, rickets and osteomalacia are often found in patients with kidney failure (Haussler and McCain, 1977).

The Dietary Essentiality of Vitamin D

The vitamin D requirement of humans can be met if their skin is exposed to a sufficient amount of sunlight or artificial ultraviolet radiation. The amount of vitamin D synthesized by this means is dependent on the area of skin exposed, the time of exposure, and the wavelength of the ultraviolet light impinging on the skin. Practical considerations are the latitude of the person's residence and the season of the year (Lawson, 1980; Webb et al., 1988). Exposure to sunlight can be further limited by customs of dress and by the institutionalization and extensive indoor residency of the ill and aged. The character of the skin also influences the efficiency of vitamin D_3 synthesis. Compared to lighter skin, skin with high melanin content requires a much longer exposure to ultraviolet light to achieve the same degree of synthesis (Clemens et al., 1982). The capacity of skin to synthesize vitamin D_3 in the elderly is approximately half that of younger people (Webb et al., 1988). Given the many factors that can affect the magnitude of ultraviolet light-dependent synthesis of vitamin D_3, vitamin D should be considered an essential dietary nutrient.

Biochemistry and Metabolism

The biochemistry and metabolism of vitamin D have been extensively reviewed (DeLuca, 1988; Fraser, 1988). Among the metabolites of vitamin D are 25-hydroxyvitamin D [25(OH)D, or calcidiol], which is formed in the liver and further hydroxylated in the kidney to yield 1,25-dihydroxyvitamin D [1,25(OH)$_2$D, or calcitriol], and 24, 25-dihydroxyvitamin D [24,25(OH)$_2$D]. In addition to ensuring adequate absorption of calcium, 1,25(OH)$_2$D contributes to plasma calcium regulation by increasing bone resorption synergistically with parathyroid hormone and stimulating the reabsorption of calcium by the kidney.

Dietary vitamin D is readily absorbed from the small intestine and transported in chylomicrons to the liver, where conversion to 25(OH)D takes place (DeLuca, 1979). Vitamin D from the liver and vitamin D synthesized in the skin are transported in the blood largely bound to a vitamin D-binding protein and albumin, as are 25(OH)D and 1,25(OH)$_2$D. The liver is the major site of vitamin D deactivation. Some of the metabolites of the vitamin excreted in bile are reabsorbed, but this process contributes little to the maintenance of vitamin D status.

Vitamin D status is reflected primarily by the concentrations of 25(OH)D and 1,25(OH)$_2$D in the blood. In surveys of large groups of healthy people, the mean value of 25(OH)D ranges from approximately 25 to 30 ng/ml (Rosen and Chesney, 1983). The concentrations of 1,25(OH)$_2$D range from 18 to 60 pg/ml of plasma in normal children and between 15 to 45 pg/ml in healthy adults. Despite the wide range of normal values, there is no seasonal variation in plasma 1,25(OH)$_2$D (Chesney et al., 1981); this implies tight regulation.

One international unit (IU) of vitamin D is defined as the activity of 0.025 μg of cholecalciferol in bioassays with rats and chicks. Thus, the biological activity of cholecalciferol is 40 IU/μg. The activity of 25(OH)D and 1,25(OH)$_2$D are approximately 1.5 and 5 times, respectively, greater than that of vitamin D.

Dietary Sources and Usual Intakes

In the United States, foods fortified with vitamin D are a major dietary source of the vitamin.[a] Processed cow's milk, which contains 10 μg of cholecalciferol (400 IU) per quart, contributes most of the vitamin ingested by children. Infant formulas are fortified with the same amount as milk. Human milk contains 0.63 to 1.25 μg of cholecalciferol per liter (Reeve et al., 1982; Tsang, 1983). The usual solid food sources are eggs, butter, and fortified margarine. The vitamin is stable in foods. Storage, processing, and cooking do not appear to affect its activity.

In the United States, the usual dietary intake has been estimated primarily for infants and children. Calculations based on reference

---

[a]Vitamin D occurs as cholecalciferol or ergocalciferol in foods and fortified food products. Since the chemical forms are generally not separately identified, the vitamin D content of foods and dietary intakes are given in micrograms of cholecalciferol for simplicity.

infants and the data of Fomon (1974) indicate that daily intakes of vitamin D from formula are 6.75 μg of cholecalciferol for the infant from birth to 3 months of age and 8.5 μg of cholecalciferol at 4 to 6 months. In contrast, the average breastfed reference newborn receives only 0.38 to 0.75 μg of cholecalciferol per day from 750 ml of human milk (AAP, 1985; Reeve et al., 1982). Children drinking three 8-oz glasses of milk daily consume about 7.5 μg of cholecalciferol plus a small amount in other foods. Data from the USDA show that the average adult male ingested 2.1 μg of cholecalciferol from milk (USDA, 1986), whereas females consumed 1.5 μg (USDA, 1987). Omdahl et al. (1982) reported that a population of 60- to 93-year-old subjects had a median dietary intake of 1.35 μg of cholecalciferol (females) and 1.95 μg of cholecalciferol/day (males); 15% of the total study population, especially women, had plasma 25(OH)D levels suggestive of deficiency.

Recommended Allowances

Establishing an RDA for vitamin D is difficult because exposure to sunlight results in synthesis of vitamin D by the skin. People regularly exposed to sunlight, under appropriate conditions, have no dietary requirement for vitamin D. However, since a substantial proportion of the U.S. population is exposed to very little sunlight, especially during certain seasons (Stryd et al., 1979), a dietary supply is needed.

Adults   Data to assess vitamin D requirements of adults are limited. Dent and Smith (1969) summarized studies of seven adult females living in the United Kingdom and suffering from nutritional osteomalacia due to vitamin D deficiency. They were either strict vegetarians or had unusual diets that rigidly excluded most fats. In all the patients, vitamin D intake was estimated to be below 1.75 μg (70 IU) per day and small additional amounts of vitamin D resulted in improved calcium utilization. On the basis of these studies and other observations on similar patients, Dent and Smith suggested that the adult vitamin D requirement was about 2.5 μg (100 IU) per day.

The relative paucity of recent controlled studies in humans and the lack of data on the variability of vitamin D requirements have led this subcommittee to keep the RDA for vitamin D for adults beyond 24 years of age at 5 μg (200 IU)—the same level recommended in 1980. It seems likely that this is a generous allowance. Data from USDA's 1977–1978 Nationwide Food Consumption Survey indicate that 1.25 to 1.75 μg/day (50 to 70 IU) is the usual dietary intake in the United States (USDA, 1983). Presumably, vitamin D stores are enriched in most people by regular exposure to sunlight, at least during certain times of the year. Clinical nutritional osteomalacia appears to be rare in the United States.

Pregnancy and Lactation   It has not been determined whether or not there is an increased need for vitamin D during pregnancy, but since calcium is deposited in the growing fetus, a daily increment of 5 μg (200 IU) is recommended for women beyond 24 years of age. Although only small amounts of vitamin D are secreted in human milk, an increment of 5 μg (200 IU) per day is recommended for lactating women beyond age 24 because of the importance of maintaining calcium balance. The vitamin D RDA for both pregnant and lactating women of all ages is 10 μg/day (400 IU).

Infants and Children   Several reports have questioned whether human milk contains sufficient vitamin D to prevent rickets in the absence of exposure to sunlight (Finberg, 1981; Greer and Tsang, 1983; Tsang, 1983). In full-term infants fed human milk, bone mineral content, total and ionized calcium in serum, and serum phosphorus and alkaline phosphatase values were similar to those in a comparison group fed infant formula containing 10 μg (400 IU) of vitamin D per quart, but serum 25(OH)D concentrations were lower in the babies fed human milk (Roberts et al., 1981). In a randomized, double-blind study, bone mineral content was less in babies fed human milk without supplemental vitamin D than in those who received 10 μg/day (400 IU) (Greer et al., 1982). In a study of premature infants, 2.5 μg (100 IU) of vitamin D daily was associated with rickets and abnormalities in alkaline phosphatase activity in some infants (Glaser et al., 1949); however, these abnormalities may have been due to dietary mineral deficiency (Steichen et al., 1981). To provide a margin of safety, the RDA is set at 7.5 μg (300 IU) for infants from birth to 6 months of age. Breastfed infants who are not exposed to sunlight should receive a daily supplement of 5 to 7.5 μg (200 to 300 IU).

The allowance for children older than 6 months of age has been set at 10 μg (400 IU) because of their increased body mass. Because peak bone mass is not achieved before the third decade, this allowance is recommended through age 24 years. This amount should be readily achievable at current levels of vitamin D fortification of foods.

Excessive Intakes and Toxicity

Vitamin D is potentially toxic, especially for young children. The effects of excessive vitamin D intake include hypercalcemia and hypercalciuria (Haussler and McCain, 1977), leading to deposition of calcium in soft tissues and irreversible renal and cardiovascular damage. Although the toxic level has not been established for all ages, consumption of as little as 45 μg (1,800 IU) of cholecalciferol per day has been associated with signs of hypervitaminosis D in young children (AAP, 1963). Since the toxic level of vitamin D may in some cases be only 5 times the RDA, and there is evidence that sunlight-stimulated production of the vitamin is active throughout the warm months, dietary supplements may be detrimental for the normal child or adult who drinks at least two glasses of vitamin D-fortified milk per day (AAP, 1963).

References

AAP (American Academy of Pediatrics). 1963. The prophylactic requirement and the toxicity of vitamin D. Pediatrics 31:512–525.

AAP (American Academy of Pediatrics). 1985. Composition of Human Milk; Normative Data. Appendix K. Pp. 363–368 in Pediatric Nutrition Handbook, 2nd ed. American Academy of Pediatrics, Elk Grove Village, Ill.

Chesney, R.W., J. Zimmerman, A. Hamstra, H.F. DeLuca, and R.B. Mazess. 1981. Vitamin D metabolite concentrations in vitamin D deficiency. Are calcitriol levels normal? Am. J. Dis. Child. 135:1025–1028.

Chick, H., E.J. Dalyell, E.M. Hume, H.M.M. Mackay, H.H. Smith, and H. Wimberger. 1923. Studies of rickets in Vienna, 1919–1922. Medical Research Council Special Report Series, No. 77. Medical Research Council, London.

Clemens, T.L., S.L. Henderson, J.S. Adams, and M.F. Holick. 1982. Increased skin pigment reduces capacity of skin to synthesize vitamin D_3. Lancet 1:74–76.

DeLuca, H.F. 1979. Vitamin D. Metabolism and Function. Springer-Verlag, Berlin. 80 pp.

DeLuca, H.F. 1988. The vitamin D story: a collaborative effort of basic science and clinical medicine. FASEB J. 2:224–236.

Dent, C.E., and R. Smith. 1969. Nutritional osteomalacia. Quart. J. Med. 38:195–209.

Edidin, D.V., L.L. Levitsky, W. Schey, N. Dumbovic, and A. Campos. 1980. Resurgence of nutritional rickets associated with breast-feeding and special dietary practices. Pediatrics 65:232–235.

Egsmose, C., B. Lund, P. McNair, B. Lund, T. Storm, and O.H. Srensen. 1987. Low serum levels of 25-hydroxyvitamin D and 1,25-dihydroxyvitamin D in institutionalized old people: influence of solar exposure and vitamin D supplementation. Age Ageing 16:35–40.

Finberg, L. 1981. Human milk feeding and vitamin D supplementation—1981. J. Pediatr. 99:228–229.

Fomon, S.J. 1974. Infant Nutrition, 2nd ed. W.B. Saunders, Philadelphia.

Fraser, D.R. 1988. Calcium-regulating hormones: vitamin D. Pp. 27–41 in B.E.C. Nordin, ed. Calcium in Human Biology. Springer-Verlag, London.

Glaser, K., A.H. Parmelee, and W.S. Hoffman. 1949. Comparative efficacy of vitamin D preparations in prophylactic treatment of premature infants. Am. J. Dis. Child. 77:1–14.

Greer, F.R., and R.C. Tsang. 1983. Vitamin D in human milk: is there enough? J. Pediatr. Gastroenterol. Nutr. 2:S227–S281.

Greer, F.R., J.E. Searcy, R.S. Levin, J.J. Steichen, P.S. Steichen-Asche, and R.C. Tsang. 1982. Bone mineral content and serum 25-hydroxyvitamin D concentrations in breast-fed infants with and without supplemental vitamin D: one year follow-up. J. Pediatr. 100:919–922.

Haussler, M.R., and T.A. McCain. 1977. Basic and clinical concepts related to vitamin D metabolism and action. N. Engl. J. Med. 297:1041–1050.

Hayward, I., M.T. Stein, and M.I. Gibson. 1987. Nutritional rickets in San Diego. Am. J. Dis. Child. 141:1060–1062.

Lawson, D.E.M. 1980. Metabolism of vitamin D. Pp. 93–126 in A.W. Norman, ed. Vitamin D: Molecular Biology and Clinical Nutrition. Marcel Dekker, New York.

Nordin, B.E.C. 1973. Metabolic Bone and Stone Disease. Williams and Wilkins Co., Baltimore. 309 pp.

Omdahl, J.L., P.J. Garry, L.A. Hunsaker, W.C. Hunt, and J.S. Goodwin. 1982. Nutritional status in a healthy population: vitamin D. Am. J. Clin. Nutr. 36:1225–1233.

Reeve, L.E., R.W. Chesney, and H.F. DeLuca. 1982. Vitamin D of human milk: identification of biologically active forms. Am. J. Clin. Nutr. 36:122–126.

Reid, I.R., D.J. Gallagher, and J. Bosworth. 1986. Prophylaxis against vitamin D deficiency in the elderly by regular sunlight exposure. Age Ageing 15:35–40.

Roberts, C.C., G.M. Chan, D. Folland, C. Rayburn, and R. Jackson. 1981. Adequate bone mineralization in breast-fed infants. J. Pediatr. 99:192–196.

Rosen, J.F., and R.W. Chesney. 1983. Circulating calcitriol concentrations in health and disease. J. Pediatrics 103:1–17.

Steichen, J.J., R.C. Tsang, F.R. Greer, M. Ho, and G. Hug. 1981. Elevated serum 1,25-dihydroxyvitamin D concentrations in rickets of very low-birth-weight infants. J. Pediatr. 99:293–298.

Stryd, R.P., T.J. Gilbertson, and M.N. Brunden. 1979. A seasonal variation study of 25-hydroxyvitamin D_3 serum levels in normal humans. J. Clin. Endocrinol. Metab. 48:771–775.

Tsang, R.C. 1983. The quandary of vitamin D in the newborn infant. Lancet 1:1370–1372.

USDA (U.S. Department of Agriculture). 1983. Table 2A-1.1. Milk, milk products; eggs; legumes, nuts, seeds. Average intake per individual per day, 1977–78. Pg. 126 in Nationwide Food Consumption Survey 1977–78. Food Intakes: Individuals in 48 States, Year 1977–78. Report No. I-1. Consumer Nutrition Division, Human Nutrition Information Service. U.S. Department of Agriculture, Hyattsville, Md.

USDA (U.S. Departament of Agriculture). 1986. Nationwide Food Consumption Survey Continuing Survey of Food Intakes by Individuals: Men 19–50 Years, 1 Day, 1985. Report No. 85-3. Nutrition Monitoring Division, Human Nutrition Information Service, U.S. Department of Agriculture, Hyattsville, Md. 94 pp.

USDA (U.S. Department of Agriculture). 1987. Nationwide Food Consumption Survey Continuing Survey of Food Intakes by Individuals: Women 19–50 Years and Their Children 1–5 Years, 4 Days, 1985. Report No. 85-4. Nutrition Monitoring Division, Human Nutrition Information Service. U.S. Department of Agriculture, Hyattsville, Md. 182 pp.

Webb, A.R., L. Kline, and M.F. Holick. 1988. Influence of season and latitude on the cutaneous synthesis of vitamin D_3: exposure to winter sunlight in Boston and Edmonton will not promote vitamin D_3 synthesis in human skin. J. Clin. Endocrinol. Metab. 67:373–378.

VITAMIN E

A requirement for vitamin E has been shown for most animal species, especially when a vitamin E-deficient diet is fed early in life. The primary signs of deficiency are reproductive failure, muscular dystrophy, and neurological abnormalities. Not until 40 years after its discovery in 1922, however, did evidence became convincing that humans also required vitamin E (Hassan et al., 1966; Oski and Barness, 1967). More recently, it has become apparent that deficiency occurs only in two classes of subjects: (1) premature, very low birth weight infants in whom low plasma vitamin E levels have been associated with some, but not all, of their medical problems (Anonymous, 1988; Bieri et al., 1983; Farrell, 1980) and (2) patients who, for a variety of reasons, do not absorb fat normally. In children, malabsorption associated with a variety of congenital conditions—cystic fibrosis, biliary atresia and other disorders of the hepatobiliary system, and lipid transport abnormalities as in abetalipoproteinemia—can produce severe neurological defects (Elias et al., 1981; Guggenheim et al., 1982; Kelleher et al., 1987; Muller, 1986). In adults, the malabsorption must persist for 5 to 10 years before subtle signs of deficiency, primarily neurological, appear (Jeffrey et al., 1987; Sokol, 1984).

Occurrence and Biological Activity

Two groups of compounds found in plant materials have vitamin E biological activity in widely varying degrees. The most important group, the tocopherols, is characterized by a ring system and a long, saturated side chain. There are four members of this group: the α-, β-, γ-, and δ-tocopherols, which differ only in the number and position of methyl groups on the ring. The second group, the tocotrienols, differ from the tocopherols by having an unsaturated side chain. The most active form of vitamin E, α-tocopherol, is also the most widely distributed in nature.

Biological activity has been determined from various animal assays, and the values are assumed to apply to humans. If the activity of α-tocopherol is designated as 100, the relative activities of the nutritionally important other compounds are β-tocopherol, 25–50; γ-tocopherol, 10–35; and α-tocotrienol, 30 (the range is due to different types of assays) (Bunyan et al., 1961; Dillard et al., 1983).

When α-tocopherol was first synthesized, the synthetic material was found to have a slightly lower biological activity than the α-tocopherol isolated from plants. This is because the molecule has several asymmetric centers that give rise to stereoisomers when synthesized. Synthetic α-tocopherol is a mixture of eight isomers, whereas the natural α-tocopherol has only one isomer. The nomenclature can be confusing, but international agreement has specified that natural α-tocopherol should be designated RRR-α-tocopherol (formerly termed d-α-tocopherol) and the synthetic compound should be designated all-*rac*-α-tocopherol (formerly dl-α-tocopherol) (Anonymous, 1987). The activity of 1 mg of the acetate form of this latter compound has been defined as equivalent to 1 IU of vitamin E. According to the *U.S. Pharmacopoeia,* the relative activity of all-*rac*-α-tocopherol is set at 74% of the activity of RRR-α-tocopherol (see Diplock, 1985, for a discussion).

For dietary purposes, vitamin E activity is expressed as RRR-α-tocopherol equivalents (α-TEs). One α-TE is the activity of 1 mg of RRR-α-tocopherol. To estimate the total α-TEs of mixed diets containing only natural forms of vitamin E, multiply the number of milligrams of β-tocopherol by 0.5, the milligrams of γ-tocopherol by 0.1, and the milligrams of α-tocotrienol by 0.3. If all-*rac*-α-tocopherol is present, the number of milligrams should be multiplied by 0.74.

Function and Metabolism

Tocopherols are known chemically as antioxidants, i.e., they prevent propagation of the oxidation of unsaturated fatty acids by trapping peroxyl free radicals. It is widely accepted that this is the basic function of vitamin E in animal tissues, where tocopherol is found in cellular membranes associated with polyunsaturated fatty acids (PUFA) in phospholipids. In vitamin E deficiency, the oxidation of PUFA is more readily propagated along the membrane, leading to cell damage and eventually symptoms, mainly neurological. Vitamin E is the primary defense against potentially harmful oxidations. This defense system is also aided by two other essential nutrients—selenium, as a component of the enzyme glutathione peroxidase (Hoekstra, 1974), and ascorbic acid (vitamin C).

Absorption of α-tocopherol is relatively inefficient, ranging from 20 to 80% in various studies. Normal bile secretion and normal pancreatic function are essential for tocopherol absorption (Gallo-Torres, 1980). Efficiency of absorption appears to decline as the dose increases; probably the small amounts consumed with each meal are absorbed to a greater extent than the larger amounts used in absorption tests. Tocopherol is secreted into the lymph in chylomicrons, taken up into the liver with chylomicron remnants, and subsequently secreted into the blood in very low density lipoproteins (VLDLs)

(Traber et al., 1988). As VLDLs are metabolized, tocopherol is transferred to low density lipoproteins (LDLs) and high density lipoproteins (HDLs) (Traber et al., 1988). In women, HDLs appear to carry more tocopherol than does LDL (Behrens et al., 1982).

Tissues take up α-tocopherol from the lipoproteins by a process not clearly understood. Binding proteins for α-tocopherol have been found in liver (Catignani, 1975) and erythrocytes (Kitabchi and Wimalesena, 1982). Liver has relatively high concentrations of tocopherol, but tissues with greater lipid content, e.g., adrenals, have higher concentrations. When expressed on the basis of lipid content, most tissues have similar concentrations (Quaife and Dju, 1949).

Blood concentrations of total tocopherols in normal adult men and women range from 0.5 to 1.2 mg/dl. Since children were found to have somewhat lower values (mean plasma concentration of 0.53 ± 0.13 mg/dl), a different standard for evaluation should be used (Levine et al., 1976). Because α-tocopherol is carried by lipoproteins, the plasma lipid content can influence the tocopherol concentration. In addition to absolute concentration, Horwitt et al. (1972) recommended that plasma vitamin E also be expressed on the basis of total plasma lipids. For practical purposes, the sum of plasma cholesterol and triglycerides is as good as total lipids (Thurnham et al., 1986). α-Tocopherol is found in the red cell membrane, where it exists in equilibrium with plasma α-tocopherol. When plasma vitamin E is considerably below normal, red cells become susceptible to excessive hemolysis (Leonard and Losowsky, 1971).

Dietary Sources and Usual Intakes

The tocopherol content of foods varies greatly, depending on processing, storage, and preparation procedures during which large losses may occur (Bauernfeind, 1980; Dicks, 1965). The richest sources in the U.S. diet are the common vegetable oils (such as soybean, corn, cottonseed, and safflower) and the products made from them (such as margarine and shortening) (USDA, 1984). Some of these oil products have more γ-tocopherol than α-tocopherol, and smaller amounts of the other tocopherols. Wheat germ is high in vitamin E, as are nuts. Meats, fish, animal fats, and most fruits and vegetables have little vitamin E (Bauernfeind, 1980), whereas green leafy vegetables supply appreciable amounts of this nutrient.

The vitamin E content of diets varies widely, depending primarily on the type and amount of fat present (i.e., animal or vegetable) and on losses that may occur during processing and cooking. Analyses of balanced adult diets ranging from 2,000 to 3,000 kcal per day indicated that the average daily intakes of α-TEs range from 7 to 11 mg (Bieri and Evarts, 1973; Bunnell et al., 1965; Horwitt, 1974; Witting and Lee, 1975). In 1985, the reported vitamin E intake among men 19 to 50 years of age in the United States (based on a 1-day recall) averaged 9.8 mg of α-TEs (USDA, 1986). The corresponding figures for women 19 to 50 years of age and their children 1 to 5 years of age (collected over 4 nonconsecutive days) were 7.1 and 5.5 mg of α-TEs, respectively (USDA, 1987). Estimates of intake should be averaged over many days because of the wide daily variation (Witting and Lee, 1975).

PUFA-Vitamin E Relationship

The requirement for vitamin E in animals increases when PUFA intake increases (Dam, 1962; Horwitt, 1962), and there is evidence that this is also true in humans (Horwitt, 1960, 1974). In extreme situations, the need for α-tocopherol may vary from as little as 5 mg to more than 20 mg/day.

Attempts have been made to specify a fixed ratio of dietary RRR-α-tocopherol to PUFA, but this has not been completely satisfactory. The tocopherol requirement for the prevention of myopathy in animals increases with increases in the intake of unsaturated fats. In *in vitro* studies, the relative peroxidizability of unsaturated fatty acids increases markedly as the number of double bonds increases. Thus, the consumption of fish oils, which are highly unsaturated and have a low tocopherol content, could raise the levels of the highly unsaturated PUFAs in the tissues without a corresponding increase in vitamin E. Furthermore, the lipids in different tissues have different fatty acid compositions. In heart tissue, for example, lipids contain greater concentrations of highly unsaturated fatty acids than do most other tissues. When the primary PUFA in the diet is linoleic acid, as in most U.S. diets, a ratio (milligrams of RRR-α-tocopherol to grams of PUFA) of approximately 0.4 has been suggested as adequate for adult humans (Bieri and Evarts, 1973; Horwitt, 1974; Witting and Lee, 1975). As intakes of the common U.S. vegetable oils increase, vitamin E intake increases as well.

The values in the Summary Table at the end of this volume should be regarded as adequate intakes in balanced diets in the United States. The adequacy of these intakes will vary, however, if the PUFA content of the diet increases greatly over intake.

Recommended Allowances

Adults An adequate level of vitamin E in the diet implies that the ratio of tocopherol to PUFA in the tissues protects the lipids from peroxidation, permits normal physiological function, and allows for individual variations of lipids in the tissues. These criteria of adequacy appear to be met by the amounts of vitamin E and PUFA consumed by normal individuals ingesting balanced diets in the United States, as reviewed in the eighth and ninth editions of the RDAs (NRC, 1974, 1980). The allowance, therefore, is based primarily on customary intakes from U.S. food sources (Bieri and Evarts, 1973; Bunnell et al., 1965; Witting and Lee, 1975). Recognizing the extent to which vitamin E is available in the U.S. diet and the facility with which it is stored in tissues, the subcommittee has established an arbitrary but practical allowance for male adults of 10 mg of α-TEs per day. Because women are generally smaller, their allowance is 8 mg/day.

Most surveys of physically active elderly populations have not shown plasma vitamin E levels to be different from those of younger adults. In a recent study of subjects over 80 years of age, however, slightly lower values were found than in a middle-aged control group. When the plasma tocopherols were normalized to plasma cholesterol, triglycerides, or total lipids, there was no difference between younger or elderly groups (Vandewoude and Vandewoude, 1987). At this time, there is no convincing evidence that the allowance for younger adults is not adequate for the elderly.

Pregnancy and Lactation Circulating tocopherol concentrations increase during pregnancy in conjunction with rising plasma lipid levels (Horwitt et al., 1972). It is assumed that pregnant women need to consume increased amounts of vitamin E to allow for growth of the fetus. The subcommittee recommends an additional 2 mg during pregnancy, increasing the allowance to 10 mg/day.

Additional requirements for the first 6 months of lactation may be calculated by assuming that 750 ml of milk is produced daily, that the tocopherol concentration in human milk is 3.2 mg/liter (Jansson et al., 1981), and by adding a coefficient of variation of 12.5% to provide a margin of safety and rounding to the nearest whole number. This indicates that 3 mg of additional α-TEs would be required daily. However, because of incomplete absorption of vitamin E from the diet, this figure has been raised to 4 mg. During the second 6 months of lactation, if 600 ml of milk were produced per day, an additional 3 mg would be required daily. These allowances are greater than those in the previous edition, reflecting the addition of an adequate margin of safety to account for individual variation in need.

Infants The recommendation for infants from birth through 6 months of age (i.e., 3 mg) has been derived by using information about the tocopherol concentration of human milk (Jansson et al., 1981), by assuming a 750 ml estimated daily volume of milk ingestion, and by adding a coefficient of variation of 12.5%, which raises average intake by 25%. Although human milk has been shown to contain all the expected isomers of tocopherol, vitamers other than α-tocopherol account only for approximately 2% of the vitamin E activity. Human milk provides about 6% of calories as PUFA (Lammi-Keefe and Jensen, 1984). When smaller volumes of milk are consumed by breastfed babies during the first week of life, sufficient tocopherol is provided by colostrum, which has a threefold higher concentration compared to mature milk (Jansson et al., 1981). The relatively high intake of PUFA by infants fed human milk or formula should be adequately met by 3 mg of vitamin E per day. For infants older than 6 months, the RDA has been increased to 4 mg in proportion to growth. These RDAs provide approximately 0.5 mg of α-TEs per kilogram infant body weights.

Premature infants present problems somewhat different from those of full-term infants of normal weight. Because of their low body stores of tocopherol, their reduced intestinal absorption (Gross and Melhorn, 1972), and the relatively greater growth rates associated with prematurity, it is more difficult for these infants to achieve and maintain normal vitamin E status (Bieri and Farrell, 1976). Thus, oral supplementation of 17 mg of vitamin E (all-*rac*-α-tocopherol) per day may be required by premature infants up to 3 months of age (Farrell et al., 1985).

Children   The requirements for vitamin E increase with increasing body weight until adulthood, but not as rapidly as during the first year of life. Thus, during the steady growth of early childhood, an intake increasing from 6 mg for the reference child of 13 kg body weight at 1 to 3 years of age to 7 mg at 7 to 10 years (28 kg) should be satisfactory for the average diet. During the adolescent growth spurt, an increase to 8 mg for females and 10 mg for males is recommended, i.e., the same amount as for adults.

Excessive Intakes and Toxicity

Compared with other fat-soluble vitamins, vitamin E is relatively nontoxic when taken by mouth. Most adults appear to tolerate oral doses of 100 to 800 mg/day (Bendich and Machlin, 1988; Farrell and Bieri, 1975) without gross signs or biochemical evidence of toxicity. In view of the lack of evidence of any definitive benefits of vitamin

E supplements for normal individuals, the subcommittee does not encourage supplementation, except as specifically noted.

References

Anonymous. 1987. Nomenclature policy: generic descriptors and trivial names for vitamins and related compounds. J. Nutr. 117:7–14.

Anonymous. 1988. Vitamin E supplementation of premature infants. Nutr. Rev. 46:122–123.

Bauernfeind, J. 1980. Tocopherols in foods. Pp. 99–167 in L.J. Machlin, ed. Vitamin E: A Comprehensive Treatise. Marcel Dekker, New York.

Behrens, W.A., J.N. Thompson, and R. Madère. 1982. Distribution of α-tocopherol in human plasma lipoproteins. Am. J. Clin. Nutr. 35:691–696.

Bendich, A., and L.J. Machlin. 1988. Safety of oral intake of vitamin E. Am. J. Clin. Nutr. 48:612–619.

Bieri, J.G., and R.P. Evarts. 1973. Tocopherols and fatty acids in American Diets. The recommended allowance for vitamin E. J. Am. Diet. Assoc. 62:147–151.

Bieri, J.G., and P.M. Farrell. 1976. Vitamin E. Vitam. Horm. 34:31–75.

Bieri, J.G., L. Corash, and V.S. Hubbard. 1983. Medical uses of vitamin E. N. Engl. J. Med. 308:1063–1071.

Bunnell, R.H., J. Keating, A. Quaresimo, and G.K. Parman. 1965. Alpha-tocopherol content of foods. Am. J. Clin. Nutr. 17:1–10.

Bunyan, J., D. McHale, J. Green, and S. Marcinkiewicz. 1961. Biological potencies of epsilon- and zeta-1-tocopherol and 5-methyltocol. Br. J. Nutr. 15:253–257.

Catignani, G.L. 1975. An α-tocopherol binding protein in rat liver cytoplasm. Biochem. Biophys. Res. Commun. 67:66–72.

Dam, H. 1962. Interrelations between vitamin E and polyunsaturated fatty acids in animals. Vit. Horm. 20:527–540.

Dicks, M.W. 1965. Vitamin E Content of Foods and Feed for Human and Animal Consumption. Agricultural Experimental Station Bulletin No. 435. University of Wyoming, Laramie.

Dillard, C.J., V.C. Gavino, and A.L. Tappel. 1983. Relative antioxidant effectiveness of α-tocopherol and γ-tocopherol in iron-loaded rats. J. Nutr. 131:2266–2273.

Diplock, A.T. 1985. Vitamin E. Pp. 154–224 in A.T. Diplock, ed. Fat-Soluble Vitamins: Their Biochemistry and Applications. Technomic Publications Co., Lancaster, Pa.

Elias, E., D.P. Muller, and J. Scott. 1981. Association of spinocerebellar disorders with cystic fibrosis or chronic childhood cholestasis and very low serum vitamin E. Lancet 2:1319–1321.

Farrell, P.M. 1980. Deficiency states, pharmacological effects, and nutrient requirments. Pp. 520–620 in L.J. Machlin, ed. Vitamin E: A Comprehensive Treatise. Basic and Clinical Nutrition, Vol. 1. Marcel Dekker, New York.

Farrell, P.M., and J.G. Bieri. 1975. Megavitamin E supplementation in man. Am. J. Clin. Nutr. 28:1381–1386.

Farrell, P.M., P.M. Zachman, and G.R. Gutcher. 1985. Fat soluble vitamins A, E, and K in the premature infant. Pp. 63–98 in R.S. Tsang, ed. Vitamin and Mineral Requirements in Preterm Infants. Marcel Dekker, New York.

Gallo-Torres, H.E. 1980. Absorption: Transport and Metabolism. Pp. 170–267 in L.J. Machlin, ed. Vitamin E: A Comprehensive Treatise. Marcel Dekker, New York.

Gross, S., and D.K. Melhorn. 1972. Vitamin E, red cell lipids and red cell stability in prematurity. Ann. N.Y. Acad. Sci. 203:141–162.

Guggenheim, M.A., S.P. Ringel, A. Silverman, B.E. Grabert, and H.E. Neville. 1982. Progressive neuromuscular disease in children with chronic cholestasis and vitamin E deficiency: clinical and muscle biopsy findings and treatment with α-tocopherol. Ann. N.Y. Acad. Sci. 393:84–93.

Hassan, H., S.A. Hashim, T.B. Van Itallie, and W.H. Sebrell. 1966. Syndrome in premature infants associated with low plasma vitamin E levels and high polyunsaturated fatty acid diet. Am. J. Clin. Nutr. 19:147–157.

Hoekstra, W.G. 1974. Biochemical role of selenium. Pp. 61–77 in W.G. Hoekstra, J.W. Suttie, H.E. Ganther, and W. Mertz, eds. Trace Element Metabolism in Animals, 2. Proceedings of the Second International Symposium. University Park Press, Baltimore, Md.

Horwitt, M.K. 1960. Vitamin E and lipid metabolism in man. Am. J. Clin. Nutr. 8:451–461.

Horwitt, M.K. 1962. Interrelations between vitamin E and polyunsaturated fatty acids in adult men. Vitam. Horm. 20:541–558.

Horwitt, M.K. 1974. Status of human requirements for vitamin E. Am. J. Clin. Nutr. 27:1182–1193.

Horwitt, M.K., C.C. Harvey, C.H. Dahm, Jr., and M.T. Searcy. 1972. Relationship between tocopherol and serum lipid levels for determination of nutritional adequacy. Ann. N.Y. Acad. Sci. 203:223–236.

Jansson, L., B. Åkesson, and L. Holmberg. 1981. Vitamin E and fatty acid composition of human milk. Am. J. Clin. Nutr. 34:8–13.

Jeffrey, G.P., D.P.R. Muller, A.K. Burroughs, S. Matthews, C. Kemp, O. Epstein, T.A. Metcalfe, E. Southam, M. Tazir-Melboucy, P.K. Thomas, and N. McIntyre. 1987. Vitamin E deficiency and its clinical significance in adults with primary biliary cirrhosis and other forms of liver disease. J. Hepatol. 4:307–317.

Kelleher, J., M.G. Miller, J.M. Littlewood, A.M. McDonald, and M.S. Losowsky. 1987. The clinical effect of correction of vitamin E depletion in cystic fibrosis. Int. J. Vitam. Nutr. Res. 57:253–259.

Kitabchi, A.E., and J. Wimalasena. 1982. Specific binding sites for D-α-tocopherol on human erythrocytes. Biochim. Biophys. Acta 684:200–206.

Lammi-Keefe, C.J., and R.G. Jensen. 1984. Lipids in human milk: a review. 2. Composition and fat-soluble vitamins. J. Pediatr. Gastroenterol. Nutr. 3:172–198.

Leonard, P.J., and M.S. Losowsky. 1971. Effect of alpha-tocopherol administration on red cell survival in vitamin E-deficient human subjects. Am. J. Clin. Nutr. 24:388–393.

Levine, S.L., A.J. Adams, M.D. Murphy, and P.M. Farrell. 1976. Survey of vitamin E status in children. Pediatr. Res. 10:356.

Muller, D.P. 1986. Vitamin E—its role in neurological function. Postgrad. Med. J. 62:107–112.

NRC (National Research Council). 1974. Recommended Dietary Allowances, 8th ed. Report of the Committee on Dietary Allowances, Committee on the Interpretation of the Recommended Dietary Allowances, Food and Nutrition Board. National Academy of Sciences, Washington, D.C. 128 pp.

NRC (National Research Council). 1980. Recommended Dietary Allowances, 9th ed. Report of the Committee on Dietary Allowances, Division of Biological Sciences, Assembly of Life Sciences, Food and Nutrition Board. National Academy of Sciences, Washington, D.C. 185 pp.

Oski, F.A., and L.A. Barness. 1967. Vitamin E deficiency: a previously unrecognized cause of hemolytic anemia in the premature infant. J. Pediatr. 70:211–220.

Quaife, M.L., and M.Y. Dju. 1949. Chemical estimation of vitamin E in tissue and tocopherol content of some normal human tissues. J. Biol. Chem. 180:263–272.

Sokol, R.J. 1984. Vitamin E deficiency in adults (letter). Ann. Int. Med. 100:769.

Thurnham. D.I., J.A. Davies, B.J. Crump, R.D. Situnayake, and M. Davis. 1986. The use of different lipids to express serum tocopherol: lipid ratios for the measurement of vitamin E status. Ann. Clin. Biochem. 23:514–520.

Traber, M.G., K.U. Ingold, G.W. Burton, and H.J. Kayden. 1988. Absorption and transport of deuterium-substituted $2R,4'R,8'R$-α-tocopherol in human lipoproteins. Lipids 23:791–797.

USDA (U.S. Department of Agriculture). 1984. Oil Crops: Outlook and Situation Report. OCS-4. Economic Research Service, U.S. Department of Agriculture, Washington, D.C. 25 pp.

USDA (U.S. Department of Agriculture). 1986. CSFII. Nationwide Food Consumption Survey Continuing Survey of Food Intakes by Individuals: Men 19–50 Years, 1 Day, 1985. Report No. 85-3. Nutrition Monitoring Division, Human Nutrition Information Service. U.S. Department of Agriculture, Hyattsville, Md. 94 pp.

USDA (U.S. Department of Agriculture). 1987. Nationwide Food Consumption Survey Continuing Survey of Food Intakes by Individuals: Women 19–50 Years and Their Children 1–5 Years, 4 Days, 1985. Report No. 85-4. Nutrition Monitoring Division, Human Nutrition Information Service. U.S. Department of Agriculture, Hyattsville, Md. 182 pp.

Vandewoude, M.F., and M.G. Vandewoude. 1987. Vitamin E status in a normal population: the influence of age. J. Am. Coll. Nutr. 6:307–311.

Witting, L.A., and L. Lee. 1975. Dietary levels of vitamin E and polyunsaturated fatty acids and plasma vitamin E. Am. J. Clin. Nutr. 28:571–576.

VITAMIN K

Vitamin K is the name for a group of compounds, all of which contain the 2-methyl-1,4-naphthoquinone moiety. In plants (phylloquinone), the substituent at C-3 is a 20-carbon phytyl group; in bacteria (menaquinones), it is a polyisoprenyl side chain with 4 to 13 5-carbon isoprenyl units. Animal tissues contain both phylloquinone and menaquinones. Menadione, a fat-soluble synthetic compound that contains no side chain, and its water-soluble derivatives are alkylated in the liver to biologically active menaquinones in humans *in vivo* (Suttie, 1985).

Compounds with vitamin K activity are essential for the formation of prothrombin and at least five other proteins (factors VII, IX, and X, and proteins C and S) involved in the regulation of blood clotting. Although vitamin K is also required for the biosynthesis of some other proteins found in the plasma, bone, and kidney, defective coagulation of the blood is the only major sign of vitamin K deficiency (Olson, 1984; Suttie, 1985).

Metabolism

Under normal conditions, vitamin K is moderately (40 to 70%) well absorbed from the jejunum and ileum, but very poorly absorbed from the colon (Shearer et al., 1974). As with other lipid-soluble vitamins, absorption depends on a normal flow of bile and pancreatic juice and is enhanced by dietary fat. Consequently, the absorption of vitamin K in fat malabsorption syndromes is very poor.

Absorbed vitamin K is transported primarily via the lymph in chylomicrons. It is initially concentrated in the liver and is then distributed widely among body tissues. Within cells, vitamin K is associated primarily with membranes, especially with those of the endoplasmic reticulum and mitochondria. Under normal physiological conditions, 30 to 40% of absorbed vitamin K is excreted via the bile into the feces as partially degraded, conjugated, water-soluble metabolites, whereas approximately 15% is excreted as water-soluble metabolites in the urine (Shearer et al., 1974). In humans, the total body pool of vitamin K is small, and its turnover is rapid (Bjornsson et al., 1980; Olson, 1984). Liver stores of vitamin K appear to consist of only about 10% phylloquinone and approximately 90% of various menaquinones, which are probably synthesized by intestinal bacteria (Shearer et al., 1988). It appears, however, that the total need for vitamin K cannot be supplied from synthesis of menaquinones by intestinal bacteria, since simple restriction of dietary vitamin K can result in alterations in clotting factors (Suttie et al., 1988).

In the liver, vitamin K plays an essential role in the posttranslational carboxylation of glutamic acid to γ-carboxyglutamyl residues in prothrombin (coagulation factor II) and in factors VII, IX, and X, and proteins C, S, and Z (Magnusson et al., 1974; Nelsestuen et al., 1974; Stenflo et al., 1974). In the absence of vitamin K, these proteins are still synthesized but are nonfunctional because they lack the γ-carboxyglutamyl residues. During the incorporation of carbon dioxide into γ-carboxyglutamyl residues, reduced vitamin K is oxidized to an epoxide intermediate and is then recycled back to the reduced vitamin by the action of several membrane-bound enzymes (Friedman et al., 1979; Hall et al., 1982; Larson et al., 1981).

Other vitamin K-dependent proteins that contain γ-carboxyglutamyl residues have also been identified in bone, kidney, and other tissues. These proteins, like the clotting proteins, bind calcium ions and seem to be related to bone crystal formation and possibly to synthesis of some phospholipids (Lev and Sundaram, 1988; Price, 1988).

Dietary Sources and Usual Intakes

The vitamin K content of commonly consumed foods is not known with precision and therefore is not given in food composition tables. Early data, mainly from bioassays, were summarized by Olson (1988). In more recent studies in which high pressure liquid chromatography was used, the phylloquinone content of common vegetables often differed by as much as threefold (higher or lower) from values found using chick bioassays (Shearer et al., 1980). Green leafy vegetables, which provide 50 to 800 μg of vitamin K per 100 g of food, are clearly the best dietary sources. Small but significant amounts of vitamin K (1 to 50 μg/100 g) are also present in milk and dairy products, meats, eggs, cereals, fruits, and vegetables.

Human milk is relatively low in vitamin K (approximately 2 μg/liter). Thus, breastfed infants may ingest only about 1 μg/day, which amounts to only 20% of the presumed requirement of 5 μg/day, or to an even smaller portion of the rather generous recommended content of 4 μg/100 kcal in infant formulas (AAP, 1976). Cow's milk contains 4 to 18 μg of vitamin K per liter (Haroon et al., 1982; Shearer et al., 1980).

Another potentially important source of vitamin K is the bacterial flora in the jejunum and ileum. The extent of utilization of menaquinones synthesized by gut microorganisms is not clear, however.

A normal mixed diet consumed daily by a healthy adult in the United States has been estimated to contain an average of 300 to 500 μg of vitamin K (Olson, 1988), although more recent studies suggest that these estimates may be too high (Suttie et al., 1988). Green leafy vegetables were consumed by only 1 of 12 persons in the United States on a specific day in 1977 (USDA, 1980); however, the *average* daily intake of vitamin K by surveyed individuals still seems to be adequate. The vitamin K intake in a single day is not a reliable indicator of its average intake by an individual over an extended period, and diets largely free of green leafy vegetables may still contain adequate amounts of vitamin K.

Recommended Allowances

Adults The major criterion for assessing the adequacy of vitamin K status in adult humans is the maintenance of plasma prothrombin concentrations in the normal range, i.e., from 80 to 120 μg/ml (Blanchard et al., 1981). Although prothrombin levels are commonly based on assays that determine clotting time, both normal and abnormal (des-γ-carboxyglutamyl) prothrombin in the plasma can now be measured directly. The ratio of the two may be a useful indicator of marginal or incipient vitamin K deficiency in the absence of an observable defect in blood clotting (Blanchard et al., 1981; Corrigan et al., 1981). The 24-hour urine excretion of γ-carboxy-glutamic acid along with plasma vitamin K concentration have also been used to assess vitamin K status (Sadowski et al., 1988).

In vitamin K-depleted adult subjects fed a diet containing small amounts of vitamin K (10 μg/day) and treated with neomycin for 4 weeks, daily intravenous dosages of 1.5 μg of vitamin K per kilogram of body weight restored normal plasma prothrombin levels, whereas 0.1 μg/kg daily did not (Frick et al., 1967). In a study of four adults fed 0.4 μg/kg daily and treated with antibiotics for 5 weeks, plasma concentrations of prothrombin fell but remained at 70% or more of normal values (O'Reilly, 1971).

Suttie et al. (1988) reported studies of 10 college-aged male subjects who consumed a self-selected diet that eliminated foods high in vitamin K (mainly green leafy vegetables and liver) for 21 days. Such a diet provided the subjects with an average of approximately 50 μg phylloquinone per day. Serum phylloquinone values decreased during this period, but prothrombin time remained in what was considered the normal range. By the end of the period of vitamin K restriction, however, there was a significant increase in the ratio of abnormal prothrombin to active prothrombin. Similarly, a decrease in urinary γ-carboxyglutamic acid was observed during the period of reduced vitamin K consumption.

Supplementation of the subjects with 50 or 500 μg of phylloquinone per day for 12 days eliminated the abnormal ratios of active to abnormal prothrombin and restored γ-carboxyglutamic acid excretion to normal values. The supplement of 50 μg of phylloquinone did not raise plasma phylloquinone levels to prerestriction levels, although the 500 μg supplement was effective in raising serum phylloquinone levels to about double normal values. This study (Suttie et al., 1988) shows that simple elimination of foods high in vitamin K from a normal diet can result in signs of vitamin K inadequacy. It also suggests that bacterial synthesis of menaquinones was not sufficient to eliminate the need for dietary vitamin K in subjects consuming approximately 50 μg of phylloquinone per day.

Given the results of Frick et al. (1967) and the more recent results of Suttie et al. (1988) discussed above, it appears that a dietary intake of about 1 μg/kg body weight per day should be sufficient to maintain normal blood clotting time in adults. Thus, the RDA for a 79-kg man is 80 μg per day, and for a 63 kg woman, it is 65 μg.

Elderly persons in good health are not known to have an increased need for vitamin K. On the other hand, 75% of an older hospital-based population had a hypoprothrombinemia that was responsive to vitamin K treatment (Hazell and Baloch, 1970). Chronic disease, drug therapy, and poor diet may well have contributed to the hypoprothrombinemic condition of this group. Trauma, physical debilitation, renal insufficiency, and chronic treatment with large doses of broad-spectrum antibiotics increase the risk of vitamin K insufficiency (Ansell et al., 1977).

Pregnancy and Lactation   Data are insufficient to establish an RDA for vitamin K during pregnancy. Because vitamin K consumed in usual diets generally exceeds the RDA established for adult women, additional increments to usual intake are not recommended. Lactation imposes little additional need, since vitamin K consumed in usual diets generally exceeds the RDA. Therefore, additional increments are not recommended.

Infants and Children   The newborn infant has low plasma prothrombin levels. Although some hypoprothrombinemic infants respond to vitamin K treatment, other factors, including immaturity of the liver, may cause hypoprothrombinemia in the newborn (Suttie, 1984). Because human milk contains low levels of vitamin K (2 µg/liter) and the intestinal flora are limited, exclusively breastfed infants who do not receive vitamin K prophylaxis at birth are at very real risk of developing fatal intracranial hemorrhage secondary to vitamin K deficiency (Lane et al., 1983). Home-delivered, breastfed infants require particular attention in this regard.

A recommended range of total intake for infants is 5 µg of phylloquinone or menaquinone per day during the first 6 months of infancy and 10 µg during the second 6 months. Newborn infants are routinely given a supplement of vitamin K by intramuscular injection to prevent hemorrhage (AAP, 1985). The usual dose is 0.5–1.0 mg for full-term infants and at least 1 mg for preterm infants. Infant formulas should contain 4 µg of vitamin K per 100 kcal (AAP, 1985). In the absence of specific information about the vitamin K requirements of children, RDA values for them are set at about 1 µg/kg body weight.

Other Considerations

In persons treated with anticoagulant drugs, such as the 4-hydroxy coumarins, vitamin K status should be carefully monitored. Accidental ingestion of large amounts of these compounds, e.g., in rat poisons, requires vitamin K therapy (Suttie, 1984). High intakes of vitamin E can produce a vitamin K-responsive hemorrhagic condition in laboratory animals and humans, particularly when humans are also being treated with anticoagulants (Olson, 1982; Suttie, 1984). Adults treated chronically with broad-spectrum antibiotics or on long-term hyperalimentation, and patients with chronic biliary obstruction or with lipid malabsorption syndromes, are particularly sensitive to vitamin K deficiency (Olson, 1982, 1984; Olson and Suttie, 1977; Suttie, 1984).

Excessive Intakes and Toxicity

Even when large amounts of vitamin K are ingested over an extended period, toxic manifestations have not been observed (Owen, 1971). However, administered menadione, but not phylloquinone, may cause hemolytic anemia, hyperbilirubinemia, and kernicterus in the newborn (Owen, 1971), primarily because of its interaction with sulfhydryl groups.

References

AAP (American Academy of Pediatrics). 1985. Pediatric Nutrition Handbook, 2nd ed. American Academy of Pediatrics, Elk Grove Village, Ill.

ASHP (American Society of Hospital Pharmacists). 1985. Phytonadione. Pp. 1709–1710 in American Hospital Formulary Service: Drug Information 85. American Society of Hospital Pharmacists, Bethesda, Md.

Ansell, J., E. Kumar, and R.D. Deykin. 1977. The spectrum of vitamin K deficiency. J. Am. Med. Assoc. 238:40–42.

Bjornsson, T.D., P.J. Meffin, S.E. Smezey, and T.F. Blaschke. 1980. Disposition and turnover of vitamin K_1 in man. Pp. 328–332 in J.W. Suttie, ed. Vitamin K Metabolism and Vitamin K-dependent Proteins. University Park Press, Baltimore.

Blanchard, R.A., B.C. Furie. M. Jorgensen, S.F. Kruger, and B. Furie. 1981. Acquired vitamin K-dependent carboxylation deficiency in liver disease. N. Engl. J. Med. 305:242–248.

Corrigan, J.J., Jr., L.M. Taussig, R. Beckerman, and J.S. Wagener. 1981. Factor II (prothrombin) coagulant activity and immunoreactive protein detection of vitamin K deficiency and liver disease in patients with cystic fibrosis. J. Pediatr. 99:254–257.

Frick, P.G., G. Riedler, and H. Brogli. 1967. Dose response and minimal daily requirement for vitamin K in man. J. Appl. Physiol. 23:387–389.

Friedman, P.A., M.A. Shia, P.M. Gallop, and A.E. Griep. 1979. Vitamin K-dependent gamma-carbon-hydrogen bond cleavage and nonmandatory concurrent carboxylation of peptide-bound glutamic acid residues. Proc. Natl. Acad. Sci. U.S.A. 76:3126–3129.

Hall, A.L., R. Kloepper, R.K.-Y Zee-Cheng, Y.J.D. Chiu, F.C. Lee, and R.E. Olson. 1982. Mechanisms of action of *tert*-butyl hydroperoxide in the inhibition of vitamin K-dependent carboxylation. Arch. Biochem. Biophys. 214:45–50.

Haroon, Y., M.J. Shearer. S. Rahim, W.G. Gunn, G. McEnergy, and P. Barkan. 1982. The content of phylloquinone (vitamin K_1) in human milk, cow's milk and infant formula foods determined by high-performance liquid chromatography. J. Nutr. 112:1105–1117.

Hazell, K., and K.H. Baloch. 1970. Vitamin K deficiency in the elderly. Gerontol. Clin. 12:10–117.

Lane, P.A., W.E. Hathaway, J.H. Githens, R.D. Krugman, and D.A. Rosenberg. 1983. Fatal intracranial hemorrhage in a normal infant secondary to vitamin K deficiency. Pediatrics 72:562–564.

Larson, A.E., P.A. Friedman. and J.W. Suttie. 1981. Vitamin K-dependent carboxylase: stoichiometry of carboxylation and vitamin K 2,2-epoxide formation. J. Biol. Chem. 256:11032–11035.

Lev, M., and K.S. Sundaram. 1988. Modulation of glycosphingolipid synthesis by vitamin K depletion in bacteria and in brain. Pp. 211–220 in J.W. Suttie, ed. Current Advances in Vitamin K Research. Elsevier, New York.

Magnusson, S., L. Sottrup-Jansen, T.E. Peterson, H.R. Morris, and A. Dell. 1974. Primary structure of the vitamin K-dependent part of prothrombin. FEBS Lett. 44:189–193.

Nelsestuen, G.L., T.H. Zythovicz, and J.B. Howard. 1974. The mode of action of vitamin K. J. Biol. Chem. 249:6347–6350.

Olson, R.E. 1982. Vitamin K. Pp. 582–594 in R.W. Colman, J. Hirsch, V.J. Marder, and W.W. Salzman, eds. Hemostasis and Thrombosis. Lippincott, New York.

Olson, R.E. 1984. The function and metabolism of vitamin K. Annu. Rev. Nutr. 4:281–337.

Olson, R.E. 1988. Vitamin K. Pp. 328–339 in M.E. Shils and V.R. Young, eds. Modern Nutrition in Health and Disease, 7th ed. Lea & Febiger, Philadelphia.

Olson, R.E., and J.W. Suttie. 1977. Vitamin K and carboxyglutamate biosynthesis. Vit. Horm. 35:59–108.

O'Reilly, R.A. 1971. Vitamin K in hereditary resistance to oral anticoagulant drugs. Am. J. Physiol. 221:1327–1330.

Owen, C.A., Jr. 1971. Pharmacology and toxicology of the vitamin K group. Pp. 492–509 in W.H. Sebrell and R.S. Harris, eds. The Vitamins, Vol. III. Academic Press, New York.

Price, P.A. 1988. Bone Gla protein and matrix Gla protein: identification of the probable structures involved in substrate recognition by the γ-carboxylase and discovery of tissue differences in vitamin K metabolism. Pp. 259–274 in J.W. Suttie, ed. Current Advances in Vitamin K Research. Elsevier, New York.

Sadowski, J.A., D.S. Bacon, S. Hood, K.W. Davidson, C.M. Ganter, Y. Haroon, and D.C. Shepard. 1988. The application of methods used for the evaluation of vitamin K nutritional status in human and animal studies. Pp. 453–463 in J.W. Suttie, ed. Current Advances in Vitamin K Research. Elsevier, New York.

Shearer, M.J., A. McBurney, and P. Barkhan. 1974. Studies on the absorption and metabolism of phylloquine (vitamin K) in man. Vit. Horm. 32:513–542.

Shearer, M.J., V. Allan, Y. Haroon, and P. Barkhan. 1980. Nutritional aspects of vitamin K in the Human. Pp. 317–327 in J.W. Suttie, ed. Vitamin K Metabolism and Vitamin K-dependent Proteins. University Park Press, Baltimore.

Shearer, M.J., P.T. McCarthy, and O.E. Crampton. 1988. The assessment of human vitamin K status from tissue measurements. Pp. 437–452 in J.W. Suttie, ed. Current Advances in Vitamin K Research. Elsevier, New York.

Stenflo, J., P. Fernlund, W. Egan, and P. Roepstorff. 1974. Vitamin K-dependent modifications of glutamic acid residues in prothrombin. Proc. Natl. Acad. Sci. U.S.A. 71:2730–2733.

Suttie, J.W. 1984. Vitamin K. Pp. 147–198 in L.J. Machlin, ed. Handbook on Vitamins, Marcel Dekker, New York.

Suttie, J.W. 1985. Vitamin K. Pp. 225–311 in A.T. Diplock, ed. The Fat Soluble Vitamins. William Heinemann, Ltd., London.

Suttie, J.W., L.L. Mummah-Schendel, D.V. Shah, B.J. Lyle, and J.L. Greger. 1988. Vitamin K deficiency from dietary vitamin K restriction in humans. Am. J. Clin. Nutr. 47:475–480.

USDA (U.S. Department of Agriculture). 1980. Nationwide Food Consumption Survey 1977–78. Food and Nutrient Intakes of Individuals in 1 Day in the United States, Spring 1977. Preliminary Report No. 2. Nutrition Monitoring Division, Human Nutrition Information Service. U.S. Department of Agriculture, Hyattsville, Md.

8

Water-Soluble Vitamins

VITAMIN C

Vitamin C (L-ascorbic acid) is a water-soluble antioxidant that can be synthesized by many mammals, but not by humans. In the diet, it is also present to some extent in its oxidized form (dehydroascorbic acid), which also has vitamin C activity (Sabry et al., 1958). Dietary deficiency eventually leads to scurvy, a serious disease characterized by weakening of collagenous structures that results in widespread capillary hemorrhaging (Hornig, 1975; Woodruff, 1975). In the United States, scurvy occurs primarily in infants fed diets consisting exclusively of cow's milk and in aged persons on limited diets.

The best defined biochemical property of vitamin C is its function as a cosubstrate in hydroxylations requiring molecular oxygen, as in the hydroxylation of proline and lysine in the formation of collagen (Barnes, 1975; Myllyla et al., 1978), of dopamine to norepinephrine (Levin et al., 1960), and of tryptophan to 5-hydroxytryptophan (Cooper, 1961). It may also be involved in reactions involving a number of other compounds, including tyrosine (La Du and Zannoni, 1961), folic acid (Stokes et al., 1975), histamine (Clemetson, 1980), corticosteroids (Wilbur and Walter, 1977), neuroendocrine peptides (Glembotski, 1987), and bile acids (Ginter, 1975). Vitamin C can also affect functions of leukocytes (Anderson and Theron, 1979) and macrophages (Anderson and Lukey, 1987), immune responses (Leibovitz and Siegel, 1978), wound healing (Levenson et al., 1971), and allergic reactions (Dawson and West, 1965). Ascorbic acid as such or as present in plant foods increases the absorption of inorganic iron when the two nutrients are ingested together (Hallberg et al., 1987).

Absorption, Transport, Storage, and Excretion

L-ascorbic acid is absorbed in the intestine by a sodium-dependent transport process (Stevenson, 1974). At low doses, absorption may be almost complete, but over the range of usual intake in food (30 to 60 mg), 80 to 90% is absorbed (Kallner et al., 1977). Absorbed ascorbic acid is present as the anion in blood plasma, unbound to plasma proteins. As the daily intake of ascorbic acid increases, the plasma concentration rises rapidly and then reaches a plateau of 1.2 to 1.5 mg/dl at an intake of 90 to 150 mg/day (Garry et al., 1987; Sauberlich et al., 1974).

Body stores of ascorbic acid in adult men reach a maximum of approximately 3,000 mg at daily intakes exceeding 200 mg. One half of this level (1,500 mg) is achieved by much lower daily intakes in the range of 60 to 100 mg. Much of the body stores is normally found within cells, in which the concentrations vary widely but are usually severalfold higher than those in blood plasma. In at least some tissues these concentrations appear to be achieved by a stereoselective transport process (Moser, 1987).

Ascorbic acid and its various metabolites are excreted mainly in the urine. At daily intakes up to 100 mg, oxalate is the major product excreted. When larger amounts are ingested, ascorbic acid is mainly excreted as such (Jaffe, 1984; Kallner et al., 1979). Little ascorbic acid is metabolized to carbon dioxide at ordinary intakes (Baker et al., 1969), but at large doses, degradation within the intestine may be substantial (Kallner et al., 1985).

Dietary Sources and Usual Intakes

Vegetables and fruits contain relatively high concentrations of vitamin C, e.g., green and red peppers, collard greens, broccoli, spinach, tomatoes, potatoes, strawberries, and oranges and other citrus fruits. Meat, fish, poultry, eggs, and dairy products contain smaller amounts, and grains contain none. Ascorbic acid in the U.S. food supply is provided almost entirely by foods of vegetable origin—38% by citrus fruits, 16% by potatoes, and 32% from other vegetables (Marsten and Raper, 1987). The rest comes from fortified and enriched products and from meat, fish, poultry, eggs, and dairy products. The average amount available per capita in the U.S. food supply increased from 98 mg in 1967–1969 to 114 mg in 1985 (Marsten and Raper, 1987). The average dietary vitamin C intake by adult men in the United States in 1985 was 109 mg (USDA, 1986). The corresponding intakes for adult women and children 1 to 5 years of age were 77 mg and 84 mg, respectively (USDA, 1987).

The dietary vitamin C may be considerably lower than the calculated amount in the food ingested, largely because of its destruction by heat and oxygen and its loss in cooking water. On the other hand, the mean total intake of vitamin C may also be considerably higher because (1) supplements of vitamin C are ingested by 35% of a representative U.S. adult population (Stewart et al., 1985), (2) food composition tables used in the U.S. Department of Agriculture surveys provide the L-ascorbic acid content only and do not include the biologically active dehydroascorbate, and (3) ascorbic acid is added to some processed foods because of its antioxidant or other properties (NRC, 1982).

Criteria for Assessing Nutritional Status

Vitamin C status is usually evaluated from signs of clinical deficiency, plasma (or blood) levels, or leukocyte concentrations. It has also been evaluated from isotopic estimates of body stores.

Clinical signs of scurvy, including follicular hyperkeratosis, swollen or bleeding gums, petechial hemorrhages, and joint pain, are associated with plasma (or serum) vitamin C values of less than 0.2 mg/dl, leukocyte concentrations of less than 2 μg/10^8 cells, and a body pool size of less than 300 mg (Hodges et al., 1969, 1971; Sauberlich, 1981). To eliminate clinical signs of scurvy in several groups of male subjects, vitamin C intakes ranging from 6.5 to 10 mg/day were required (Baker et al., 1971; Bartley et al., 1953; Hodges et al., 1969, 1971).

Recommended Allowances

Adults The dietary allowances for vitamin C must be set, somewhat arbitrarily, between the amount necessary to prevent overt symptoms of scurvy (approximately 10 mg/day in adults) and the amount beyond which the bulk of vitamin C is not retained in the body, but rather is excreted as such in the urine (approximately 200 mg/day). Between these limits, body stores vary directly with intake, albeit not linearly. Since vitamin C is poorly retained in the body in the absence of continuous intake, the RDA has traditionally been set at a level that will prevent scorbutic symptoms for several weeks on a diet lacking vitamin C. Observed depletion rates in a small group of well-nourished adult men with a body pool of approximately 1,500 mg were exponential and averaged 3.2% daily (range, 2.2 to 4.1% in nine subjects), which would yield a body pool of vitamin C of 300 mg (the amount below which scorbutic symptoms can occur) in about

30 days (Baker et al., 1971). In 6 of 11 healthy, well-nourished young women fed ascorbate-free diets, scorbutic symptoms developed within 24 days (bleeding, red, or tender gums) in association with blood levels consistent with body stores below 300 mg (Sauberlich et al., in press). By means of steady state analysis of ascorbate kinetics in men, Kallner et al. (1979) found the turnover time to vary from about 56 days at low intakes (approximately 15 mg/day) to about 14 days at intakes of approximately 80 mg/day. Above 80 mg/day, urinary excretion of unmetabolized ascorbate increased rapidly. Kallner and colleagues reported that a three-pool model was required to fit the observed kinetic data and postulated that one of these pools reflected ascorbate bound within cells. They also failed to observe a clear-cut renal threshold for ascorbate. Since the turnover time varied with tissue stores, Kallner (1987) proposed that the depletion rates observed in earlier studies might be erroneously low. Saturation of tissue binding, and maximal rates of metabolism and renal tubular absorption, seemed to be approached at turnover rates of 60 to 80 mg daily, equivalent to body stores of about 1,500 mg.

The subcommittee has set the RDA for adult men at 60 mg/day, the same as in the previous edition. This amount is based upon (1) the observed variation in depletion rates and turnover rates; (2) the average depletion rates and the steady state turnover rates at a pool size of 1,500 mg; (3) the less than complete absorption of ascorbic acid, estimated at 85% for usual intakes; and (4) the variable loss of ascorbic acid in food preparation. This level of intake will prevent signs of scurvy for at least 4 weeks. Given the development of early scorbutic symptoms in adult women considered to be well nourished after somewhat less than 4 weeks of depletion, the subcommittee recommends the same RDA for adult women as for men.

An intake of 60 mg is easily provided in ordinary mixed diets. In the previous edition of the RDAs, an intake of 45 mg/day for adult men was considered to provide an average pool size of 1,500 mg, and an intake of 60 mg/day was recommended to provide a margin of safety. Higher values, in fact, have been suggested to yield a pool size of 1,500 mg (Kallner, 1987), which would result in a recommended allowance of about 100 mg/day. It was the view of the subcommittee, however, that an allowance of 60 mg/day for both men and women provides an adequate margin of safety.

Persons 65 years and older ingest more vitamin C on the average (90 to 150 mg/day) than the mean intake for all ages (Garry et al., 1982; USDA, 1984). Low plasma concentrations are, however, observed frequently in some groups of elderly persons (Cheng et al., 1985; Newton et al., 1985). Such low levels are believed to reflect inadequate intake in the groups examined. Therefore, no increment in the RDA for the elderly is recommended.

Cigarette smokers have lower concentrations of ascorbic acid in serum (Johnson et al., 1984; Pelletier, 1975; Schectman et al., 1989; Smith and Hodges, 1987) and leukocytes (Brook and Grimshaw, 1968). The lower serum levels are only partially explained by the reduced vitamin C intakes of smokers (Schectman et al., 1989). The metabolic turnover of men who smoked 20 or more cigarettes daily was found to be increased to a level 40% greater than that of non-smoking men (Kallner et al., 1981). From calculations based on all these observations, the vitamin C requirement of smokers has been estimated to be as much as twice that of nonsmokers. The subcommittee recommends that regular cigarette smokers ingest at least 100 mg of vitamin C daily.

Pregnancy and Lactation   During pregnancy, the concentration of vitamin C and several other solutes in blood plasma decreases (Morse et al., 1975), probably as a result of the hemodilution that accompanies pregnancy (Hytten, 1980; Rivers and Devine, 1975). Fetal and infant plasma levels of vitamin C are 50% higher than those of the mother (Khattab et al., 1970; Salmenpera, 1984), however, indicative both of active transport across the placenta and of a higher relative pool size in the fetus and infant.

If the requirement for vitamin C per unit body weight is comparable to that of nonpregnant adults, the increment in requirement for the fetus near term would be small (approximately 3 to 4 mg/day). Requirements are likely to be somewhat higher because the catabolic rate in the fetus is probably greater. To offset losses from the mother's body pool during pregnancy, a 10 mg/day increment in the maternal vitamin C RDA is recommended during pregnancy.

The concentration of vitamin C in human milk varies widely (3 to 10 mg/dl), depending upon the dietary intake of the nutrient as well as other factors (Bates et al., 1983; Byerley and Kirksey, 1985; Salmenpera, 1984; Sneed et al., 1981; Tarjan et al., 1965). Assuming a concentration of 3 mg/dl, and average milk volumes of 750 and 600 ml in the first and second 6 months, respectively, the subcommittee estimates the average maternal losses are 22 and 18 mg/day. Allowing for variation in milk production (2 SDs, or 25%), and an intestinal absorption efficiency of 85%, a daily increment of 35 mg is recommended during the first 6 months of lactation and 30 mg thereafter.

Infants and Children   Breastfed infants with vitamin C intakes of 7 to 12 mg/day and bottle-fed infants with vitamin C intakes of 7 mg/

day have been protected from scurvy (Goldsmith, 1961; Rajalakshmi et al., 1965; Van Eekelan, 1953). There are no other data on which to base an RDA. Accordingly, the subcommittee recommends 30 mg/day during the first 6 months of life on the basis of the vitamin C content of milk, which should provide an adequate margin of safety. Premature infants may exhibit transient tyrosinemia (Irwin and Hutchins, 1976) and may therefore require a larger amount. The RDA beyond 6 months of age is gradually increased to the adult level.

Other Considerations

Usual daily dietary intakes of vitamin C (25 to 75 mg) can enhance the intestinal absorption of dietary nonheme iron by two- to fourfold (Cook and Monsen, 1977; Rossander et al., 1979). No effect on iron status as assessed from serum ferritin concentration was observed, however, in two studies in which vitamin C supplements were given with meals for several weeks (Cook et al., 1984). In one of these studies (Cook et al., 1984), intestinal adaptation to high intakes was excluded as a cause of apparent lack of change in iron stores. The significance of these observations in omnivorous, meat-eating subjects is unclear (Hallberg et al., 1987), but they do not exclude an effect of vitamin C on iron status in vegetarians or in other individuals with more limited intake of heme iron.

Ascorbic acid may prevent the formation of carcinogenic nitrosamines by reducing nitrites. The ingestion of fruits and vegetables rich in vitamin C has been associated with a reduced incidence of some cancers, but there is no evidence that vitamin C is responsible for any such effects (NRC, 1989).

Pharmacologic Intakes and Toxicity

Daily intakes of ascorbic acid of 1 g or more have been reported to reduce the frequency and severity of symptoms of the common cold and other respiratory illnesses (Pauling, 1971). In controlled, double-blind trials, however, the effect of ascorbic acid was considerably smaller than had previously been reported (Anderson, 1975) or was not reproducible (Coulehan et al., 1976). Several reviewers (Chalmers, 1975; Dykes and Meier, 1975) have concluded that any benefits of large doses of ascorbic acid for these conditions are too small to justify recommending routine intake of large amounts by the entire population.

Large doses of ascorbic acid have also been reported to lower serum cholesterol in some hypercholesterolemic subjects (Ginter et al.,

1977), but these observations have not been confirmed by others (Peterson et al., 1975). A number of effects of large doses of ascorbic acid on other medical conditions have been reported, but there is no general agreement about their value.

Many persons habitually ingest 1 g or more of ascorbic acid without developing apparent toxic manifestations. A number of adverse effects have, however, been reported (Barnes, 1975; Hornig and Moser, 1981; Rivers, 1987), and the risk of sustained ingestion of such amounts is unknown. Routine use of large doses of ascorbic acid is therefore not recommended.

References

Anderson, R., and P.T. Lukey, 1987. A biological role for ascorbate in the selective neutralization of extracellular phagocyte-derived oxidants. Ann. N.Y. Acad. Sci. 498:229–247.

Anderson, R., and A. Theron. 1979. Effects of ascorbate on leucocytes. Part III. In vitro and in vivo stimulation of abnormal neutrophil motility by ascorbate. S. Afr. Med. J. 56:429–433.

Anderson, T.W. 1975. Large-scale trials of vitamin C. Ann. N.Y. Acad. Sci. 258:498–504.

Baker, E.M., R.E. Hodges, J. Hood, H.E. Sauberlich, and S.C. March. 1969. Metabolism of ascorbic-1-^{14}C acid in experimental human scurvy. Am. J. Clin. Nutr. 22:549–558.

Baker, E.M., R.E. Hodges, J. Hood, H.E. Sauberlich, S.C. March, and J.E. Canham. 1971. Metabolism of ^{14}C- and ^{3}H-labeled L-ascorbic acid in human scurvy. Am. J. Clin. Nutr. 24:444–454.

Barnes, M.J. 1975. Function of ascorbic acid in collagen metabolism. Ann. N.Y. Acad. Sci. 258:264–277.

Bartley, W., H.A. Krebs, and J.R.P. O'Brien. 1953. Vitamin C Requirement of Human Adults. A Report by the Vitamin C Subcommittee of the Accessory Food Factors Committee. Medical Research Council Special Report Series No. 280. Her Majesty's Stationery Office, London.

Bates, C.J., A.M. Prentice, A. Prentice, W.H. Lamb, and R.G. Whitehead. 1983. The effect of vitamin C supplementation on lactating women in Keneba, a West African rural community. Int. J. Vitam. Nutr. Res. 53:68–76.

Brook, M., and J.J. Grimshaw. 1968. Vitamin C concentration of plasma and leukocytes as related to smoking habit, age, and sex of humans. Am. J. Clin. Nutr. 21:1254–1258.

Byerley, L.O., and A. Kirksey. 1985. Effects of different levels of vitamin C intake on the vitamin C concentration in human milk and the vitamin C intakes of breast-fed infants. Am. J. Clin. Nutr. 81:665–671.

Chalmers, T.C. 1975. Effects of ascorbic acid on the common cold: an evaluation of the evidence. Am. J. Med. 58:532–536.

Cheng, L., M. Cohen, and H.N. Bhagavan. 1985. Vitamin C and the elderly. Pp. 157–185 in R.R. Watson, ed. CRC Handbook of Nutrition in the Aged. CRC Press, Boca Raton, Fla.

Clemetson, C.A.B. 1980. Histamine and ascorbic acid in human blood. J. Nutr. 110:662–668.

Cook, J.D., and E.R. Monson. 1977. Vitamin C, the common cold, and iron absorption. Am. J. Clin. Nutr. 30:235–241.

Cook, J.D., S.S. Watson, K.M. Simpson, D.A. Lipschitz, and B.S. Skikne. 1984. The effect of high ascorbic acid supplementation on body iron stores. Blood 64:721–726.

Cooper, J.R. 1961. The role of ascorbic acid in the oxidation of tryptophan to 5-hydroxytryptophan. Ann. N.Y. Acad. Sci. 92:208–211.

Coulehan, J.L., S. Eberhard, L. Kapner, F. Taylor, K. Rogers, and P. Garry. 1976. Vitamin C and acute illness in Navajo school children. N. Engl. J. Med. 295:973–977.

Dawson, W., and G.B. West. 1965. The influence of ascorbic acid on histamine metabolism in guinea pigs. Br. J. Pharmacol. 24:725–734.

Dykes, M.H.M., and P. Meier. 1975. Ascorbic acid and the common cold: evaluation of its efficacy and toxicity. J. Am. Med. Assoc. 231:1073–1079.

Garry, P.J., J.S. Goodwin, W.C. Hunt, and B.A. Gilbert. 1982. Nutritional status in a healthy elderly population: vitamin C. Am. J. Clin. Nutr. 36:332–339.

Garry, P.J., D.J. Vanderjagt, and W.C. Hunt. 1987. Ascorbic acid intakes and plasma levels in healthy elderly. Ann. N.Y. Acad. Sci. 498:90–99.

Ginter, E. 1975. Ascorbic acid in cholesterol and bile acid metabolism. Ann. N.Y. Acad. Sci. 258:410–421.

Ginter, E., O. Cerna, J. Budlovsky, V. Balaz, F. Hubra, V. Roch, and E. Sasko. 1977. Effect of ascorbic acid on plasma cholesterol in humans in a long-term experiment. Int. J. Vitam. Nutr. Res. 47:123–134.

Glembotski, C.C. 1987. The role of ascorbic acid in the biosynthesis of the neuroendocrine peptides α-MSH and TRH. Ann. N.Y. Acad. Sci. 498:54–61.

Goldsmith, G.A. 1961. Human requirements for vitamin C and its use in clinical medicine. Ann. N.Y. Acad. Sci. 92:230–245.

Hallberg, L., M. Brune, and L. Rossander-Hulthén. 1987. Is there a physiological role of vitamin C in iron absorption? Pp. 324–332 in J.J. Burns, J.M. Rivers, and L.J. Machlin, eds. Third Conference on Vitamin C. Annals of the New York Academy of Sciences, Vol. 498. New York Academy of Sciences, New York.

Hodges, R.E., E.M. Baker, J. Hood, H.E. Sauberlich, and S.C. March. 1969. Experimental scurvy in man. Am. J. Clin. Nutr. 22:535–548.

Hodges, R.E., J. Hood, J.E. Canham, H.E. Sauberlich, and E.M. Baker. 1971. Clinical manifestations of ascorbic acid deficiency in man. Am. J. Clin. Nutr. 24:432–443.

Hornig, D. 1975. Metabolism of ascorbic acid. World Rev. Nutr. Diet. 23:225–258.

Hornig, D.H., and U. Moser. 1981. The safety of high vitamin C intakes in man. Pp. 225–248 in J.N. Counsell and D.H. Hornig, eds. Vitamin C (ascorbic acid). Applied Science, London.

Hytten, F.E. 1980. Nutrition. Pp. 163–192 in F. Hytten and G. Chamberlain, eds. Clinical Physiology in Obstetrics. Blackwell, Oxford.

Irwin, M.I., and B.K. Hutchins. 1976. A conspectus of research on vitamin C requirements of man. J. Nutr. 106:823–879.

Jaffe, G.M. 1984. Vitamin C. Pp. 199–244 in L.J. Machlin, ed. Handbook of Vitamins: Nutritional, Biochemical, and Clinical Aspects. Marcel Dekker, New York.

Johnson, C., C. Wotecki, and R. Murphy. 1984. Smoking, vitamin supplement use, and other factors affecting serum vitamin C. Fed. Proc. 43:666.

Kallner, A. 1987. Requirement for vitamin C based on metabolic studies. Ann. N.Y. Acad. Sci. 498:418–423.

Kallner, A., D. Hartmann, and D. Hornig. 1977. On the absorption of ascorbic acid in man. Int. J. Vitam. Nutr. Res. 47:383–388.

Kallner, A., D. Hartmann, and D. Hornig. 1979. Steady-state turnover and body pool of ascorbic acid in man. Am. J. Clin. Nutr. 32:530–539.

Kallner, A.B., D. Hartmann, and D.H. Hornig. 1981. On the requirements of ascorbic acid in man: steady-state turnover and body pool in smokers. Am. J. Clin. Nutr. 34:1347–1355.

Kallner, A., D. Hornig, and R. Pellikka. 1985. Formation of carbon dioxide from ascorbate in man. Am. J. Clin. Nutr. 41:609–613.

Khattab, A.K., S.A. al-Nagdy, K.A. Mourad, and H.I. el-Azghal. 1970. Foetal maternal ascorbic acid gradient in normal Egyptian subjects. J. Trop. Pediatr. 16:112–115.

La Du, B.N., and V.G. Zannoni. 1961. The role of ascorbic acid in tyrosine metabolism. Ann. N.Y. Acad. Sci. 92:175–191.

Leibovitz, B., and B.V. Siegel. 1978. Ascorbic acid, neutrophil function, and the immune response. Int. J. Vitam. Nutr. Res. 48:159–164.

Levenson, S.M., G. Manner, and E. Seifter. 1971. Aspects of the adverse effects of dysnutrition on wound healing. Pp. 132–156 in S. Margen, ed. Progress in Human Nutrition, Vol. 1. AVI Publishing, Westport, Conn.

Levin, E.Y., B. Levenberg, and S. Kaufman. 1960. The enzymatic conversion of 3,4-dihydroxyphenylethylamine to norepinephrine. J. Biol. Chem. 235:2080–2086.

Marston, R., and N. Raper. 1987. Nutrient content of the U.S. food supply. Natl. Food Rev. Winter–Spring, NFR-36: 18–23.

Morse, E.H., R.P. Clark, D.E. Keyser, S.B. Merrow, and D.E. Bee. 1975. Comparison of the nutritional status of pregnant adolescents with adult pregnant women. I. Biochemical findings. Am. J. Clin. Nutr. 28:1000–1013.

Moser, U. 1987. Uptake of ascorbic acid by leukocytes. Ann. N.Y. Acad. Sci. 498:200–215.

Myllyla, R., E.R. Kuutti-Savolainen, and K.I. Kivirikko. 1978. The role of ascorbate in the prolyl hydroxylase reaction. Biochem. Biophys. Res. Commun. 83:441–448.

Newton, H.M.V., C.J. Schorah, N. Habibzadeh, D.B. Morgan, and R.P. Hullin. 1985. The cause and correction of low blood vitamin C concentrations in the elderly. Am. J. Clin. Nutr. 42:656–659.

NRC (National Research Council). 1982. Diet, Nutrition, and Cancer. Report of the Committee on Diet, Nutrition, and Cancer, Assembly of Life Sciences. National Academy Press, Washington, D.C. 496 pp.

NRC (National Research Council). 1989. Diet and Health: Implications for Reducing Chronic Disease Risk. Report of the Committee on Diet and Health, Food and Nutrition Board. National Academy Press, Washington, D.C. 750 pp.

Pauling, L. 1971. The significance of the evidence about ascorbic acid and the common cold. Proc. Natl. Acad. Sci. U.S.A. 68:2678–2681.

Pelletier, O. 1975. Vitamin C and cigarette smokers. Ann. N.Y. Acad. Sci. 258:156–168.

Peterson, V.E., P.A. Crapo, J. Weininger, H. Ginsberg, and J. Olefsky. 1975. Quantification of plasma cholesterol and triglyceride levels in hypercholesterolemic subjects receiving ascorbic acid supplements. Am. J. Clin. Nutr. 28:584–587.

Rajalakshmi, R., A.D. Doedhar, and C.V. Ramarkrishnan. 1965. Vitamin C secretion during lactation. Acta Paediatr. Scand. 54:375–382.

Rivers, J.M. 1987. Safety of high-level vitamin C ingestion. Ann. N.Y. Acad. Sci. 498:445–454.

Rivers, J.M., and M.M. Devine. 1975. Relationships of ascorbic acid to pregnancy, and oral contraceptive steroids. Ann. N.Y. Acad. Sci. 258:465–482.

Rossander, L., L. Hallberg, and E. Bjorn-Rasmussen. 1979. Absorption of iron from breakfast meals. Am. J. Clin. Nutr. 32:2484–2489.

Sabry, J.H., K.H. Fisher, and M.L. Dodds. 1958. Human utilization of dehydroascorbic acid. J. Nutr. 64:457–466.

Salmenpera, L. 1984. Vitamin C nutrition during prolonged lactation: optimal in infants while marginal in some mothers. Am. J. Clin. Nutr. 40:1050–1056.

Sauberlich, H.E. 1981. Ascorbic acid (vitamin C). Pp. 673–684 in R.F. Babbe, ed. Clinics in Laboratory Medicine, Vol. 1. Symposium on Laboratory Assessment of Nutritional Status. W.B. Saunders, Philadelphia.

Sauberlich, H.E., J.H. Skala, and R.P. Dowdy. 1974. Pp. 13–22 in Laboratory Tests for the Assessment of Nutritional Status. CRC Press, Cleveland, Ohio.

Sauberlich, H.E., M.J. Kretsch, P.C. Taylor, H.L. Johnson, and J.H. Skalam. In press. Ascorbic acid and erythorbic acid metabolism in nonpregnant women. Am. J. Clin. Nutr.

Schectman, G., J.C. Byrd, and H.W. Gruchow. 1989. The influence of smoking on vitamin C status in adults. Am. J. Public Health 79:158–162.

Smith, J.L., and R.E. Hodges. 1987. Serum levels of vitamin C in relation to dietary and supplemental intake of vitamin C in smokers and nonsmokers. Ann. N.Y. Acad. Sci. 498:144–152.

Sneed, S.M., C. Zane, and M.R. Thomas. 1981. The effects of ascorbic acid, vitamin B_6, vitamin B_{12}, and folic acid supplementation on the breast milk and maternal nutrition status of low socioeconomic lactating women. Am. J. Clin. Nutr. 34:1338–1346.

Stevenson, N.R. 1974. Active transport of L-ascorbic acid in the human ileum. Gastroenterology 67:952–956.

Stewart, M.L., J.T. McDonald, A.S. Levy, R.E. Schucker, and D.P. Henderson. 1985. Vitamin/mineral supplement use: a telephone survey of adults in the United States. Am. J. Diet. Assoc. 85:1585–1590.

Stokes, P.L., V. Melikian, R.L. Leeming, H. Portman-Graham, J.A. Blair, and W.T. Cooke. 1975. Folate metabolism in scurvy. Am. J. Clin. Nutr. 28:126–129.

Tarjan, R., M. Kramer, K. Szoke, K. Lindner, T. Szarvas, and E. Dworshak. 1965. The effect of different factors on the composition of human milk. II. The composition of human milk during lactation. Nutr. Dieta 7:136–154.

USDA (U.S. Department of Agriculture). 1984. Nationwide Food Consumption Survey. Nutrient Intakes: Individuals in 48 States, Year 1977–78. Report No. I-2. Consumer Nutrition Division, Human Nutrition Information Service. U.S. Department of Agriculture, Hyattsville, Md. 439 pp.

USDA (U.S. Department of Agriculture). 1986. Nationwide Food Consumption Survey. Continuing Survey of Food Intakes by Individuals: Men 19–50 Years, 1 Day, 1985. Report No. 85-3. Nutrition Monitoring Division, Human Nutrition Information Service. U.S. Department of Agriculture, Hyattsville, Md. 94 pp.

USDA (U.S. Department of Agriculture). 1987. Nationwide Food Consumption Survey. Continuing Survey of Food Intakes of Individuals: Women 19–50 Years and Their Children 1–5 Years, 4 Days, 1985. Report No. 85-4. Nutrition Monitoring Division, Human Nutrition Information Service. U.S. Department of Agriculture, Hyattsville, Md. 182 pp.

Van Eekelen, M. 1953. Occurrence of vitamin C in foods. Proc. Nutr. Soc. 12:228–232.

Wilbur, V.A., and B.L. Walker. 1977. Dietary ascorbic acid and the time of response of the guinea pig to ACTH administration. Nutr. Rep. Int. 16:789–794.

Woodruff, C.W. 1975. Ascorbic acid—scurvy. Prog. Food Nutr. Sci. 1:493–506.

THIAMIN

Thiamin as thiamin pyrophosphate (TPP) is a coenzyme required for the oxidative decarboxylation of α-keto acids and for the activity of transketolase in the pentose phosphate pathway. At usual levels in the diet, thiamin is rapidly absorbed, largely in the proximal small intestine. It is excreted in the urine, both intact as thiamin acetic acid and as metabolites of its cleavage products—the pyrimidine and thiazolic moieties (Hansen and Munro, 1970; McCormick, 1988; Ziporin et al., 1965).

General Signs of Deficiency

Thiamin deficiency is associated with abnormalities of carbohydrate metabolism related to a decrease in oxidative decarboxylation. During severe deficiencies, plasma and tissue levels of pyruvate are increased. Reduced TPP saturation of erythrocyte transketolase has also been observed in animals and humans fed diets low in thiamin (Sauberlich et al., 1979). Clinical signs of deficiency have been noted when less than 7% (70 μg) of a 1 mg dose of thiamin is excreted in the urine in a dose-retention test (Horwitt et al., 1948).

The clinical condition associated with the prolonged intake of a diet low in thiamin is traditionally called beriberi, whose primary symptoms involve the nervous and cardiovascular systems. The characteristic signs include mental confusion, anorexia, muscular weakness, ataxia, peripheral paralysis, ophthalmoplegia, edema (wet beriberi), muscle wasting (dry beriberi), tachycardia, and enlarged heart (Horwitt et al., 1948; Inouye and Katsura, 1965; Platt, 1967; Williams et al., 1942). In even a moderate deficiency, addition of a glucose load (100 g) can raise the plasma levels of lactic and pyruvic acids above those noted in control subjects (Williams et al., 1943), and may increase liver and heart muscle glycogen (Hawk et al., 1954). Indeed, carbohydrate loading can be an important precipitant of the thiamin-responsive neuropathy characteristic of the Wernicke-Korsakoff syndrome (Watson et al., 1981). Moreover, the development of wet beriberi in both its acute and chronic forms is favored by a high carbohydrate intake and increased physical activity (Burgess, 1958; Platt, 1958), a finding consistent with the fact that addition of even a 1-minute mild exercise period 60 minutes after a glucose load increases the differences in plasma lactic and pyruvic acids between controls and thiamin-depleted subjects (Horwitt et al., 1948). In infants, deficiency symptoms appear more suddenly than they do in adults and are usually more severe, often involving cardiac failure (McCormick, 1988).

Thiamin deficiency occurs most frequently in areas where the diet consists mainly of unenriched white rice and white flour, or when low dietary levels of thiamin are associated with consumption of large amounts of raw fish whose intestinal microbes contain thiaminase (Hilker and Somogyi, 1982). In the United States, thiamin deficiency is observed most frequently among alcoholics in whom decreased consumption and absorption and increased requirement all appear to play a role in the development of the deficiency (Leevy and Baker, 1968). Other persons at risk are renal patients undergoing long-term dialysis (Raskin and Fishman, 1976), patients fed intravenously for long periods (Nadel and Burger, 1976), patients with chronic febrile infections (Gilbert et al., 1969), and relatively few people with thiamin-responsive inborn errors of metabolism (McCormick, 1988).

Dietary Sources and Usual Intakes

Dietary sources of thiamin include unrefined cereal grains, brewer's yeast, organ meats (liver, heart, kidney), lean cuts of pork, legumes, and seeds/nuts. Enriched and fortified grains, cereals, and bakery products contribute large amounts of thiamin to the U.S. diet; among different groups of adults, thiamin intake from these sources averaged from 29 to 44% of the RDA according to USDA's 1977–1978 Nationwide Food Consumption Survey (Cook and Welsh, 1986).

The average thiamin intake of adult men in the United States in 1985 was 1.75 mg (0.68 mg/1,000 kcal) (USDA, 1986). The corresponding intakes for adult women and children 1 to 5 years of age were 1.05 mg (0.69 mg/1,000 kcal) and 1.12 mg (0.79 mg/1,000 kcal), respectively (USDA, 1987).

Recommended Allowances

Allowances for thiamin have been based on assessment of the effects of varying levels of dietary thiamin on the occurrence of clinical signs of deficiency, on the excretion of thiamin or its metabolites, and on erythrocyte transketolase activity.

Adults Clinical signs of thiamin deficiency have been observed in adult men and women with intakes of about 0.12 mg/1,000 kcal or less (Elsom et al., 1942; Foltz et al., 1944; Horwitt et al., 1948; Williams et al., 1942, 1943). Various thiamin intakes per 1,000 kcal— 0.3 mg (Sauberlich et al., 1979), 0.35 mg (Elsom et al., 1942), 0.33 to 0.45 mg (Foltz et al., 1944), 0.41 mg (Glickman et al., 1946), 0.37 to 0.45 mg (Hathaway and Strom, 1946), and 0.5 mg (Williams et al.,

1942)—were reported to be consistent with good health during the periods of observation. Anderson et al. (1986) found that thiamin status (as measured by transketolase activity) was better predicted when the dietary intake of thiamin was expressed as mg/day rather than as mg/1,000 kcal. They recommended a minimum thiamin intake of 1.22 mg/day for men and 1.03 mg/day for women.

At low levels of intake, very little thiamin is excreted; excretion increases at higher dietary levels. A critical intake point appears to be approximately 0.2 mg/1,000 kcal, below which urinary excretion is low and clinical signs of thiamin deficiency may appear (Horwitt et al., 1948; Mickelson et al., 1947; Oldham et al., 1946; Pearson, 1962; Williams et al., 1942, 1943). Studies comparing urinary excretion of thiamin at varying levels of intake and measurements of urinary excretion of thiamin in dietary deficiency cases suggest that the minimum requirement is approximately 0.33 to 0.35 mg/1,000 kcal (Bamji, 1970; Melnick, 1942; Ziporin et al., 1965). An intake of more than 0.5 mg/1,000 kcal may be required to ensure tissue saturation (Hathaway and Strom, 1946; Reuter et al., 1967; Williams et al., 1942, 1943), but there is no evidence that so-called tissue saturation is required for good health.

When dietary intake cannot be monitored or urine collected, TPP concentrations in the blood can be measured either directly (Warnock et al., 1978) or indirectly (Berit-Kjosen and Seim, 1977). When healthy subjects were studied under controlled experimental conditions, good correlations of urinary excretions with the erythrocyte transketolase activity and TPP stimulation of transketolase were recorded (Sauberlich et al., 1970, 1979; Wood et al., 1980). Normal red-cell transketolase activities with and without added TPP have been observed in subjects consuming 0.4 mg/1,000 kcal (Reuter et al., 1967) and 0.5 mg/1,000 kcal (Bamji, 1970; Haro et al., 1966), but 0.6 to 0.8 mg/1,000 kcal of thiamin (Kraut et al., 1966) or 1.1 mg/1,000 kcal (Reuter et al., 1967) were necessary to obtain maximum activity. There is no indication, however, that the lower transketolase activity at an intake below 0.4 mg/1,000 kcal was attended by any ill effect.

No evidence that thiamin requirements are increased by aging was observed in a 3-year study of 18 young and 21 old male adults (Horwitt et al., 1948). Although blood thiamin levels or transketolase assays have shown low thiamin status in some older adults, Iber et al. (1982) considered that the thiamin RDA of 0.5 mg/1,000 kcal is sufficient for those over 60 years of age.

On the basis of all these data, a thiamin allowance for adults of 0.5 mg/1,000 kcal, as recommended in the 1980 RDAs, is believed to provide an adequate margin of safety for all adults. A minimum of 1.0 mg/day is recommended, even for those consuming less than 2,000 kcal daily. Although thiamin is essential for the metabolism of carbohydrate and certain amino acids, but not for fat and the remaining protein fraction, it is difficult in practice to separate energy intake into these components; hence, the thiamin recommendation is expressed by convention in terms of total caloric intake.

Pregnancy and Lactation   Studies of urinary excretion of thiamin, blood thiamin levels, and erythrocyte transketolase activity all indicate that the requirement for thiamin in women increases during pregnancy (Heller et al., 1974; Kaminetzky et al., 1973; Lockhart et al., 1943; Oldham et al., 1950; Toverud, 1940). This increase appears to occur early in pregnancy and to remain constant throughout (Heller et al., 1974; Kaminetzky et al., 1973). On the basis of an increased energy intake of 300 kcal/day during pregnancy and an adult allowance of 0.5 mg of thiamin per 1,000 kcal, an additional 0.4 mg/day is recommended throughout pregnancy to accommodate maternal and fetal growth and increased maternal caloric intake.

Thiamin requirements also increase during lactation. The lactating woman secretes approximately 0.2 mg of thiamin/day in milk (Nail et al., 1980). To account for both the thiamin loss in milk and increased energy consumption during lactation, an increment of 0.5 mg is recommended throughout lactation.

Infants   Information on the thiamin requirements of infants is limited. In one study of the relationship between thiamin intake and excretion, Holt et al. (1949) concluded that the thiamin requirement of seven 1- to 10-month-old infants ranged from 0.14 to 0.20 mg/day. Studies of the thiamin content of human milk suggest that the minimum daily requirement to protect against deficiency is approximately 0.17 mg/day. This estimate is based on a mean concentration of 0.23 ± 0.03 mg of thiamin/liter of human milk (Nail et al., 1980) and a mean consumption of 750 ml of human milk per day by the infant. Thiamin concentrations were measured in women with unsupplemented (1.26 ± 0.17 mg of thiamin per day) and supplemented (3.33 ± 0.77 mg of thiamin per day) intakes of thiamin. Adequate thiamin status also was documented in both groups of women, i.e., urinary thiamin levels exceeded 0.1 mg/day. An allowance for thiamin was estimated from the mean thiamin concentration plus 2 SDs in human milk—0.3 mg/liter, or 0.4 mg/1,000 kcal. The American Academy of Pediatrics also estimates the allowance for thiamin for infants at 0.4 mg/1,000 kcal (AAP, 1985).

Children and Adolescents   Few studies have been conducted to determine the thiamin requirements of children and adolescents. In one study by Boyden and Erikson (1966), urinary excretion of thiamin and whole blood thiamin levels in a group of preadolescent children indicated that intakes approximating 0.3 mg/1,000 kcal were adequate. In a study of the urinary thiamin excretion of 16- to 18-year-old girls, Hart and Reynolds (1957) concluded that a daily intake of 0.3 mg/1,000 kcal was inadequate. Dick et al. (1958) reported that thiamin excretion of boys 14 to 17 years old fed diets containing 3,582 kcal/day and six different levels of thiamin indicated that their mean daily requirement for thiamin was 0.38 ± 0.059 mg/1,000 kcal. Thus, the mean plus 2 SDs would be 0.50 mg/1,000 kcal. Therefore, the thiamin allowance recommended for children and teenagers, like that for adults, is 0.5 mg/1,000 kcal, which provides for variability in requirements. This appears to provide an adequate margin of safety in the absence of clinical and biochemical evidence of deficiency.

Excessive Intakes and Toxicity

Excess thiamin is easily cleared by the kidneys. Although there is some evidence of toxicity from large doses given parenterally (McCormick, 1988), there is no evidence of thiamin toxicity by oral administration; oral doses of 500 mg taken daily for a month were found to be nontoxic (Hawk et al., 1954).

References

AAP (American Academy of Pediatrics). 1985. Composition of human milk: normative data. Appendix K. Pp. 363–368 in Pediatric Nutrition Handbook, 2nd ed. American Academy of Pediatrics, Elk Grove Village, Ill.

Anderson, S.H., C.A. Vickery, and A.D. Nicol. 1986. Adult thiamine requirements and the continuing need to fortify processed cereals. Lancet 2:85–89.

Bamji, M.S. 1970. Transketolase activity and urinary excretion of thiamin in the assessment of thiamin-nutrition status of Indians. Am. J. Clin. Nutr. 23:52–58.

Berit-Kjosen, M.S., and S.H. Seim. 1977. The transketolase assay of thiamine in some diseases. Am. J. Clin. Nutr. 30:1591–1596.

Boyden, R.E., and S.E. Erickson. 1966. Metabolic patterns in preadolescent children: thiamine utilization in relation to nitrogen intake. Am. J. Clin. Nutr. 19:398–406.

Burgess, R.C. 1958. Beriberi. I. Epidemiology. Fed. Proc. Suppl. 17:3–8.

Cook, D.A., and S.O. Welsh. 1986. The effect of enriched and fortified grain products on nutrient intake. Cereal Foods World 32:191–196.

Dick, E.C., S.D. Chen, M. Bert, and J.M. Smith. 1958. Thiamine requirement of eight adolescent boys, as estimated from urinary thiamine excretion. J. Nutr. 66:173–188.

Elsom. K.O., J.G. Reinhold, J.T.L. Nicholson, and C. Chornock. 1942. Studies of the B vitamins in the human subject. V. The normal requirement for thiamine; some factors influencing its utilization and excretion. Am. J. Med. Sci. 203:569–577.

Foltz, E.E., C.J. Barborka, and A.C. Ivy. 1944. The level of vitamin B-complex in the diet at which detectable symptoms of deficiency occur in man. Gastroenterology 2:323–344.

Gilbert, V.E., M.C. Susser, and A. Nolte. 1969. Deficient thiamin pyrophosphate and blood alpha-ketoglutarate-pyruvate relationships during febrile human infections. Metabolism 18:789–799.

Glickman, N., R.W. Keeton, H.H. Mitchell, M.K. Fahnestock. 1946. The tolerance of man to cold as affected by dietary modifications; high versus low intake of certain water-soluble vitamins. Am. J. Physiol. 146:538–558.

Hansen, R.G., and H.N. Munro, eds. 1970. Proceedings of a Workshop on Problems of Assessment and Alleviation of Malnutrition in the United States. Held at Nashville, Tennessee, January 13–14, 1970. Nutrition and Health Program, Vanderbilt University, Regional Medical Programs. Health Services and Mental Health Administration, Washington, D.C. 186 pp.

Haro, E.N., M. Brin, and W.W. Faloon. 1966. Fasting in obesity. Thiamine depletion as measured by erythrocyte transketolase changes. Arch. Intern. Med. 117:175–181.

Hart, M., and M.S. Reynolds. 1957. Thiamine requirement of adolescent girls. J. Home Econ. 49:35–37.

Hathaway, M.L., and J.E. Strom. 1946. A comparison of thiamine synthesis and excretion in human subjects on synthetic and natural diets. J. Nutr. 32:1–8.

Hawk, P.D., B.L. Oser, and W.H. Summerson, eds. 1954. Vitamins and deficiency diseases. Pp. 1104–1296 in Practical Physiological Chemistry, 13th ed. Blakiston Company, Inc., New York.

Heller, S., R.M. Salkeld, and W.F. Korner. 1974. Vitamin B_1 status in pregnancy. Am. J. Clin. Nutr. 27:1221–1224.

Hilker, D.M., and J.C. Somogyi. 1982. Antithiamins of plant origin: their chemical nature and mode of action. Ann. N.Y. Acad. Sci. 378:137–145.

Holt, L.E., Jr., R.L. Nemir, S.E. Snyderman, A.A. Albanese, K.C. Ketron, L.P. Guy, and R. Carretero. 1949. The thiamine requirement of the normal infant. J. Nutr. 37:53–66.

Horwitt, M.K., E. Liebert, O. Kreisler, and P. Wittman. 1948. Investigations of Human Requirements for B-Complex Vitamins. Bulletin of the National Research Council No. 116. Report of the Committee on Nutritional Aspects of Ageing, Food and Nutrition Board, Division of Biology and Agriculture. National Academy of Sciences, Washington, D.C. 106 pp.

Iber, F.L., J.P. Blass, M. Brin, and C.M. Leevy. 1982. Thiamin in the elderly—relation to alcoholism and to neurological degenerative disease. Am. J. Clin. Nutr. 36:1067–1082.

Inouye, K., and E. Katsura. 1965. Etiology and pathology of beriberi. Pp. 1–28 in N. Shimazono and E. Katsura, eds. Review of Japanese Literature on Beriberi and Thiamine. Vitamin B Research Committee of Japan. Igaku Shoin, Tokyo.

Kaminetzky, H.A., A. Langer, H. Baker, O. Frank, A.D. Thomson, E.D. Munves, A. Opper, F.C. Behrle, and B. Glista. 1973. The effect of nutrition in teen-age gravidas on pregnancy and status of the neonate. I. A nutritional profile. Am. J. Obstet. Gynecol. 115:639–644.

Kraut, H., L. Wildemann, and M. Bohm. 1966. Untersuchungen zum Thiaminbedarf des Menschen. Int. Z. Vitamininforsch. 36:157–193.

Leevy, C.M., and H. Baker. 1968. Vitamins and alcoholism. Am. J. Clin. Nutr. 21:1325–1328.

Lockhart, H.S., S.B. Kirkwood, and R.S. Harris. 1943. The effect of pregnancy and puerperium on the thiamine status of women. Am. J. Obstet. Gynecol. 46:358–365.

McCormick, D.B. 1988. Thiamin. Pp. 355–361 in M.E. Shils and V.R. Young, eds. Modern Nutrition in Health and Disease, 7th ed. Lea & Febiger, Philadelphia.

Melnick, D. 1942. Vitamin B_1 (thiamin) requirement of man. J. Nutr. 24:139–151.

Mickelsen, O., W.O. Caster, and A. Keys. 1947. A statistical evaluation of the thiamin and pyramin excretions of normal young men on controlled intakes of thiamine. J. Biol. Chem. 168:415–431.

Nadel, A.M., and P.C. Burger. 1976. Wernicke encephalopathy following prolonged intravenous therapy. J. Am. Med. Assoc. 235:2403–2431.

Nail, P.A., M.R. Thomas, and B.S. Eakin. 1980. The effect of thiamin and riboflavin supplementation on the level of those vitamins in human breast milk and urine. Am. J. Clin. Nutr. 33:198–204.

Oldham, H.G., M.V. Davis, and L.J. Roberts. 1946. Thiamine excretions and blood levels of young women on diets containing varying levels of the B vitamins, with some observations on niacin and pantothenic acid. J. Nutr. 32:163–180.

Oldham, H., B.B. Sheft, and T. Porter. 1950. Thiamine and riboflavin intakes and excretions during pregnancy. J. Nutr. 41:231–245.

Pearson, W.N. 1962. Biochemical appraisal of the vitamin nutritional status in man. J. Am. Med. Assoc. 180:49–55.

Platt, B.S. 1958. Beriberi. II. Clinical features of endemic beriberi. Fed. Proc. Suppl. 17:8–20.

Platt, B.S. 1967. Thiamine deficiency in human beriberi and in Wernicke's encephalopathy. Pp. 135–143 in G.E.W. Wolstenholme and M. O'Connor, eds. Thiamine Deficiency: Biochemical Lesions and Their Clinical Significance. Ciba Foundation Study Group No. 28. Churchill Livingstone, London.

Raskin, N.H., and R.A. Fishman. 1976. Neurologic disorders in renal failure (second of two parts). N. Engl. J. Med. 294:204–210.

Reuter, H.C., B. Gassmann, and M. Bohm. 1967. Thiamine requirement in humans. Int. J. Vit. Res. 37:315–328.

Sauberlich, H.E., Y.F. Herman, and C.O. Stevens. 1970. Thiamin requirement of the adult human. Am. J. Clin. Nutr. 23:671–672.

Sauberlich, H.E., Y.F. Herman, C.O. Stevens, and R.H. Herman. 1979. Thiamin requirement of the adult human. Am. J. Clin. Nutr. 32:2237–2248.

Toverud, K.U. 1940. Excretion of aneurin in pregnant and lactating women and in infants. Int. Z. Vitaminforsch. 10:255–267.

USDA (U.S. Department of Agriculture). 1986. Nationwide Food Consumption Survey Continuing Survey of Food Intakes by Individuals: Men 19–50 Years, 1 Day, 1985. Report No. 85-3. Nutrition Monitoring Division, Human Nutrition Information Service. U.S. Department of Agriculture, Hyattsville, Md. 94 pp.

USDA (U.S. Department of Agriculture). 1987. Nationwide Food Consumption Survey Continuing Survey of Food Intakes by Individuals: Women 19–50 Years and Their Children 1–5 Years, 4 Days, 1985. Report No. 85-4. Nutrition Monitoring Division, Human Nutrition Information Service, U.S. Department of Agriculture, Hyattsville, Md. 182 pp.

Warnock, L.G., C.R. Prudhomme, and C. Wagner. 1978. The determination of thiamin pyrophosphate in blood and other tissues, and its correlation with erythrocyte transketolase activity. J. Nutr. 108:421–427.

Watson, A.J.S., J.F. Walker, G.H. Tomkin, M.M.R. Finn, and J.A.B. Keogh. 1981. Acute Wernicke's encephalopathy precipitated by glucose loading. Isr. J. Med. Sci. 150:301–303.

Williams, R.D., H.L. Mason, B.F. Smith, and R.M. Wilder. 1942. Induced thiamin (vitamin B_1) deficiency and the thiamine requirement of man: further observations. Arch. Inter. Med. 69:721–738.

Williams, R.D., H.L. Mason, and R.M. Wilder. 1943. The minimum daily requirement of thiamine of man. J. Nutr. 25:71–97.

Wood, B., A. Gijsbers, A. Goode, S. Davis, J. Mulholland, and K. Breen. 1980. A study of partial thiamin restriction in human volunteers. Am. J. Clin. Nutr. 33:848–861.

Ziporin, Z.Z., W.T. Nunes, R.C. Powell, P.P. Waring, and H.E. Sauberlich. 1965. Thiamine requirement in the adult human as measured by urinary excretion of thiamine metabolites. J. Nutr. 85:297–304.

RIBOFLAVIN

Riboflavin is a water-soluble vitamin that functions primarily as a component of two flavin coenzymes—flavin mononucleotide (FMN) and flavin adenine dinucleotide (FAD)—that catalyze many oxidation-reduction reactions. Among the enzymes that require riboflavin is the FMN-dependent oxidase responsible for conversion of phosphorylated pyridoxine to functional coenzyme and the FAD-dependent hydroxylase involved in the conversion of tryptophan to niacin (McCormick, 1988).

Riboflavin is readily absorbed, largely in the proximal small intestine, and is excreted with its metabolites in the urine. In adults who ingest levels of riboflavin that are about at the RDA, only one-half to two-thirds of urinary flavin is riboflavin; the rest is found in several different oxidation products (Chastain and McCormick, 1987).

Under controlled conditions, riboflavin excreted over a 24-hour period offers the most reliable index of riboflavin nutrition. In men, urinary excretion of less than 10% of riboflavin intake may reflect potential riboflavin deficiency (Horwitt et al., 1950). When urine collections are difficult to obtain, the estimates of the riboflavin present in erythrocytes can provide some indication of riboflavin nutrition (Bates et al., 1981; Bessey et al., 1956).

Erythrocyte glutathione reductase (EGR), an enzyme that requires FAD as a coenzyme, has also been used to assess riboflavin deficiency (Tillotson and Baker, 1972). In erythrocytes from persons consuming a riboflavin-deficient diet, EGR activity increases when FAD is added *in vitro*, indicating that the apoenzyme is not saturated with the coenzyme. The ratio of EGR activity in erythrocytes with and without added FAD is considered the activity coefficient. Sauberlich et al.

(1972) suggested that an EGR activity coefficient above 1.2 may be an indication of riboflavin deficiency.

General Signs of Deficiency

Deficiency symptoms have been reported to include oral-buccal cavity lesions (e.g., cheilosis, angular stomatitis), a generalized seborrheic dermatitis, scrotal and vulval skin changes, and a normocytic anemia. Because riboflavin is essential to the functioning of vitamins B_6 and niacin, some symptoms attributed to riboflavin deficiency are actually due to the failure of systems requiring these other nutrients to operate effectively (McCormick, 1988).

Dietary Sources and Usual Intakes

Animal protein sources such as meats, poultry, fish, and, especially, dairy products are good sources of riboflavin. Grain products naturally contain relatively low levels of riboflavin; however, enriched and fortified grains, cereals, and bakery products supply large amounts. Among adults in the United States, riboflavin intake from these plant sources averaged from 20 to 26% of the RDA in 1977–1978 (Cook and Welsh, 1987). Green vegetables such as broccoli, turnip greens, asparagus, and spinach are good sources.

The USDA found that adult men in the United States consumed an average of 2.08 mg of riboflavin per day in 1985 (USDA, 1986); the intake for adult women was 1.34 mg, and for their children 1 to 5 years of age, 1.57 mg (USDA, 1987).

Recommended Allowances

Adults Data on which the RDA for riboflavin is based come primarily from several long-term feeding studies in a few humans conducted more than 40 years ago. These studies clearly show that a riboflavin intake of 0.55 mg or less per day results in clinically recognizable signs of riboflavin deficiency (Horwitt et al., 1950; Sebrell et al., 1941). Symptoms appeared after the subjects had been fed the low riboflavin diets for 89 days or longer. In other studies, no signs of deficiency were observed in men receiving 0.31 mg/1,000 kcal (Keys et al., 1944) and women receiving 0.35 mg/1,000 kcal (Williams et al., 1943) for periods ranging from 84 days to 288 days. Similarly, only 1 of 22 male subjects receiving from 0.75 to 0.85 mg of riboflavin per day for more than 2 years showed signs of riboflavin deficiency (Horwitt et al., 1950).

Subjects fed 0.75 to 0.85 mg of riboflavin per day excreted only marginally more urinary riboflavin than subjects receiving approximately 0.55 mg per day. But riboflavin excretion increased markedly when daily intake was increased from 1.1 to 1.6 mg/day in diets providing 2,200 kcal/day (Horwitt et al., 1950). In women, the proportion of ingested riboflavin excreted was shown to increase markedly at intakes above 1 mg/day in diets providing 1,850 kcal per day (Oldham et al., 1950). Bessy et al. (1956) found that erythrocyte riboflavin levels were maintained when 1.6 mg/day was consumed by men but were low when 0.55 mg/day was consumed.

The data (summarized above) from controlled, long-term studies in humans fed deficient or low riboflavin intakes suggest that at riboflavin intakes of approximately 1 mg/day (0.5 mg/1,000 kcal), urinary riboflavin is only slightly greater than that observed when riboflavin deficiency signs are observed. When riboflavin intakes exceed this level, a higher proportion of consumed riboflavin is excreted via the urine.

These data have led previous RDA committees to consider that consumption of 0.6 mg of riboflavin per 1,000 kcal should supply the needs for essentially all healthy people and therefore to recommend a minimum intake of 1.2 mg/day per adult. The present subcommittee concluded that there are no new data that justify changes in the earlier basic recommendation for riboflavin. In the RDA table, variations in riboflavin intake at various ages are due primarily to changes in recommended caloric intakes at the ages listed.

Several factors are known to change indices of riboflavin status. More riboflavin is retained when nitrogen balance is positive, and more is excreted when nitrogen balance is negative (Pollack and Bookman, 1951; Windmueller et al., 1964). Increased energy expenditure has been related to increased riboflavin requirement. Periods of hard work have been shown to decrease urinary excretion of riboflavin in young men (Tucker et al., 1960), and moderate exercise has been shown to increase the EGR activity ratio and to decrease riboflavin excretion in young women consuming levels of riboflavin at about the RDA (Belko et al., 1983). In the studies of Belko et al. (1983), however, subjects consuming diets containing 1.0 to 1.2 mg of riboflavin per day had urinary riboflavin levels higher than those associated with riboflavin inadequacy, even after exercise. For this reason, the subcommittee has not recommended an increased RDA for riboflavin for people who undertake heavy exercise.

Pregnancy and Lactation　As pregnancy progresses, women tend to excrete less riboflavin than do nonpregnant women eating similar diets (Brzezinski et al., 1952; Jansen and Jansen, 1954). The EGR activity ratio also tends to increase during pregnancy (Bates et al., 1981; Heller et al., 1974). In view of the increased tissue synthesis for both fetal and maternal development, an additional riboflavin intake of 0.3 mg/day is recommended during pregnancy.

During lactation, the requirement is assumed to increase by an amount at least equal to that excreted in milk (Brzezinski et al., 1952), which has a mean riboflavin content of approximately 35 μg/100 ml (Roderuck et al., 1946; Toverud et al., 1950). At an average milk production of 750 ml/day and 600 ml/day during the first and second 6 months of lactation, riboflavin secretion is 0.26 mg/day and 0.21 mg/day, respectively. Since the utilization of the riboflavin for milk production is assumed to be 70% (WHO, 1965), and the coefficient of variation of milk production is 12.5%, an additional daily intake of 0.5 mg is recommended for the first 6 months of lactation and 0.4 mg thereafter.

Infants and Children   Although clinical signs of ariboflavinosis are rare, the riboflavin allowance for children is an important consideration, since inadequacy may lead to growth inhibition. Snyderman et al. (1949) noted that an intake of 0.4 mg of riboflavin daily was sufficient for the maintenance of adequate blood and urine levels in infants weighing 5.9 to 9 kg. This corresponds to an intake of 0.53 mg/1,000 kcal for reference infants of these weights whose energy intakes are average. The amount of riboflavin consumed by the average breastfed infant ingesting 750 ml/day is 0.26 mg, or 0.48 mg/1,000 kcal. The allowance for the reference infant from birth to 6 months of age is set at 0.6 mg/1,000 kcal. This level allows for a margin of safety and is recommended for children of all ages and for adults.

Excessive Intakes and Toxicity

No cases of toxicity from ingestion of riboflavin have been reported, since the capacity of the normal human gastrointestinal tract to absorb this modestly soluble vitamin is rather limited (McCormick, 1988).

References

Bates, C.J., A.M. Prentice, A.A. Paul, B.A. Sutcliffe, M. Watkinson, and R.G. Whitehead. 1981. Riboflavin status in Gambian pregnant and lactating women and its implications for Recommended Dietary Allowances. Am. J. Clin. Nutr. 34:928–935.

Belko, A.Z., E. Obarzanek, H.J. Kalkwarf, M.A. Rotter, S. Bogusz, D. Miller, J.D. Haas, and D.A. Roe. 1983. Effects of exercise on riboflavin requirements of young women. Am. J. Clin. Nutr. 37:509–517.

Bessey, O.A., M.K. Horwitt, and R.H. Love. 1956. Dietary deprivation of riboflavin and blood riboflavin levels in man. J. Nutr. 58:367–383.

Brzezinski, A., Y.M. Bromberg, and K. Braun. 1952. Riboflavin excretion during pregnancy and early lactation. J. Lab. Clin. Med. 39:84–90.

Chastain, J.L., and D.B. McCormick. 1987. Flavin catabolites: identification and quantitation in human urine. Am. J. Clin. Nutr. 46:832–834.

Cook, D.A., and S.O. Welsh. 1987. The effect of enriched and fortified grain products on nutrient intake. Cereal Foods World 32:191–196.

Heller, S., R.M. Salked, and W.F. Korner. 1974. Riboflavin status in pregnancy. Am. J. Clin. Nutr. 27:1225–1230.

Horwitt, M.K., C.C. Harvey, O.W. Hills, and E. Liebert. 1950. Correlation of urinary excretion of riboflavin with dietary intake and symptoms of ariboflavinosis. J. Nutr. 41:247–264.

Jansen, A.P., and B.C. Jansen. 1954. Riboflavin-excretion with urine in pregnancy. Int. Z. Vitaminforsch. 25:193–199.

Keys, A., A.F. Henschel, O. Mickelson, J.M. Brozek, and J.H. Crawford. 1944. Physiological and biochemical functions in normal young men on a diet restricted in riboflavin. J. Nutr. 27:165–178.

McCormick, D.B. 1988. Riboflavin. Pp. 362–369 in M.E. Shils and V.R. Young, eds. Modern Nutrition in Health and Disease. Lea & Febiger, Philadelphia.

Oldham, H., B.B. Shett, and T. Porter. 1950. Thiamin and riboflavin intakes and excretions during pregnancy. J. Nutr. 41:231–245.

Pollack, H., and J.J. Bookman. 1951. Riboflavin excretion as a function of protein metabolism in the normal, catabolic, and diabetic human being. J. Lab. Clin. Med. 38:561–573.

Roderuck, C., N.M. Colryell, H.H. Williams, and I.G. Macy. 1946. Metabolism of women during reproductive cycle; utilization of riboflavin during lactation. J. Nutr. 32:267–283.

Sauberlich, H.E., J.H. Judd, Jr., G.E. Nichoalds, H.P. Broquist, and W.J. Darby. 1972. Application of the erythrocyte glutathione reductase assay in evaluating riboflavin nutritional status in a high school population. Am. J. Clin. Nutr. 25:756–762.

Sebrell, W.H., Jr., R.E. Butler, J.G. Wooley, and H. Isbell. 1941. Human riboflavin requirement estimated by urinary excretion of subjects on controlled intake. Publ. Health Rep. 56:510–519.

Snyderman, S.E., K.G. Ketron, H.B. Burch, O.H. Lowry, O.A. Bessey, L.P. Guy, and L.E. Holt, Jr. 1949. The minimum riboflavin requirement of the infant. J. Nutr. 39:219–232.

Tillotson, J.A., and E.M. Baker. 1972. An enzymatic measurement of the riboflavin status in man. Am. J. Clin. Nutr. 25:425–431.

Toverud, K.U., G. Stearns, and I.G. Macy. 1950. Maternal Nutrition and Child Health: An Interpretative Review. Bulletin of the National Research Council No. 123. Prepared for the Committee on Maternal and Child Feeding of the Food and Nutrition Board. National Academy of Sciences, Washington, D.C. 174 pp.

Tucker, R.G., O. Mickelson, and A. Keys. 1960. The influence of sleep, work diuresis, heat acute starvation, thiamine intake and bed rest on human riboflavin excretion. J. Nutr. 72:251–261.

USDA (U.S. Department of Agriculture). 1986. Nationwide Food Consumption Survey Continuing Survey of Food Intakes by Individuals: Men 19–50 Years, 1 Day,

1985. Report No. 85-3. Nutrition Monitoring Division, Human Nutrition Information Service, U.S. Department of Agriculture, Hyattsville, Md. 94 pp.

USDA (U.S. Department of Agriculture). 1987. Nationwide Food Consumption Survey Continuing Survey of Food Intakes by Individuals: Women 19–50 Years and Their Children 1–5 Years, 4 Days, 1985. Report No. 85-4. Nutrition Monitoring Division, Human Nutrition Information Service, U.S. Department of Agriculture, Hyattsville, Md. 182 pp.

WHO (World Health Organization). 1965. Nutrition in Pregnancy and Lactation. Report of a WHO Expert Committee. Technical Report Series No. 302. World Health Organization, Geneva.

Williams, R.D., H.L. Mason, P.L. Cusick, and R.M. Wilder. 1943. Observations on induced riboflavin deficiency and the riboflavin requirement of man. J. Nutr. 25:361–377.

Windmueller, H.G., A.A. Anderson, and O. Mickelsen. 1964. Elevated riboflavin levels in urine of fasting human subjects. Am. J. Clin. Nutr. 15:73–76.

NIACIN

Niacin is a water-soluble vitamin whose requirement by humans and many animal species is normally met in part by the conversion of dietary tryptophan to niacin. The term niacin is used here in the generic sense for both nicotinic acid and nicotinamide (niacinamide). Nicotinamide functions in the body as a component of two coenzymes, nicotinamide adenine dinucleotide (NAD) and nicotinamide adenine dinucleotide phosphate (NADP). These coenzymes are present in all cells and participate in many metabolic processes, including glycolysis, fatty acid metabolism, and tissue respiration. Metabolism of nicotinamide nucleotides is regulated at both the cellular (Gholson, 1966) and the systemic levels (Dietrich et al., 1968) by a series of enzyme activations and inhibitions involving the synthesis and degradation of the niacin coenzymes. Determination of the urine levels of two of the many metabolites, N^1-methylnicotinamide and its 2-pyridone, have proved useful in estimating the nutritional adequacy of the niacin-tryptophan supply in the diet (Lee et al., 1969).

Pellagra is a multiple deficiency disease characterized by dermatitis, diarrhea, inflammation of the mucous membranes, and, in severe cases, dementia (Harris, 1941). It was a widespread problem in the southern United States in the early part of this century and still is in parts of Africa and Asia. This deficiency syndrome has been found to be associated with diets providing only low levels of niacin equivalents and other B vitamins, and flares up when the skin is subjected to strong sunlight. Some cases respond to niacin alone, others only to yeast or mixtures of niacin and other B vitamins (Sebrell and Butler, 1939).

Niacin, which is found in high concentrations in meats, is stable in foods and can withstand reasonable periods of heating, cooking, and storage with little loss. In some foods, however, the bioavailability of the niacin may be low (see below). Even when tryptophan intake is limited, a portion of it appears to be diverted into the niacin pathway (Brown et al., 1958; Goldsmith et al., 1961; Horwitt et al., 1956; Nakagawa et al., 1973; Vivian et al., 1958).

Tryptophan to Niacin Interconversion

For calculating the adequacy of a diet as a source of niacin, a factor is needed for estimating the contribution of tryptophan to meeting the need for niacin. In four studies in which niacin status was judged by urinary excretion of niacin metabolites, the quantities of supplementary tryptophan required to give the same response as 1 mg of niacin ranged from 39 to 86 mg (Goldsmith et al., 1961; Horwitt et al., 1956; Patterson et al., 1980; Vivian, 1964). The convention is to consider 60 mg of tryptophan as equivalent to 1 mg of niacin, and to regard each to be 1 niacin equivalent (NE) for calculating both dietary contributions and recommended allowances (Horwitt et al., 1981). The extent of conversion is, to some extent, under hormonal control and appears to increase during pregnancy or when contraceptive pills are used.

Dietary Sources and Usual Intakes

Some foods such as milk and eggs contain very little niacin but have sufficient tryptophan to more than offset the lack of niacin. Meat contains high levels of both preformed niacin and tryptophan. Tryptophan intake can be approximated by assuming that proteins contain at least 1.0% tryptophan, i.e., that 60 g of protein provide 600 mg of tryptophan or 10 NEs (Horwitt et al., 1981). If more precision is desired, the following closer approximations of tryptophan content may be used: corn products, 0.6%; other grains, fruits, and vegetables, 1.0%; meats, 1.1%; milk, 1.4%; and eggs, 1.5% of the protein in each food. In the average U.S. diet, 65% of the protein comes from meat, milk, and eggs.

Some foodstuffs contain niacin in chemical combinations that result in its bioavailability being low (Carter and Carpenter, 1982; Darby et al., 1975; Gopalan and Jaya Rao, 1975; Mason et al., 1973). In mature cereal grains, as much as 70% of the niacin may be biologically unavailable because of the structure of the compounds in which it is bound. In considering cereal-based diets, therefore, it may be necessary to make an allowance for poor bioavailability unless the cereal has been treated with lime, a process that increases niacin availability

(Goldsmith et al., 1956). In typical U.S. diets, some 25 to 40% of the preformed niacin comes from grain products (USDA, 1984). If all this is provided by niacin naturally present in the grains, and one allowed for only 30% of this being available, the estimates for total intakes of NEs referred to above would have to be reduced by an average of 5 mg. In practice, much of the niacin comes from fully available, synthetic niacin added to fortify milled grain products. Values in most tables of food composition do not take into account the bioavailability of niacin, nor do they include an estimate of NEs. The latter values must then be calculated from information on the tryptophan content of foods.

Average diets in the United States for women ages 19 to 50 supply 700 mg of tryptophan daily, and for men 19 to 50, 1,100 mg. The corresponding values for preformed niacin are 16 and 24 mg, respectively. Thus, the calculated intakes of total NEs are 27 mg for women and 41 mg for men (USDA, 1984). The most recent estimates for the intakes of low-income women have given essentially the same values as those given above for all women in the earlier survey (USDA, 1987).

Recommended Allowances

Adults   There have been only a few studies in which subjects have been fed diets deficient in NEs but otherwise complete. Essentially all the information used in estimating niacin requirements for humans comes from studies conducted more than 30 years ago on adult men and women (Goldsmith et al., 1952, 1955, 1956; Horwitt et al., 1956). In one of these, niacin deficiency was observed in people receiving 4.9 NE/1,000 kcal and as much as 8.8 NE/day (Goldsmith, 1956). When these subjects were fed diets containing approximately 200 mg of tryptophan and varying levels of niacin, there was a significant increase in urinary niacin metabolites whenever they were given 8 to 10 mg of niacin (Goldsmith et al., 1955). These results suggest that a daily intake of 11.3 to 13.3 NEs (200 mg of tryptophan + 8 to 10 mg of niacin) is adequate to prevent depletion of body stores of niacin. In another study (Horwitt et al., 1956), no signs of pellagra were observed in 15 subjects receiving 4.4 NE/1,000 kcal or 9.2 to 12.3 NEs daily for 38 to 87 weeks.

Niacin recommendations over the past 20 years have been 6.6 NEs per 1,000 kcal and not less than 13 NEs at caloric intakes of less than 2,000 kcal for adults of all ages. The adequacy of this allowance has recently been confirmed in young men (Jacob et al., 1989). Allowances for adults are therefore unchanged.

Pregnancy and Lactation   The increased conversion of tryptophan to niacin derivatives during pregnancy (Brown et al., 1961; Darby et al., 1953; Wertz et al., 1958) appears to be under hormonal control—a consequence of the increase in estrogen formation during pregnancy (Wolf, 1971). The increase in the urinary excretion of N^1-methylnicotinamide, also observed in pregnant women (Horwitt et al., 1981), reflects an enchanced capacity for the biosynthesis of nicotinate ribonucleotide from tryptophan. Despite the possible involvement of a biological mechanism that increases the ability of pregnant women to convert tryptophan to niacin derivatives, an increased niacin intake during pregnancy is recommended because of increased energy requirements. The allowance provides for an increase of 2 NEs daily.

The average lactating woman will secrete approximately 1.0 to 1.3 mg of preformed niacin daily (AAP, 1985; USDA, 1976; Wertz et al., 1958) in 750 ml of milk. Taking this into account and the recommended increase in energy expenditure to support lactation, the subcommittee recommends an additional 5 NEs per day throughout lactation.

Infants and Children   There are no data on the niacin requirements of children from infancy through adolescence. It is known, however, that human milk contains approximately 1.5 mg of niacin and 210 mg of tryptophan per liter (AAP, 1985). This supplies 3.7 NEs per 750 ml of milk, or about 7 NEs per 1,000 kcal. Milk from a well-nourished mother appears to be adequate to meet the niacin needs of the infant. The niacin allowance recommended for formula-fed infants up to 6 months of age is 8 NEs per 1,000 kcal.

The niacin allowances for children more than 6 months of age are based on the same standard as for adults, i.e., 6.6 NE/1,000 kcal and are increased in proportion to energy intake. Needs of teenagers are considered to be similar to those of adults. There is no evidence from epidemiological records of pellagra outbreaks that the young are more at risk than adults.

Excessive Intakes and Toxicity

Ingestion of nicotinic acid, but not of the amide, may produce vascular dilatation, or flushing. The ingestion of a pharmacological dose ranging from 3 to 9 g of nicotinic acid daily results in various metabolic effects, including increased utilization of muscle glycogen stores, decreased serum lipids, and decreased mobilization of fatty acids from adipose tissue during exercise (Darby et al., 1975).

References

AAP (Amercian Academy of Pediatrics). 1985. Composition of human milk: normative data. Appendix K. Pp. 363–368 in Pediatric Nutrition Handbook, 2nd ed. American Academy of Pediatrics, Elk Grove Village, Ill.

Brown, R.R., V.M. Vivian, M.S. Reynolds, and J.M. Price. 1958. Some aspects of tryptophan metabolism in human subjects. II. Urinary tryptophan metabolites on low-niacin diet. J. Nutr. 66:599–606.

Brown, R.R., M.J. Thornton, and J.M. Price. 1961. The effect of vitamin supplementation on urinary excretion of tryptophan metabolites by pregnant women. J. Clin. Invest. 40:617–623.

Carter, E.G.A., and K.J. Carpenter. 1982. The bioavailability for humans of bound niacin from wheat bran. Am. J. Clin. Nutr. 36:855–861.

Darby, W.J., W.J. McGanity, M.P. Martin, E. Bridgforth, P.M. Densen, M.M. Kaser, P.J. Ogle, J.A. Newbill, A. Stockell, M.E. Ferguson, O. Touster, G.S. McClellan, C. Williams, and R.O. Cannon. 1953. The Vanderbilt Cooperative Study of maternal and infant nutrition. IV. Dietary, laboratory and physical findings in 2,129 delivered pregnancies. J. Nutr. 51:565–597.

Darby, W.J., K.W. McNutt, and E.N. Todhunter. 1975. Niacin. Nutr. Rev. 33:289–297.

Dietrich, L.S., L. Martinez, and L. Franklin. 1968. Role of the liver in systemic pyridine nucleotide metabolism. Naturwissenschaften 55:231–232.

Gholson, R.D. 1966. The pyridine nucleotide cycle. Nature 212:933–935.

Goldsmith, G.A. 1956. Experimental niacin deficiency. J. Am. Diet. Assoc. 32:312–316.

Goldsmith, G.A., H.P. Sarett, U.D. Register, and J. Gibbens. 1952. Studies on niacin requirement in man. I. Experimental pellagra in subjects on corn diets low in niacin and tryptophan. J. Clin. Invest. 31:533–542.

Goldsmith, G.A., H.L. Rosenthal, J. Gibbens, and W.G. Unglaub. 1955. Studies of niacin requirement in man. II. Requirement on wheat and corn diets low in tryptophan. J. Nutr. 56:371–386.

Goldsmith, G.A., J. Gibbens, W.G. Unglaub, and O. N. Miller. 1956. Studies on niacin requirement in man. III. Comparative effects of diets containing lime-treated and untreated corn in the production of experimental pellagra. Am. J. Clin. Nutr. 4:151–160.

Goldsmith, G.A., O.N. Miller, and W.G. Unglaub. 1961. Efficiency of tryptophan as a niacin precursor in man. J. Nutr. 73:172–176.

Gopalan, C., and K.S. Jaya Rao. 1975. Pellagra and amino acid imbalance. Vitam. Horm. 33:505–542.

Harris, S. 1941. Clinical Pellagra. Mosby, St. Louis, Mo.

Horwitt, M.K., C.C. Harvey, W.S. Rothwell, J.L. Cutler, and D. Haffron. 1956. Tryptophan-niacin relationships in man: studies with diets deficient in riboflavin and niacin, together with observations on the excretion of nitrogen and niacin metabolites. J. Nutr. 60 Suppl. 1:1–43.

Horwitt, M.K., A.E. Harper, and L.M. Henderson. 1981. Niacin-tryptophan relationships for evaluating niacin equivalents. Am. J. Clin. Nutr. 34:423–427.

Jacob, R.A., M.E. Swendseid, R.W. McKee, C.S. Fu, and R.A. Clemens. 1989. Biochemical markers for assessment of niacin status in young men: urinary and blood levels of niacin metabolites. J. Nutr. 119:591–598.

Lee, Y.C., R.K. Gholson, and N. Raica. 1969. Isolation and identification of two new nicotinamide metabolites. J. Biol. Chem. 244:3277–3282.

Mason, J.B., N. Gibson, and E. Kodicek. 1973. The chemical nature of the bound nicotinic acid of wheat bran; studies of nicotinic acid-containing macromolecules. Br. J. Nutr. 30:297–311.

Nakagawa, I., T. Takahashi, A. Sasaki, M. Kajimoto, and T. Suzuki. 1973. Efficiency of conversion of tryptophan to niacin in humans. J. Nutr. 103:1195–1199.

Patterson, J.I., R.R. Brown, H. Linkswiler, and A.E. Harper. 1980. Excretion of tryptophan-niacin metabolites by young men: effects of tryptophan, leucine, and vitamin B_6 intakes. Am. J. Clin. Nutr. 33:2157–2167.

Sebrell, W.H., and R.E. Butler. 1939. Riboflavin deficiency in man (ariboflavinosis). Public Health Rep. 54:2121–2131.

USDA (U.S. Department of Agriculture). 1976. Composition of Foods: Dairy and Egg Products, Raw, Processed, Prepared. Agriculture Handbook No. 8–1. U.S. Government Printing Office, Washington, D.C. 144 pp.

USDA (U.S. Department of Agriculture). 1984. Nationwide Food Consumption Survey. Nutrient Intakes: Individuals in 48 States, Year 1977–78. Report No. I-2. Consumer Nutrition Division, Human Nutrition Information Service. U.S. Department of Agriculture, Hyattsville, Md. 439 pp.

USDA (U.S. Department of Agriculture). 1987. Nationwide Food Consumption Survey. Continuing Survey of Food Intakes of Individuals: Low-Income Women 19–50 Years and Their Children 1–5 Years, 1 Day, 1986. Report No. 86-2. Nutrition Monitoring Division, Human Nutrition Information Service. U.S. Department of Agriculture, Hyattsville, Md. 166 pp.

Vivian, V.M. 1964. Relationship between tryptophan-niacin metabolism and changes in nitrogen balance. J. Nutr. 82:395–400.

Vivian, V.M., M.M. Chaloupka, and M.S. Reynolds. 1958. Some aspects of tryptophan metabolism in human subjects. I. Nitrogen balances, blood pyridine nucleotides and urinary excretion of N^1-methylnicotinamide and N^1-methyl-2-pryridone-5-carboxamide on a low-niacin diet. J. Nutr. 66:587–598.

Wertz, A.W., M.E. Lojkin, B.S. Bouchard, and M.B. Derby. 1958. Tryptophan-niacin relationships in pregnancy. J. Nutr. 64:339–353.

Wolf, H. 1971. Hormonal alterations of efficiency of conversion of tryptophan to urinary metabolites of niacin in man. Am. J. Clin. Nutr. 24:792–799.

VITAMIN B_6

Vitamin B_6 comprises three chemically, metabolically, and functionally related forms—pyridoxine (pyridoxol, PN), pyridoxal (PL), and pyridoxamine (PM). These forms are converted in the liver, erythrocytes, and other tissues to pyridoxal phosphate (PLP) and pyridoxamine phosphate (PMP), which serve primarily as coenzymes in transamination reactions. PLP also participates in decarboxylation and racemization of A-amino acids, in other metabolic transformations of amino acids, and in the metabolism of lipids and nucleic acids. In addition, it is the essential coenzyme for glycogen phosphorylase. The phosphoric acid esters of the active forms of vitamin B_6 are hydrolyzed before release from cells. Also, PL can be further oxidized to pyridoxic acid and other inactive oxidation products, which are excreted in the urine.

The various dietary forms of vitamin B_6 are absorbed by intestinal mucosal cells through a nonsaturable process. Cellular B_6 is metabolically phosphorylated, and two of the phospho-forms (PNP and PMP) are oxidized to PLP. PLP is largely present in the plasma as a PLP-albumin complex and in erythrocytes in association with hemoglobin.

The requirement for vitamin B_6 increases as the intake of protein increases (Baker et al., 1964; Canham et al., 1969; Donald et al., 1971; Linkswiler, 1978; Miller and Linkswiler, 1967; Schultz and Leklem, 1981). This relationship is believed to reflect the major role of PLP in amino acid metabolism.

Vitamin B_6 nutritional status can be assessed both clinically and biochemically by a variety of methods. Assessment methods include (1) direct measurements of the vitamer forms of B_6 in the blood or urine (e.g., the level of coenzyme PLP in the plasma or the urinary excretion of 4-pyridoxic acid [4-PA], a metabolically inactive end product); (2) load tests (e.g., measurement of urinary tryptophan metabolites such as xanthurenic and kynurenic acids following an oral load of 2–5 g L-tryptophan); and (3) indirect functional tests that measure the activity of several vitamin B_6-dependent enzymes (e.g., erythrocyte alanine aminotransferase in plasma or erythrocytes). Vitamin B_6 nutriture is best assessed by a combination of these assessment methods (e.g., plasma PLP levels, urinary excretion of 4-PA, and the response of urinary metabolites to a 2-g tryptophan load test) (Leklem and Reynolds, 1981).

General Signs of Deficiency

Vitamin B_6 deficiency rarely occurs alone and is most commonly seen in people who are deficient in several B-complex vitamins. Clinical signs of deficiency include epileptiform convulsions, dermatitis, and anemia (McCormick, 1988). Deficiency in infants leads to a variety of neurological symptoms as well as abdominal distress (Bessey et al., 1957; Coursin, 1954; Kirksey and Roepke, 1981). As protein intake increases, the onset of deficiency becomes more rapid.

Dietary Sources and Usual Intakes

The richest sources of vitamin B_6 are chicken, fish, kidney, liver, pork, and eggs, each of which provides more than 0.4 mg per 100-g serving. Other good sources are unmilled rice, soy beans, oats, whole-wheat products, peanuts, and walnuts. Dairy products and red meats are relatively poor sources. Losses of vitamin B_6 through food processing can be considerable. From 15 to 70% is lost in freezing fruits and vegetables, 50 to 70% in processing luncheon meats, and 50 to 90% in milling cereal, but little is lost in processing dairy products (Schroeder, 1971; Tarr et al., 1981).

Data on the vitamin B_6 content of foods and its bioavailability are incomplete. Studies in animals and humans have shown, however, that bioavailability varies widely (Gregory and Kirk, 1978; Haskell, 1978; Kabir et al., 1983; Leklem et al., 1980; Nelson et al., 1977).

Approximately 40 drugs (e.g., isonicotinic acid hydrazide and penicillamine) are known to affect the metabolism or bioavailability of vitamin B_6 (Bauernfeind and Miller, 1978; Bhagavan, 1985). Oral contraceptives alter tryptophan metabolism, and their use is associated with low plasma PLP values, but it is not clear that these low PLP values are associated with increased risk of vitamin B_6 deficiency (Leklem et al., 1975; NRC, 1980).

In 1985, the average vitamin B_6 intake of adult men in the United States was 1.87 mg (0.019 mg/g protein) (USDA, 1986). The corresponding intake for adult women was 1.16 mg (0.019 mg/g protein), and, for children 1 to 5 years old, 1.22 mg (0.023 mg/g protein) (USDA, 1987).

Recommended Allowances

Adults Many studies on adult men have shown that 0.010 to 0.015 mg of vitamin B_6 per gram of protein either prevented or eliminated the appearance of biochemical indicators of deficiency when protein intakes ranged from 54 to 165 g/day (Linkswiler, 1978; Miller and Linkswiler, 1967; Park and Linkswiler, 1970). Among women, Brown et al. (1975) reported that subjects needed from 0.8 to 2.0 mg of vitamin B_6 per day when protein intake was 78 g (0.010 to 0.016 mg/g). Schultz and Leklem (1981), who measured urinary excretion of 4-PA and vitamin B_6 as well as plasma PLP levels in 41 adult females, reported acceptable levels of each indicator at dietary intakes of 1.25 and 1.5 mg (0.0125 and 0.015 mg/g of protein).

A dietary vitamin B_6 ratio of 0.016 mg/g protein appears to ensure acceptable values for most indices of nutritional status in adults of both sexes. The RDA is established in relation to the upper boundary of acceptable levels of protein intake, i.e., twice the RDA for protein (NRC, 1989), which is 126 g/day for men and 100 g/day for women. The RDA for vitamin B_6 is, accordingly, 2.0 mg/day for men and 1.6 mg/day for women. These allowances are adequate for the reported average protein intakes of approximately 100 g/day for men (USDA, 1986) and 60 g/day for women (USDA, 1987), but may not be sufficient for those whose habitual protein intake is at or above the reported 90th percentile of consumers. Because vitamin B_6 and protein tend to occur together naturally in foods, vitamin B_6 levels are likely to be adequate if protein is consumed at high levels in normal foodstuffs.

The RDA for vitamin B_6 in this edition is somewhat lower than in the ninth edition, being based on a figure of 0.016 mg/g protein rather than 0.020 mg/g. The subcommittee concluded the latter figure is higher than can be justified by the requirements studies cited above.

Pregnancy and Lactation The extra protein allowance for pregnancy should be accompanied by additional vitamin B_6. Several investigators have observed that pregnant women have lower levels of both vitamin B_6 and PLP in plasma (Cleary et al., 1975; Contractor and Shane, 1970; Hamfelt and Tuvemo, 1972; Roepke and Kirksey, 1979; Schuster et al., 1984) as well as decreased alanine aminotransferase activity and higher activity coefficients (stimulation of enzyme activity by the addition of PLP *in vitro*) (Lumeng et al., 1976; Schuster et al., 1981) compared to nonpregnant controls. It is uncertain whether these indices of vitamin B_6 status reflect inadequate intake or normal physiological changes of pregnancy. In the absence of new data and the lack of any information on the requirements of the fetus, the subcommittee supports the recommendation in the ninth edition of the RDA that pregnant women increase their vitamin B_6 intake by 0.6 mg/day.

The concentration of vitamin B_6 in human milk is approximately 0.01 to 0.02 mg/liter during the first days of lactation and gradually increases to 0.10 to 0.25 mg/liter (Coursin, 1955; Karlin, 1959; Kirksey and West, 1978; West and Kirksey, 1976). The vitamin B_6 content of milk reflects the nutritional status of the mother (Karlin, 1959; Kirksey and West, 1978; Roepke and Kirksey, 1979; Thomas et al., 1979; West and Kirksey, 1976). The ratio of vitamin B_6 to protein in human milk averaged 13 μg/g at a consumption of less than 2.5 mg of vitamin B_6 per day (Kirksey and West, 1978; West and Kirksey, 1976). In the absence of more recent information, the subcommittee maintains the recommendation in the ninth edition: an additional allowance of 0.5 mg of vitamin B_6 per day during lactation.

Infants and Children The vitamin B_6 content and vitamin-to-protein ratio is generally low in milk from nonsupplemented women, and there is evidence of vitamin B_6 deficiency symptoms in infants breastfed by women whose intakes are less than 2.0 mg/day and whose milk contains less than 0.1 mg of vitamin B_6 per day (Kirksey et al., 1981; Kirksey and Udipi, 1985; McCoy et al., 1985). In healthy babies, vitamin B_6 intakes of 0.3 mg/day protected against abnormal excretion of tryptophan metabolites following a load test (Bessey et al., 1957). General experience with proprietary formulas suggests that metabolic requirements are satisfied if the vitamin is present in amounts of 0.015 mg/g of protein or 0.04 mg/100 kcal (AAP, 1976; McCoy, 1978). The present subcommittee maintains the vitamin B_6 recommendations of the ninth edition of the RDA—0.3 mg/day during the first 6 months of infancy and 0.6 mg/day for older infants.

Studies on the nutritional status of children and adolescents in relation to their intake of vitamin B_6 are limited. In a study of 35 3- to 4-year-old boys and girls, Fries et al. (1981) found 3 subjects whose intakes were less than the RDAs of 0.9 and 1.3 mg and whose blood levels of PLP were indicative of vitamin B_6 inadequacy. Lewis and Nunn (1977) reported that 2- to 9-year-old children with an average daily intake of 1.10 mg of vitamin B_6 (0.02 mg/g of protein) excreted 48% as 4-PA in their urine, suggesting intakes in excess of need. Kirksey et al. (1978) reported a calculated mean intake of 1.24 ± 0.70 mg for 12- to 14-year-old females. Since there are no new data to justify changes in the vitamin B_6 recommendations for children and adolescents, the present subcommittee maintains the RDA of 0.02 mg/g protein from the ninth edition of the RDA. Allowances in the Summary Table for these age groups are based on average protein intakes, as determined by the Nationwide Food Consumption Survey (USDA, 1984).

Excessive Intakes and Toxicity

The acute toxicity of vitamin B_6 is low (McCormick, 1988). When taken in gram quantities for months or years (as it might be when self-administered or prescribed by physicians to treat premenstrual syndrome and several types of mental disorders), however, vitamin B_6 can cause ataxia and a severe sensory neuropathy (Schaumburg, 1983). Pyridoxine toxicity was the apparent cause of neurological symptoms in 103 women attending a private clinic who took an average of 117 ± 92 mg of this nutrient for more than 6 months to more than 5 years (Dalton and Dalton, 1987). These women recovered completely from their symptoms within 6 months of discontinuing the supplements.

References

AAP (American Academy of Pediatrics). 1985. Recommended ranges of nutrients in formulas. Appendix I. Pp. 356–357 in Pediatric Nutrition Handbook, 2nd ed. American Academy of Pediatrics, Elk Grove Village, Ill.

Baker, E.M., J.E. Canham, W.T. Nunes, H.E. Sauberlich, and M.E. McDowell. 1964. Vitamin B_6 requirement for adult men. Am. J. Clin. Nutr. 15:59–66.

Bauernfeind, J.C., and O.N. Miller. 1978. Vitamin B_6: Nutritional and pharmaceutical usage, stability, bioavailability, antagonists, and safety. Pp. 78–110 in Human Vitamin B_6 Requirements. Proceedings of a Workshop, June 11–12, 1976. Letterman Army Institute of Research, Presidio of San Francisco, California. A Report of the Committee on Dietary Allowances, Food and Nutrition Board. National Academy of Sciences, Washington, D.C.

Bessey, O.A., D.J. Adam, and A.E. Hansen. 1957. Intake of vitamin B_6 and infantile convulsions: a first approximation of requirements of pyridoxine in infants. Pediatrics 20:33–44.

Bhagavan, H.N. 1985. Interaction between vitamin B_6 and drugs. Pp. 401–415 in R.D. Reynolds and J.E. Leklem, eds. Vitamin B_6: Its Role in Health and Disease. Alan R. Liss, New York.

Brown, R.R., D.P. Rose, J.E. Leklem, H. Linkswiler, and R. Anand. 1975. Urinary 4-pyridoxic acid, plasma pyridoxal phosphate, and erythrocyte amino-transferase levels in oral contraceptive users receiving controlled intakes of vitamin B_6. Am. J. Clin. Nutr. 28:10–19.

Canham, J.E., E.M. Baker, R.S. Harding, H.E. Sauberlich, and I.C. Plough. 1969. Dietary protein—its relationship to vitamin B_6 requirements and function. Ann. N.Y. Acad. Sci. 166:16–29.

Cleary, R.E., L. Lumeng, and T.K. Li. 1975. Maternal and fetal plasma levels of pyridoxal phosphate at term: adequacy of vitamin B-6 supplementation during pregnancy. Am. J. Obstet. Gynecol. 121:25–28.

Contractor, S.F., and B. Shane. 1970. Blood and urine levels of vitamin B-6 in mother and fetus before and after loading of mother with vitamin B-6. Am. J. Obstet. Gynecol. 107:635–640.

Coursin, D.B. 1954. Convulsive seizures in infants with pyridoxine-deficient diet. J. Am. Med. Assoc. 154:406–408.

Coursin, D.B. 1955. Symposium on frontiers of human nutrition in relation to milk; vitamin B_6 (pyridoxine) in milk. Q. Rev. Pediatr. 10:2–9.

Dalton, K., and M.J.T. Dalton. 1987. Characteristics of pyridoxine overdose neuropathy syndrome. Acta Neurol. Scand. 76:8–11.

Donald, E.A., L.D. McBean, M.H.W. Simpson, M.F. Sun, and H.E. Aly. 1971. Vitamin B_6 requirement of young adult women. Am. J. Clin. Nutr. 24:1028–1041.

Fries, M.E., B.M. Chrisley, and J.A. Driskell. 1981. Vitamin B-6 status of a group of preschool children. Am. J. Clin. Nutr. 34:2706–2710.

Gregory, J.F., and J.R. Kirk. 1981. The bioavailability of vitamin B_6 in foods. Nutr. Rev. 39:1–8.

Hamfelt, A., and T. Tuvemo. 1972. Pyridoxal phosphate and folic acid concentration in blood and erythrocyte aspartate aminotransferase activity during pregnancy. Clin. Chim. Acta 41:287–298.

Haskell, B.F. 1978. Analysis of vitamin B_6. Pp. 61–71 in Human Vitamin B_6 Requirements. Proceedings of a Workshop, June 11–12, 1976. Letterman Army Institute of Research, Presidio of San Francisco, California. A Report of the

Committee on Dietary Allowances, Food and Nutrition Board. National Academy of Sciences, Washington, D.C.

Kabir, H., J. Leklem, and L.T. Miller. 1983. Measurement of glycosylated vitamin B_6 in foods. J. Food Sci. 40:1422–1425.

Karlin, R. 1959. Effect of excess administration of pyridoxine on the vitamin B_6 content of human milk. Bull. Soc. Chim. Biol. 41:1085–1091.

Kirksey, A., and J.L.B. Roepke. 1981. Vitamin B-6 nutriture of mothers of three breast-fed neonates with central nervous system disorders. Fed. Proc. 40:864.

Kirksey, A., and S.A. Udipi. 1985. Vitamin B-6 in human pregnancy and lactation. Pp. 57–77 in R.D. Reynolds and J.E. Leklem, eds. Vitamin B-6: Its Role in Health and Disease. Alan R. Liss, New York.

Kirksey, A., and K.D. West. 1978. Relationship between vitamin B_6 intake and the content of the vitamin in human milk. Pp. 238–251 in Human Vitamin B_6 Requirements. Proceedings of a Workshop, June 11–12, 1976. Letterman Army Institute of Research, Presidio of San Francisco, California. A Report of the Committee on Dietary Allowances, Food and Nutrition Board. National Academy of Sciences, Washington, D.C.

Kirksey, A., K. Keaton, R.P. Abernathy, and J.L. Greger. 1978. Vitamin B_6 nutritional status of a group of female adolescents. Am. J. Clin. Nutr. 31:946–954.

Kirksey, A., J.L.B. Roepke, and L.M. Styslinger. 1981. The vitamin B-6 content in human milk. Pp. 269–288 in J.E. Leklem and R.D. Reynolds, eds. Methods in Vitamin B-6 Nutrition: Analysis and Status Assessment. Plenum Press, New York.

Leklem, J.E., and R.D. Reynolds. 1981. Recommendations for status assessment of vitamin B-6. Pp. 389–392 in J.E. Leklem and R.D. Reynolds, eds. Methods in Vitamin B-6 Nutrition: Analysis and Status Assessment. Plenum Press, New York.

Leklem, J.E., R.R. Brown, D.P. Rose, and H.M. Linkswiler. 1975. Vitamin B_6 requirements of women using oral contraceptives. Am. J. Clin. Nutr. 28:535–541.

Leklem, J.E., L.T. Miller, A.D. Perera, and D.E. Peffers. 1980. Bioavailability of vitamin B-6 from wheat bread in humans. J. Nutr. 110:1819–1828.

Lewis, J.S., and K.P. Nunn. 1977. Vitamin B_6 intakes and 24-hr 4-pyridoxic acid excretions of children. Am. J. Clin. Nutr. 30:2023–2027.

Linkswiler, H.M. 1978. Vitamin B_6 requirements of men. Pp. 279–290 in Human Vitamin B_6 Requirements. National Academy of Sciences, Washington, D.C.

Lumeng, L., R.E. Cleary, R. Wagner, Y. Pao-Lo, and T.K. Li. 1976. Adequacy of vitamin B-6 supplementation during pregnancy: a prospective study. Am. J. Clin. Nutr. 29:1376–1383.

McCormick, D. 1988. Vitamin B_6. Pp. 376–382 in M.E. Shils and V.R. Young, eds. Modern Nutrition in Health and Disease, 7th ed. Lea & Febiger, Philadelphia.

McCoy, E.E. 1978. Vitamin B_6 requirements of infants and children. Pp. 257–271 in Human Vitamin B_6 Requirements. Proceedings of a Workshop, June 11–12, 1976. Letterman Army Institute of Research, Presidio of San Francisco, California. A Report of the Committee on Dietary Allowances, Food and Nutrition Board. National Academy of Sciences, Washington, D.C.

McCoy, E., K. Strynadka, and K. Brunet. 1985. Vitamin B-6 intake and whole blood levels of breast and formula fed infants. Serial whole blood vitamin B-6 levels in premature infants. Pp. 79–96 in R.D. Reynolds and J.E. Leklem, eds. Vitamin B-6: Its Role in Health and Disease. Alan R. Liss, New York.

Miller, L.T., and H.M. Linkswiler. 1967. Effect of protein intake on the development of abnormal tryptophan metabolism by men during vitamin B_6 depletion. J. Nutr. 93:53–59.

Nelson, E.W., C.W. Burgin, and J.J. Cerda. 1977. Characterization of food binding of vitamin B$_6$ in orange juice. J. Nutr. 107:2128–2134.

NRC (National Research Council). 1980. Recommended Dietary Allowances, 9th revised ed. Report of the Committee on Dietary Allowances, Food and Nutrition Board, Division of Biological Sciences, Assembly of Life Sciences. National Academy of Sciences, Washington, D.C. 185 pp.

NRC (National Research Council). 1989. Diet and Health: Implications for Reducing Chronic Disease Risk. Report of the Committee on Diet and Health, Food and Nutrition Board. National Academy Press, Washington, D.C. 750 pp.

Park, Y.K., and H. Linkswiler. 1970. Effect of vitamin B$_6$ depletion in adult man on the excretion of cystathionine and other methionine metabolites. J. Nutr. 100:110–116.

Roepke, J.L.B., and A. Kirksey. 1979. Vitamin B-6 nutriture during pregnancy and lactation. I. Vitamin B-6 intake, levels of the vitamin in biological fluids, and condition of the infant at birth. Am. J. Clin. Nutr. 32:2249–2256.

Schaumberg, H., J. Kaplan, A. Windebank, N. Vick, S. Ragmus, D. Pleasure, and M.J. Brown. 1983. Sensory neuropathy from pyrisoxine abuse. N. Engl. J. Med. 309:445–448.

Schroeder, H.A. 1971. Losses of vitamins and trace minerals resulting from processing and preservation of foods. Am. J. Clin. Nutr. 24:562–573.

Schultz, T.D., and J.E. Leklem. 1981. Urinary 4-pyridoxic acid, urinary vitamin B-6 and plasma pyridoxal phosphate as measures of vitamin B-6 status and dietary intake of adults. Pp. 297–320 in J.E. Leklem and R.D. Reynolds, eds. Methods in Vitamin B-6 Nutrition: Analysis and Status Assessment. Plenum Press, New York.

Schuster, K., L.B. Bailey, and C.S. Mahan. 1981. Vitamin B-6 status of low-income adolescent and adult pregnant women and the condition of their infants at birth. Am. J. Clin. Nutr. 32:1731–1735.

Schuster, K., L.B. Bailey, and C.S. Mahan. 1984. Effect of maternal pyridoxine-HCl supplementation on the vitamin B-6 status of mother and infant on pregnancy outcome. J. Nutr. 114:977–988.

Tarr, J.B., T. Tamura, and E.L.R. Stokstad. 1981. Availability of vitamin B$_6$ and pantothenate in an average American diet in man. Am. J. Clin. Nutr. 34:1328–1337.

Thomas, M.R., J. Kawamoto, S.M. Sneed, and R. Eaken. 1979. The effects of vitamin C, vitamin B$_6$ and vitamin B$_{12}$ supplementation on the breast milk and maternal status of well nourished women. Am. J. Clin. Nutr. 32:1679–1685.

USDA (U.S. Department of Agriculture). 1984. Nationwide Food Consumption Survey. Nutrient Intakes: Individuals in 48 States, Year 1977–78. Report No. I-2. Consumer Nutrition Division, Human Nutrition Information Service. U.S. Department of Agriculture, Hyattsville, Md. 439 pp.

USDA (U.S. Department of Agriculture). 1986. Nationwide Food Consumption Survey. Continuing Survey of Food Intakes by Individuals: Men 19–50 Years, 1 Day, 1985. Report No. 85-3. Nutrition Monitoring Division, Human Nutrition Information Service. U.S. Department of Agriculture, Hyattsville, Md. 94 pp.

USDA (U.S. Department of Agriculture). 1987. Nationwide Food Consumption Survey. Continuing Survey of Food Intakes by Individuals: Women 19–50 Years and Their Children 1–5 Years, 4 Days, 1985. Report No. 85-4. Nutrition Monitoring Division, Human Nutrition Information Service. U.S. Department of Agriculture, Hyattsville, Md. 182 pp.

West, K.D., and A. Kirksey. 1976. Influence of vitamin B_6 intake on the content of the vitamin in human milk. Am. J. Clin. Nutr. 29:961–969.

FOLATE

Folate and folacin are generic descriptors for compounds that have nutritional properties and chemical structures similar to those of folic acid (pteroylglutamic acid, or PGA). Metabolically active forms of folate have reduced (tetrahydro) pteridine rings and several glutamic acids attached (polyglutamates). Folate activity is measured by microbiological assay and by radioisotope dilution and binding methods.

Folates function metabolically as coenzymes that transport single carbon fragments from one compound to another in amino acid metabolism and nucleic acid synthesis. Deficiency of the vitamin leads to impaired cell division and to alterations of protein synthesis— effects most noticeable in rapidly growing tissues.

Different forms of folate vary in stability under various conditions, but in general, heat, oxidation, and ultraviolet light may cleave the folate molecule, rendering it inactive.

Dietary Sources and Usual Intakes

Folate is widely distributed in foods. Liver, yeast, leafy vegetables, legumes, and some fruits are especially rich sources. As much as 50% of food folate may be destroyed during household preparation, food processing, and storage. Comprehensive data on folate in food are published in the *Agriculture Handbooks No. 8* (USDA, 1976–1989). However, food analysis methods present difficulty, and values in these tables may be as much as 20% low due to incomplete recovery (Phillips and Wright, 1983).

Folacin is reported to have been essentially unchanged from 1960 to 1985, averaging 280 to 300 μg in the U.S. food supply per capita per day (USDA, 1988). In Canada, the mean folate intake is reported to be 205 μg/day for men and 149 μg/day for women (Health and Welfare Canada, 1977).

Bioavailability

Naturally occurring folates in foods have one or more glutamic acid residues as part of the molecule. Only monoglutamates are absorbed directly from the intestine, but folylpolyglutamate hydrolase enzymes associated with the intestinal mucosa release absorbable monoglutamates from polyglutamates. Approximately three-fourths of the folate in a mixed diet is present as polyglutamate (Butterworth et al., 1963). Estimates of the efficiency of absorption of food folates and the availability of polyglutamates relative to monoglutamates are quite variable, depending upon amount and type of test substance and other aspects of methodology (Rodriguez, 1978). Differences in the relative absorption of folate measurable in different foods may also relate to the presence of folate hydrolase inhibitors, binders, or other unknown factors (Colman et al., 1975a; Tamura and Stokstad, 1973). Efficiency of absorption of folate may also increase when folate status is low (Iyenger and Babu, 1975).

Overall, approximately 90% of folate monoglutamate and 50 to 90% of folate polyglutamate ingested separately from food is absorbed, but this percentage is decreased in the presence of many foods, irrespective of whether the folate was derived from or added to the food (Colman et al., 1975b; Tamura and Stokstad, 1973). Food composition and intestinal absorption data indicate that the bioavailability of folate in the typical U.S. diet is about one-half that of crystalline folic acid, which is efficiently absorbed (Sauberlich et al., 1987).

Assessment of Folate Status

Well-nourished individuals excrete daily up to 40 µg of folate in the urine (Herbert, 1968) and approximately 200 µg in feces (Herbert et al., 1984). The folate content of bile is approximately 5 times that of serum, but enterohepatic recirculation tends to conserve the body pool of folate (Steinberg, 1984). Krumdieck et al. (1978) found that after an equilibration period following an oral dose of radioactive folate, radioactive fecal and urinary losses were approximately equal. Nonradioactive fecal loss greatly exceeds urinary folate excretion, indicating that feces also contain folate synthesized by intestinal bacteria. Fecal folate is therefore not a reliable indicator of turnover, intake, or absorption.

Herbert et al. (1962) estimated the adult male's total folate pool to be 7.5 ± 2.5 mg, a coefficient of variation of 33%. Liver folate is a major part of this total (Chanarin, 1979). Among 370 male and 190 female subjects, distributed among age groups ranging from 1 to more than 80 years old, autopsy data revealed an average hepatic folate concentration of about 7 µg/g liver (range, 3 to 16 µg/g) which did not vary greatly by age or sex (Hoppner and Lampi, 1980). Morphologic evidence of folate deficiency is not manifest until liver levels fall below 1 µg/g (Gailani et al., 1970). Red cell folate reflects liver folate fairly closely (Chanarin, 1979), and average daily dietary folate intake correlates significantly with red cell folate (Bates et al., 1980).

In experimental human folate deficiency, serum and erythrocyte folate levels fall below accepted limits (3 ng/ml and 160 ng/ml, respectively) and evidence of defective DNA synthesis is seen as hypersegmentation of cells and abnormality in the sensitive deoxyuridine (dU) suppression test. Overtly megaloblastic bone marrow and macrocytic anemia are late consequences of deficiency (Herbert and Colman, 1988).

Recommended Allowances

Two general approaches have been used to estimate dietary allowances for folate (Anderson and Talbot, 1981; Rodriguez, 1978). One involves determining a minimum requirement for pure folic acid and increasing this amount to cover bioavailability, individual variation, and the need for adequate reserves. A second approach is evaluation of the average intake of food folate among persons in good folate status.

Adults and Adolescents   The daily requirement for absorbed folate has been judged to be approximately 50 μg for adults, on the basis of observations that daily parenteral administration of this amount of PGA successfully treats uncomplicated folate deficiency anemia (Zalusky and Herbert, 1961). Dietary intake of about 100 μg/day has been reported to prevent development of folate deficiency (Banerjee et al., 1975; Herbert, 1962). Sauberlich et al. (1987) have concluded that women depleted of folate require 200 to 250 μg/day of dietary folate to maintain stable plasma levels or to restore them toward normal under experimental conditions (including blood sampling). Their graphic portrayal of plasma values indicates that levels were stabilized in four subjects given 80 μg pure PGA plus 20 μg of dietary folate. Forty adult males living in a metabolic ward on a strictly controlled diet containing an average of 200 μg of folate/day (~ 3 μg/kg body weight) maintained normal serum and red cell folate levels for 6 months (Milne et al., 1983).

The minimum folate requirement can be estimated theoretically from the rate of loss of folate when none is fed. Loss of folate from the liver varies from 35 to 47 μg daily during folate depletion (Gailani et al., 1970). If extrahepatic stores are approximately half those in liver and are lost at the same rate, total daily folate loss in an adult eating essentially no folate would average about 60 μg, or roughly 1 μg/kg body weight.

Approximately 85% (range, 50 to 94%) of a 10 to 200 μg oral dose of folic acid is absorbed (Anderson et al., 1960; Jeejeebhoy et al., 1968; Waslien, 1977). Thus, a minimum requirement of approximately 1 μg/kg body weight, adjusted with a conservative estimate of 50% bioavailability of food folate and with a further adjustment for individual variabilty (coefficient of variation approximately 30%), suggests an allowance of approximately 3 μg/kg body weight for adults.

One can also approach the issue of folate allowances from population intakes. The average folate intake of both U.S. and Canadian populations is roughly 3 μg/kg body weight. Approximately 10% of people from these populations are reported to have low folate stores but no signs of deficiency (Senti and Pilch, 1984). Therefore, the average dietary intakes must provide about 90% of the adult population with sufficient absorbable folate for daily metabolic needs and also for substantial folate storage.

The elderly are considered in the same category as other adults with respect to folate needs (Rosenberg et al., 1982). On diets estimated to contain 135 μg folate per day, all of 21 elderly men and women living at home sustained erythrocyte folate greater than 100 ng/ml and were hematologically normal; 9 had levels less than 150 ng/ml (Bates et al., 1980).

The RDA for folate is accepted to be approximately 3 μg/kg body weight for men, nonpregnant, nonlactating women, and adolescents. The RDA is 200 μg for adult males and 180 μg for adult females. This allowance should provide for liver storage adequate to protect against development of a folate deficiency during short periods of inadequate intake.

Pregnancy and Lactation Pregnancy increases the incidence of folate deficiency among populations with low or marginal intakes of the vitamin (Colman et al., 1975c; Giles, 1966; Lawrence and Klipstein, 1967). Even for populations consuming nutritionally sound diets, folic acid supplements ranging from 100 to 1,000 μg/day have been recommended by different investigators (Chanarin et al., 1968; Colman et al., 1974, 1975b). Baumslag et al. (1970) reported a reduced incidence of premature births in women given supplementary folic acid; an oral PGA supplement of 500 μg/day was associated with a 50% reduction in the incidence of small-for-date births among 134 pregnant women in India (Iyengar and Rajalakshmi, 1975).

A daily oral supplement of 100 μg of PGA prevented any fall in the mean erythrocyte folate of British women during pregnancy (Chanarin et al., 1968). The dietary folate content in the United

Kingdom was subsequently reported to be about 190 μg/day (Bates et al., 1982). Thus, in women who started pregnancy with moderate folate stores, folate deficiency probably was prevented by the equivalent of 200 μg of PGA per day (100 μg supplement plus 50% of the average population intake of dietary folate). In women with poor folate stores and whose diet was essentially devoid of folate, the progression of folate deficiency was as effectively prevented by administering a supplement of 300 μg of PGA daily in maize meal (a food that reduced availability by 44%, i.e., the effective dose was 168 μg of PGA) as it was by higher doses of more efficient vehicles (Colman et al., 1975b).

On the basis of a 50% food folate absorption, the RDA for folate is set at 400 μg/day during pregnancy to build or maintain maternal folate stores and to keep pace with the increased folate need to support rapidly growing tissue. This level can be met by a well-selected diet without food fortification or oral supplementation.

In the past, the demand of lactation on maternal folate reserves was estimated to be 20 μg/day, varying with the folate content and volume of milk (Matoth et al., 1965). This estimate was based on daily production of 850 ml of milk with an average folate content of 50 μg per liter. Ek (1983) reported that supplementation was unnecessary to maintain folate status in women in the socioeconomic middle class in Sweden. On the basis of daily production of 750 ml of milk, a coefficient of variation of 12.5%, and 50% absorption of food folate, the allowance for folate during lactation is set at the RDA of 180 μg plus 100 μg/day, a total of 280 μg/day during the first 6 months. The increment during the second 6 months, based on average milk production of 600 ml/day and the same adjustments, is 80 μg/day, a total of 260 μg/day.

Infants and Children Although serum folate in infants at birth is 3 times maternal folate, body stores at birth are small and are rapidly depleted by the requirements for growth, especially in premature infants. Full-term infants have higher liver stores of folate (Salmi, 1963). By 2 weeks of age, serum and erythrocyte folate fall below adult values and remain there during the entire first year of life (WHO, 1968). In a study of 20 infants aged 2 to 11 months, Asfour et al. (1977) demonstrated the nutritional adequacy of diets providing 3.6 μg of folate per kilogram of body weight per day over 6- to 9-month periods. Waslien (1977) concluded that 3.5 μg of folate per kilogram of body weight per day appeared adequate for infants up to 2 years of age.

Human and cow milk both contain about 50 μg of folate per liter; the concentration of folate in human colostrum and early milk is much lower. The needs of infants are adequately met by milk from humans or cows, but not by goat milk, which contains only 10 μg/liter (Herbert, 1981).

Milk contains a factor that is essentially unaffected by pasteurization and that facilitates folate uptake by gut cells (Colman et al., 1981a, 1981b). Presumably, this factor facilitates both absorption of dietary folate and reabsorption of bile folate. Boiling, or the preparation of evaporated milk, destroys an average of 50% of the folate in cow's milk, so that infants receiving boiled formulas prepared from pasteurized, sterilized, or powdered cow's milk should be given additional folate to ensure an adequate intake (Ghitis, 1966). If the diet consists of goat's milk, folic acid supplementation should be given in any case.

Megaloblastic anemia due to dietary folate deficiency is rare in children. Those who drink vegetable or fruit juice or eat fresh uncooked fruits or vegetables each day maintain adequate folate status; deficiency has been observed among children whose entire diet consists of fine-particulate foods cooked for a long time (Herbert, 1981).

On the basis of the above considerations, the allowance for folate is set at 3.6 μg/kg per day for healthy infants from birth to age 1 year. This value should provide an adequate margin of safety and is comparable to the folate content of human milk. The folate RDA for healthy children between 1 and 10 years of age is interpolated from the allowances for infants and adolescents.

Excessive Intakes and Toxicity

Folic acid and the anticonvulsant drug phenytoin inhibit uptake of each other at the gut cell membrane and possibly at the brain cell membrane (Chanarin, 1979; Colman and Herbert, 1979). Very large doses of folic acid (100 or more times the RDA) may precipitate convulsions in persons whose epilepsy is in continuous control by phenytoin (Colman and Herbert, 1979). In laboratory animals, very large doses of folic acid given parenterally may precipitate in the kidneys, producing kidney damage and hypertrophy (Colman and Herbert, 1979). No untoward effects have been reported in women given 10 mg/day of folic acid continuously for 4 months (Butterworth et al., 1988). However, without evidence of benefit and with some potential for toxicity, excessive intakes of supplemental folate are not recommended.

Changes in Folate Allowances Compared to Ninth Edition

Recognition that diets containing about half as much folate as the previous RDA maintain adequate folate status (including liver stores greater than 3 μg/g) provides the basis for lowering the folate RDA in the present edition. The new RDA is consistent with the safe level of folate intake recommended by the FAO (1988).

References

Anderson, S.A., and J.M. Talbot. 1981. A Review of Folate Intake, Methodology, and Status. Life Sciences Research Office. Federation of American Societies for Experimental Biology, Bethesda, Md.

Anderson, B., E.H. Belcher, I. Chanarin, and D.L. Mollin. 1960. The urinary and faecal excretion of radioactivity after oral doses of ^{3}H-folic acid. Br. J. Haematol. 6:439–455.

Asfour, R., N. Wahbea, C. Waslien, S. Guindi, and W.J. Darby, Jr. 1977. Folacin requirements of children. III. Normal infants. Am. J. Clin. Nutr. 30:1098–1105.

Banerjee, D.K., A. Maitra, A.K. Basu, and J.B. Chatterjea. 1975. Minimal daily requirement of folic acid in normal Indian subjects. Indian J. Med. Res. 63:45–53.

Bates, C.J., M. Fleming, A.A. Paul, A.E. Black, and A.R. Mandal. 1980. Folate status and its relation to vitamin C in healthy elderly men and women. Age Ageing 9:241–248.

Bates, C.J., A.E. Black, D.R. Phillips, A.J. Wright, and D.A. Southgate. 1982. The discrepancy between normal folate intakes and the folate RDA. Human Nutr. Appl. Nutr. 36:422–429.

Baumslag, N., T. Edelstein, and J. Metz. 1970. Reduction of incidence of prematurity by folic acid supplementation in pregnancy. Br. Med. J. 1:16–17.

Butterworth, C.E., Jr., R. Santini, Jr., and W.B. Frommeyer, Jr. 1963. The pteroylglutamate composition of American diets as determined by chromatographic fractionation. J. Clin. Invest. 42:1929–1939.

Butterworth, C.E., K. Hatch, P. Cole, H.E. Sauberlich, T. Tamura, P.E. Cornwell, and S.J. Soong. 1988. Zinc concentration in plasma and erythrocytes of subjects receiving folic acid supplementation. Am. J. Clin. Nutr. 47:484–486.

Chanarin, I. 1979. The Megaloblastic Anaemias, 2nd ed. Blackwell, Oxford.

Chanarin, I., D. Rothman, A. Ward, and J. Perry. 1968. Folate status and requirement in pregnancy. Br. Med. J. 2:390–394.

Colman, N., and V. Herbert. 1979. Dietary assessments with special emphasis on prevention of folate deficiency. Pp. 23–33 in M.I. Botez and E.H. Reynolds, eds. Folic Acid in Neurology, Psychiatry, and Internal Medicine. Raven Press, New York.

Colman, N., M. Barker, R. Green, and J. Metz. 1974. Prevention of folate deficiency in pregnancy by food fortification. Am. J. Clin. Nutr. 27:339–344.

Colman, N., R. Green, and J. Metz. 1975a. Prevention of folate deficiency by food fortification. II. Absorption of folic acid from fortified staple foods. Am. J. Clin. Nutr. 28:459–464.

Colman, N., J.V. Larsen, M. Barker, E.A. Barker, R. Green, and J. Metz. 1975b. Prevention of folate deficiency by food fortification. III. Effect in pregnant subjects of varying amounts of added folic acid. Am. J. Clin. Nutr. 28:465–470.

Colman, N., E.A. Barker, M. Barker, R. Green, and J. Metz. 1975c. Prevention of folate deficiency by food fortification. IV. Identification of target groups in addition to pregnant women in an adult rural population. Am. J. Clin. Nutr. 28:471–476.

Colman, N., N. Hettiarachchy, and V. Herbert. 1981a. Detection of a milk factor that facilitates folate uptake by intestinal cells. Science 211:1427–1429.

Colman, N., J.-F. Chen, W. Gavin, and V. Herbert. 1981b. Factors affecting enhancement by milk of folate uptake into intestinal cells. Blood 58 Suppl. 1:26a.

Ek, J. 1983. Plasma, red cell, and breast milk folacin concentrations in lactating women. Am. J. Clin. Nutr. 38:929–935.

FAO (Food and Agriculture Organization). 1988. Requirements of Vitamin A, Iron, Folate and Vitamin B12. Report of a Joint FAO/WHO Expert Consultation. FAO Food and Nutrition Series No. 23. Food and Agriculture Organization, Rome. 107 pp.

Gailani, S.D., R.W. Carey, J.F. Holland, and J.A. O'Malley. 1970. Studies of folate deficiency in patients with neoplastic diseases. Cancer Res. 30:327–333.

Ghitis, J. 1966. The labile folate of milk. Am. J. Clin. Nutr. 18:452–457.

Giles, C. 1966. An account of 335 cases of megaloblastic anemia of pregnancy and the puerperium. J. Clin. Pathol. 19:1–11.

Health and Welfare Canada. 1977. Food Consumption Patterns. Bureau of Nutritional Sciences, Department of National Health and Welfare. Canadian Government Publishing Centre, Ottawa.

Herbert, V. 1962. Experimental nutritional folate deficiency in man. Trans. Assoc. Am. Physicians 75:307–320.

Herbert, V., N. Cuneen, L. Jaskiell, and C. Kapff. 1962. Minimal daily adult folate requirement. Arch. Intern. Med. 110:649–652.

Herbert, V. 1968. Nutritional requirements for vitamin B12 and folic acid. Am. J. Clin. Nutr. 21:743–752.

Herbert, V. 1981. Nutritional anemias of childhood—Folate, B12: the megaloblastic anemias. Pp. 133–144 in R.M. Suskind, ed. Textbook of Pediatric Nutrition. Raven Press, New York.

Herbert, V., and N. Colman. 1988. Folic acid and vitamin B12. Pp. 388–416 in M. E. Shils and V. Young, eds. Modern Nutrition in Health and Disease, 7th ed. Lea & Febiger, Philadelphia.

Herbert, V., G. Drivas, C. Manusselis, B. Mackler, J. Eng, and E. Schwartz. 1984. Are colon bacteria a major source of cobalamin analogues in human tissues? 24-h human stool contains only about 5 μg cobalamin but about 100 μg apparent analogue (and 200 μg folate). Trans. Assoc. Am. Physicians 97:161–171.

Hoppner, K., and B. Lampi. 1980. Folate levels in human liver from autopsies in Canada. Am. J. Clin. Nutr. 33:862–864.

Iyengar, L., and S. Babu. 1975. Folic acid absorption in pregnancy. Br. J. Obstet. Gynaecol. 82:20–23.

Iyengar, L., and K. Rajalakshmi. 1975. Effect of folic acid supplement on birth weights of infants. Am. J. Obstet. Gynecol. 122:332–336.

Jeejeebhoy, K.N., H.G. Desai, A.V. Borkar, V. Deshpande, and S.M. Pathare. 1968. Tropical malabsorption syndrome in West India. Am. J. Clin. Nutr. 21:994–1006.

Krumdieck, C.L., K. Fukushima, T. Fukushima, T. Shiota, and C.E. Butterworth, Jr. 1978. A long-term study of the excretion of folate and pterins in a human subject after ingestion of ^{14}C folic acid, with observations on the effect of diphenylhydantoin administration. Am. J. Clin. Nutr. 31:88–93.

Lawrence, C., and F.A. Klipstein. 1967. Megaloblastic anemia of pregnancy in New York City. Ann. Intern. Med. 66:25–34.

Matoth, Y., A. Pinkas, and C. Sroka. 1965. Studies on folic acid in infancy. III. Folates in breast fed infants and their mothers. Am. J. Clin. Nutr. 16:356–359.

Milne, D.B., L.K. Johnson, J.R. Mahalko, and H.H. Sandstead. 1983. Folate status of adult males living in a metabolic unit: possible relationships with iron nutriture. Am. J. Clin. Nutr. 37:768–773.

Phillips, D.R., and A.J.A. Wright. 1983. Studies on the response of *Lactobacillus casei* to folate vitamin in foods. Br. J. Nutr. 49:181–186.

Rodriguez, M.S. 1978. A conspectus of research on folacin requirements of man. J. Nutr. 108:1983–2103.

Rosenberg, I.H., B.B. Bowman, B.A. Cooper, C.H. Halsted, and J. Lindenbaum. 1982. Folate nutrition in the elderly. Am. J. Clin. Nutr. 36:1060–1066.

Salmi, H.A. 1963. Comparative studies on vitamin B_{12} in developing organisms and placenta. Human and animal investigations with reference to the effects of low vitamin B_{12} diet on tissue vitamin B_{12} concentrations in rat. Ann. Acad. Sci. Fenn. 103:1–91.

Sauberlich, H.E., M.J. Kretsch, J.H. Skala, H.L. Johnson, and P.C. Taylor. 1987. Folate requirement and metabolism in nonpregnant women. Am. J. Clin. Nutr. 46:1016–1028.

Senti, F.R., and S.M. Pilch, eds. 1984. Assessment of the Folate Nutritional Status of the U.S. Population Based on Data Collected in the Second National Health and Nutrition Examination Survey, 1976–1980. Life Sciences Research Office, Federation of American Societies for Experimental Biology, Bethesda, Md. 96 pp.

Steinberg, S.E. 1984. Mechanisms of folate homeostasis. Am. J. Physiol. 246:G319-G324.

Tamura, T., and E.L.R. Stokstad. 1973. The availability of food folate in man. Br. J. Haematol. 25:513–532.

USDA (U.S. Department of Agriculture). 1976–1989. USDA Agricultural Handbook Series 8. Composition of Foods—Raw, Processed, and Prepared. Nutrient Data Research, Human Nutrition Information Service. U.S. Department of Agriculture, Hyattsville, Md. (various pagings)

USDA (U.S. Department of Agriculture). 1988. The Nutrient Content of the U.S. Food Supply. Tables of Nutrients and Food Provided by the U.S. Food Supply. Human Nutrition Information Service Report No. 299–21. U.S. Department of Agriculture, Hyattsville, Md. 72 pp.

Waslien, C.I. 1977. Folacin requirements of infants. Pp. 232–246 in Folic Acid: Biochemistry and Physiology in Relation to the Human Nutrition Requirement. Report of the Food and Nutrition Board, National Research Council. National Academy of Sciences, Washington, D.C.

WHO (World Health Organization). 1968. Nutritional Anaemias. Report of a Scientific Group. WHO Technical Report Series No. 405. World Health Organization, Geneva.

Zalusky, R., and V. Herbert. 1961. Megaloblastic anemia in scurvy with response to 50 micrograms of folic acid daily. N. Engl. J. Med. 265:1033–1038.

VITAMIN B_{12}

The terms vitamin B_{12} and cobalamin refer to all members of a group of large cobalt-containing corrinoids that can be converted to methylcobalamin or 5′-deoxyadenosylcobalamin, the two cobalamin coenzymes active in human metabolism. Cyanocobalamin is the commercially available form of vitamin B_{12} used in vitamin pills and pharmaceuticals. This form is water soluble and heat stable and, when given either orally or parenterally, is converted by the removal of cyanide to the forms that are metabolically active in humans. In plasma and tissue, the predominant forms are methylcobalamin, adenosylcobalamin, and hydroxocobalamin (Dolphin, 1982). Animal products are the primary dietary source of the vitamin. The dominant forms in meat are adenosyl- and hydroxocobalamin, whereas dairy products, including human milk, contain mainly methyl- and hydroxocobalamin (Gimsing and Nex, 1983).

Dietary Sources and Usual Intakes

Bacteria, fungi, and algae can synthesize vitamin B_{12}, but yeasts, higher plants, and animals cannot. In the human diet, vitamin B_{12} is supplied primarily by animal products, where it has accumulated from bacterial synthesis. Plant foods are essentially devoid of vitamin B_{12} except for adventitious inclusion of microbially formed B_{12} in soil or water.

The average dietary vitamin B_{12} intake of adult men in the United States was 7.84 μg/day in 1985 (USDA, 1986). The corresponding intakes for adult women and their children 1 to 5 years of age were 4.85 μg and 3.80 μg/day, respectively. About 5 to 30% of the reported vitamin B_{12} in foods may be microbiologically active noncobalamin corrinoids rather than true vitamin B_{12} (Herbert et al., 1984).

An additional nondietary source of small amounts of absorbable vitamin B_{12} may be bacteria in the small intestine of humans (Albert et al., 1980). A 24-hour human stool contains approximately 5 μg of cobalamin and about 100 μg of non-B_{12} analogs, produced in part by bacteria in the colon (Herbert et al., 1984). Cobalamin does not, however, appear to be absorbed from the colon (Dolphin, 1982).

General Signs of Deficiency

Vitamin B_{12} deficiency results in macrocytic, megaloblastic anemia, in neurological symptoms due to demyelination of the spinal cord and brain and the optic and peripheral nerves, and in other less specific symptoms (e.g., sore tongue, weakness). Neuropsychiatric manifestations of vitamin B_{12} deficiency are seen in the absence of anemia, particularly in the elderly (Lindenbaum et al., 1988). Dietary deficiency of vitamin B_{12} is rare; more than 95% of the vitamin B_{12}

deficiency seen in the United States is due to inadequate absorption (Herbert, 1984).

The coenzyme methylcobalamin catalyzes a transmethylation from a folic acid cofactor to homocysteine to form methionine. This reaction releases the unmethylated folate cofactor for other single carbon transfer reactions important to nucleic acid synthesis. This reaction is a site of B_{12}-folate interaction and may relate to the similarity in B_{12} and folate deficiency signs (Herbert and Colman, 1988). The other cobalamin coenzyme, deoxyadenosylcobalamin, catalyzes the conversion of methylmalonyl-coenzyme A to succinyl-coenzyme A, a reaction in the pathway for the degradation of certain amino acids and odd-chain fatty acids. Blockage of this reaction in B_{12} deficiency leads to the characteristic increased urinary excretion of methylmalonic acid.

Metabolism

The intestinal absorption of vitamin B_{12} takes place at receptor sites in the ileum, mediated by a highly specific binding glycoprotein (Castle's intrinsic factor), which is secreted in the stomach. In crossing the intestinal mucosa, vitamin B_{12} is transferred to the plasma transport protein transcobalamin II, which delivers the vitamin to cells. Absorption may also occur by simple diffusion, a process that probably accounts for the absorption of only 1 to 3% of the vitamin consumed in ordinary diets. This mechanism becomes biologically important when pharmacologic amounts (30 μg or more) of the free vitamin are ingested (Herbert and Colman, 1988).

At intakes of 0.5 μg or less, approximately 70% of the available vitamin is absorbed (Heyssel et al., 1966). The percentage absorbed decreases as the intake of vitamin B_{12} increases, although the absolute amount of B_{12} absorbed increases. A maximum of about 1.5 μg is absorbed from single oral doses ranging from 5 to 50 μg (Chanarin, 1979). Intrinsic factor-mediated B_{12} absorption appears to be a saturable process, but absorption of 1.5 μg in one meal does not preclude absorption of normal amounts of the vitamin some hours later (FAO, 1988).

An effective enterohepatic circulation recycles the vitamin from bile and other intestinal secretions, accounting in part for its long biological half-life. In pernicious anemia, vitamin B_{12} is not absorbed from the diet or reabsorbed from the bile due to lack of intrinsic factor activity. The importance of reabsorption of cobalamin excreted in the bile is illustrated by the fact that vegetarians who eat no animal products (but may receive small amounts from bacterial sources and contaminants) develop vitamin B_{12} deficiency only after 20 to 30 years, but in pernicious anemia or with other absorptive defects, vitamin B_{12} deficiency may develop in as short a time as 2 to 3 years (Chanarin, 1979; Herbert, 1984).

Pool Size and Turnover

Adams (1962) estimated total body vitamin B_{12} content to be 2.2 mg, based on analysis of tissues obtained at autopsy. This pool size (2 to 2.5 mg) was confirmed by Hall (1964) and Linnell et al. (1974). Reizenstein et al. (1966) calculated the body pool to be 3.0 mg as measured by radioisotope dilution.

The daily loss of vitamin B_{12} is approximately 0.1% (range, 0.05 to 0.2%) of the body pool, regardless of pool size (Heyssel et al., 1966). Using a whole-body counting technique, Heinrich (1964) found the half-life of a tracer dose to be 1,360 days and estimated the daily loss to be 2.55 μg, and Reizenstein et al. (1966) calculated a daily loss of 1.2 μg from two healthy subjects. Hall (1964) reported half-life to range from 480 to 1,284 days and the average daily loss of radiolabeled vitamin B_{12} to be 1.3 μg, almost equally divided between urine and feces.

Basis for Establishing Allowances

In patients with pernicious anemia, daily injections of 0.1 μg of cyanocobalamin are reported to produce suboptimal hematologic responses (Sullivan and Herbert, 1965), whereas doses of 0.5 to 1.0 μg/day have maintained patients with pernicious anemia in complete hematologic and neurologic remission (Herbert, 1968). Patients with pernicious anemia or those who have undergone total gastrectomy are not, however, good models for determining normal dietary requirements, because they are unable to reabsorb the B_{12} excreted in the bile. Nonetheless, they do provide information on the gross requirement for absorbed B_{12}.

Other evidence derives from studies of persons whose diets are low or deficient in vitamin B_{12}. Deficiency can be, but rarely is, produced by a strict vegetarian (i.e., vegan) diet devoid of meat, eggs, and dairy products. An Indian woman resident of London developed deficiency with a diet containing 0.5 μg of vitamin B_{12} per day (Stewart et al., 1970). Intakes in four other deficiency cases ranged from 0.07 to 0.25 μg/day (Baker and Mathin, 1981). Only 21 of 431 Australian vegetarians had unacceptable blood levels of B_{12} at an average intake of 0.26 ± 0.23 μg/day (mean ± SD), and none of these developed deficiency symptoms over a 1-year period of evaluation (Armstrong et al., 1974). An intake of 0.3 to 0.65 μg/day in food produced satisfactory hematologic responses in vitamin B_{12}-deficient Indian patients (Baker and Mathin, 1981). Although serum concentrations of vitamin B_{12} remained below normal in these cases, bone marrow became normoblastic, and there was no anemia.

These findings suggest that the adult requirement for vitamin B_{12} is approximately 0.5 μg/day for persons with low serum B_{12} concentrations and whose pool size is presumed to be small. The evidence of the long lag period before symptoms of deficiency appear when absorption is impaired suggests that the usual pool size of omnivores (2 to 3 mg) exceeds daily needs by perhaps three orders of magnitude. To maintain the usual pool size with turnover rates as reported above (half-life of 480 to 1,360 days) would require 1 to 3 μg/day. Estimates of requirement are necessarily dependent on a judgment as to desirable pool size.

Recommended Allowances

Adults   A dietary intake of 1 μg daily can be expected to sustain average normal adults. To allow for biological variation and the maintenance of normal serum concentrations and substantial body stores, the vitamin B_{12} RDA for adults is set at 2.0 μg. The subcommittee has concluded that a substantial body store is desirable in view of the increasing prevalence of achlorhydria and pernicious anemia beyond age 60 (Chanarin, 1979). Dietary intake will frequently exceed the RDA, but this is not considered a justification for either raising the allowance or modifying the diet.

The results of various surveys have indicated that although serum vitamin B_{12} levels decline in the elderly (Carmel and Karnaze, 1985), they tend to remain in the normal range (Garry et al., 1984). The evidence reported by Herbert (1985) suggests that the decline in the mean serum B_{12} level is due to the gradual appearance among the elderly of B_{12} malabsorption. Such malabsorption would require injection of vitamin B_{12}, rather than an increase in the RDA for B_{12} in the elderly. Measurement of cobalamin in serum among the elderly will identify those who require medical intervention (Herbert, 1985; Herzlich et al., 1985).

Pregnancy and Lactation   From analysis of the vitamin B_{12} content of stillborn infants from normally nourished mothers, FAO (1988) estimated that fetal demands are approximately 0.1 to 0.2 μg/day. The placenta concentrates vitamin B_{12}, and the serum B_{12} levels of newborns are double that of their mothers (Giugliani et al., 1985). Normally, maternal body stores are sufficient to meet the needs of pregnancy, and it is unlikely that any increment in vitamin B_{12} intake is needed. An additional allowance of 0.2 μg/day can, however, be justified.

Vitamin B_{12} in human milk parallels the concentration in serum. At 6 months postpartum, 0.6 μg/liter was found in the milk of well-nourished women in the United States (Thomas et al., 1980). This would mean a loss of 0.45 μg in 750 ml of human milk, or 0.56 μg/ day at the upper level of production. An additional allowance of 0.6 μg/day is recommended for lactating women.

Symptoms of vitamin B_{12} deficiency have been observed in some breastfed infants of women who are strict vegetarians (Higginbottom et al., 1978; Specker et al., 1988). Pregnant and lactating women adhering to diets devoid of animal-source foods should be advised to take supplementary vitamin B_{12} at RDA levels (i.e., 2.2 and 2.6 μg/ day, respectively).

Infants and Children   Since overt vitamin B_{12} deficiency does not occur in infants breastfed by women with adequate serum vitamin B_{12} levels (Lampkin et al., 1966), and vitamin B_{12}-deficient infants of B_{12}-deficient vegetarian mothers show a full therapeutic response to oral doses of 0.1 μg/day (Jadhav et al., 1962), the RDA for the young infant has been set at 0.3 μg/day (i.e., 0.05 μg/kg body weight) to allow a substantial margin for storage. The RDAs for older infants and preadolescent children have been based on progressive increases with increasing body size (at 0.05 μg/kg body weight) until the RDA for adults (2 μg) is reached.

Excessive Intakes and Toxicity

No clear toxicity has been reported from daily oral ingestion of up to 100 μg. Similarly, no benefit has been reported in nondeficient people from such large quantities.

Changes in Vitamin B_{12} Allowances Compared to Ninth Edition

The present RDAs for vitamin B_{12} are one-third to one-half lower than those given in the ninth edition. They are, however, approximately double the safe level of intake of vitamin B_{12} established by the FAO (1988). The difference in recommendations based on the same body of evidence reflects the present subcommittee's conservative stance on the desirability of maintaining a substantial body pool of vitamin B_{12}.

References

Adams, J.F. 1962. The measurement of the total assayable vitamin B_{12} in the body. P. 397 in C. Heinrich, ed. Vitamin B_{12} und Intrinsic Faktor. Ferdinand Enke, Stuttgart, Federal Republic of Germany.

Albert, M.J., V.I. Mathan, and S.J. Baker. 1980. Vitamin B_{12} synthesis by human small intestinal bacteria. Nature 283:781–782.

Armstrong, B.K., R.E. Davis, D.J. Nicol, A.J. van Merwyk, and C.J. Larwood. 1974. Hematological, vitamin B_{12}, and folate studies on Seventh-Day Adventist vegetarians. Am. J. Clin. Nutr. 27:712–718.

Baker, S.J., and V.I. Mathan. 1981. Evidence regarding the minimal daily requirement of dietary vitamin B_{12}. Am. J. Clin. Nutr. 34:2423–2433.

Carmel, R., and D.S. Karnaze. 1985. The deoxyuridine suppression test identifies subtle cobalamin deficiency in patients without typical megaloblastic anemia. J. Am. Med. Assoc. 253:1284–1287.

Chanarin, I. 1979. The Megaloblastic Anaemias, 2nd ed. Blackwell, Oxford.

Dolphin, D., ed. 1982. B_{12}. Vol. 2. Biochemistry and Medicine. John Wiley & Sons, New York. 505 pp.

FAO (Food and Agriculture Organization). 1988. Requirements of Vitamin A, Iron, Folate, and Vitamin B_{12}. Report of a Joint FAO/WHO Expert Consultation. FAO Food and Nutrition Series No. 23. Food and Agriculture Organization, Rome. 107 pp.

Garry, P.J., J.S. Goodwin, and W.C. Hunt. 1984. Folate and vitamin B_{12} status in a healthy elderly population. J. Am. Geriatr. Soc. 32:719–726.

Gimsing, P., and E. Nex. 1983. The forms of cobalamin in biological materials. Pp. 7–30 in C.A. Hall, ed. The Cobalamins. Churchill Livingstone, Edinburgh.

Giugliani, E.R.J., S.M. Jorge, and A.L. Gonçalves. 1985. Serum vitamin B_{12} levels in parturients, in the intervillous space of the placenta and in full-term newborns and their interrelationships with folate levels. Am. J. Clin. Nutr. 41:330–335.

Hall, C.A., 1964. Long term excretion of Co^{57}-vitamin B_{12} and turnover within plasma. Am. J. Clin. Nutr. 14:156–162.

Heinrich, H.C. 1964. Metabolic basis of the diagnosis and therapy of vitamin B_{12} deficiency. Semin. Hematol. 1:199–249.

Herbert, V. 1968. Nutritional requirements for vitamin B_{12} and folic acid. Am. J. Clin. Nutr. 21:743–752.

Herbert, V. 1984. Vitamin B_{12}. Pp. 347–364 in Nutrition Reviews' Present Knowledge in Nutrition, 5th ed. The Nutrition Foundation, Washington, D.C.

Herbert, V. 1985. Biology of disease: megaloblastic anemias. Lab. Invest. 52:3–19.

Herbert, V.D., and N. Colman. 1988. Folic acid and vitamin B_{12}. Pp. 388–416 in M.E. Shils and V.R. Young, eds. Modern Nutrition in Health and Disease, 7th ed. Lea & Febiger, Philadelphia.

Herbert, V., G. Drivas, C. Manusselis, M. Mackler, J. Eng, and E. Schwartz. 1984. Are colon bacteria a major source of cobalamin analogues in human tissues? 24-h human stool contains only about 5 μg of cobalamin but about 100 μg of apparent analogue (and 200 μg folate). Trans. Assoc. Amer. Phys. 97:161–171.

Herzlich, B., G. Drivas, and V. Herbert. 1985. A new serum test which may reliably diagnose vitamin B_{12} deficiency: total desaturation of serum transcobalamin II (TC II). Clin. Res. 33:605A.

Heyssel, R.M., R.C. Bozian, W.J. Darby, and M.C. Bell. 1966. Vitamin B_{12} turnover in man. The assimilation of vitamin B_{12} from natural foodstuff by man and estimates of minimal dietary requirements. Am. J. Clin. Nutr. 18:176–184.

Higginbottom, M.C., L. Sweetman, and W.L. Nuhan. 1978. A syndrome of methylmalonic aciduria, homocystinuria, megaloblastic anemia and neurologic abnormalities in a vitamin B_{12}-deficient breast-fed infant of a strict vegetarian. N. Eng. J. Med. 299:317–323.

Jadhav, M., J.K.G. Webb, S. Vaishnava, and S.J. Baker. 1962. Vitamin B_{12} deficiency in Indian infants: a clinical syndrome. Lancet 2:903–907.

Lampkin, B.D., N.A. Shore, and D. Chadwick. 1966. Megaloblastic anemia of infancy secondary to maternal pernicious anemia. N. Engl. J. Med. 274:1168–1171.

Lindenbaum, J., E.B. Healton, D.G. Savage, J.C.M. Brust, T.J. Garrett, E.R. Podell, P.D. Marcell, S.P. Stabler, and R.H. Allen. 1988. Neuropsychiatric disorders caused by cobalamin deficiency in the absence of anemia or macrocytosis. N. Engl. J. Med. 318:1720–1728.

Linnell, J.C., A.V. Hoffbrand, H.A.A. Hussein, I.J. Wise, and D.M. Matthews. 1974. Tissue distribution of coenzyme and other forms of vitamin B_{12} in control subjects and patients with pernicious anemia. Clin. Sci. Mol. Med. 46:163–172.

Reizenstein, P.C., G. Ek, and C.M.E. Matthews. 1966. Vitamin B12 kinetics in man. Implications of total-body B12 determinations, human requirements, and normal and pathological cellular B12 uptake. Phys. Med. Biol. 2:295–306.

Specker, B.L., D. Miller, E.J. Norman, H. Greene, and K.C. Hayes. 1988. Increased urinary methylmalonic acid excretion in breast-fed infants of vegetarian mothers and identification of an acceptable dietary source of vitamin B12. Am. J. Clin. Nutr. 47:89–92.

Stewart, J.S., P.D. Roberts, and A.V. Hoffbrand. 1970. Response of dietary vitamin-B_{12} deficiency to physiological oral doses of cyanocobalamin. Lancet 2:542–545.

Sullivan, L.W., and V. Herbert. 1965. Studies on the minimum daily requirements for vitamin B_{12}. Hematopoietic responses to 0.1 microgram of cyanocobalamin or coenzyme B_{12} and comparison of their relative potency. N. Engl. J. Med. 272:340–346.

Thomas, M.R., S.M. Sneed, C. Wei, P.A. Nail, M. Wilson, and E.E. Sprinkle III. 1980. The effects of vitamin C, vitamin B_6, vitamin B_{12}, folic acid, riboflavin, and thiamin on the breast milk and maternal status of well-nourished women at 6 months postpartum. Am. J. Clin. Nutr. 33:2151–2156.

USDA (U.S. Department of Agriculture). 1986. Nationwide Food Consumption Survey Continuing Survey of Food Intakes by Individuals: Men 19–50 Years, 1 Day, 1985. Report No. 85-3. Nutrition Monitoring Division, Human Nutrition Information Service. U.S. Department of Agriculture, Hyattsville, Md. 94 pp.

USDA (U.S. Department of Agriculture). 1987. Nationwide Food Consumption Survey Continuing Survey of Food Intakes by Individuals: Women 19–50 Years and Their Children 1–5 Years, 4 Days, 1985. Report No. 85-4. Nutrition Monitoring Division, Human Nutrition Information Service. U.S. Department of Agriculture, Hyattsville, Md. 182 pp.

BIOTIN

Biotin is a sulfur-containing vitamin essential for several species, including humans. It is a component of various foods and is synthesized in the lower gastrointestinal tract by microorganisms and some fungi. The chemically related compounds oxybiotin and biocytin are also biologically active for some species. (For a more detailed discussion of the role of biotin in human nutrition, see Bonjour, 1985.)

Biotin is an integral part of enzymes that transport carboxyl units and fix carbon dioxide in animal tissue. The conversion of biotin to the active coenzyme is dependent on magnesium and adenosine triphosphate (ATP) (Bonjour, 1984). Two biotin enzymes, pyruvate carboxylase and acetyl-coenzyme A (CoA) carboxylase, play essential roles in gluconeogenesis and fatty acid synthesis, respectively. Extensive fatty infiltration of the liver and kidney, hypoglycemia, and depressed gluconeogenesis in the liver of biotin-deficient chicks provide further evidence of the importance of biotin in carbohydrate and lipid metabolism (Bannister, 1976). Two other biotin enzymes, propionyl-CoA carboxylase and 3-methylcrotonyl CoA carboxylase, are required for propionate metabolism and the catabolism of branched-chain amino acids. Low activity of biotin enzymes results in the urinary excretion of organic acids (the nature of which is determined by the metabolic step that is blocked), skin rash, and hair loss. Multiple carboxylase deficiencies are usually due to defective holocarboxylase synthetase, which is required for the conversion of inactive apocarboxylase to form active carboxylases through the addition of biotin (Sweetman, 1981). This inborn error of metabolism can be overcome by large doses (10 to 40 mg) of biotin (Wolf and Feldman, 1982). Another genetic defect results in a deficiency of biotinidase, an enzyme that releases protein-bound biotin and cleaves biocytin so that the biotin can be recycled (Wolf and Feldman, 1982).

General Signs of Deficiency

In adult humans and most animals, biotin deficiency can be produced by the ingestion of large amounts of avidin—the biotin-binding glycoprotein found only in raw egg white (Baugh et al., 1968). Biotin deficiency is characterized by anorexia, nausea, vomiting, glossitis, pallor, mental depression, alopecia and a dry scaly dermatitis, and an increase in serum cholesterol and bile pigments. Symptoms of hair loss have been observed in two adults on long-term total parenteral nutrition (TPN) without added biotin following extensive gut resection, which decreases the amount produced by intestinal biosynthesis (Innis and Allardyce, 1983), and in children on TPN (McClain, 1983). Symptoms were alleviated with 200 to 300 μg of biotin per day. Hair loss in an infant on TPN for 5 months was reversed by administering 10 mg of biotin (Mock et al., 1981). Evidence indicates that the seborrheic dermatitis of infants under 6 months of age is due to nutritional biotin deficiency. In such cases, blood levels and urinary excretion of the vitamin are depressed. Prompt improvement occurs with therapeutic doses of the vitamin—approximately 5 mg/day (Bonjour, 1985).

Dietary Sources and Usual Intakes

The best sources of biotin are liver (100 to 200 μg/100 g), egg yolk (16 μg/100 g), soy flour (60 to 70 μg/100 g), cereals (3 to 30 μg/100 g), and yeast (100 to 200 μg/100 g). Fruit and meat are poor sources, each containing from 0.6 to 2.3 μg of biotin per 100 g (Guilarte, 1985; Hoppner and Lampi, 1983; Paul and Southgate, 1978). The bioavailability of biotin varies considerably, depending on whether it is present in the biologically available unbound form as it is in most foods or in the unavailable bound form in wheat.

Information on the biotin content of food provided in tables of food composition is not complete. As a result, intake of biotin is seldom considered in nutrient consumption studies. In a study by Marshall et al. (1985), biochemical analyses of duplicate samples of U.S. diets indicated that biotin intakes were 28 to 42 μg/day. Dietary biotin consumed in Western Europe is estimated to range from 50 to 100 μg/day (Bonjour, 1985).

Intestinal Synthesis

Biotin is synthesized by intestinal microorganisms, but the extent of its availability for absorption is not established. The combined urinary and fecal excretion of biotin can exceed the dietary intake. Thus, fecal excretion apparently comprises biotin synthesized in the gut as well as unabsorbed dietary biotin. The urine contains biotin absorbed from the diet, from body stores, and, possibly, from intestinal synthesis. Urinary values range from less than 6 to 50 μg/day (Baker, 1985; Marshall et al., 1985).

Information on blood levels is so variable that it is of little diagnostic value. Men whose diets contained 28 to 42 μg/day had serum biotin levels ranging from 627 to 737 pg/ml (Marshall et al., 1985). Serum, urinary, and dietary biotin were correlated.

Estimated Safe and Adequate Daily Dietary Intakes

Adults The lack of definitive studies of biotin requirements make it difficult to estimate an allowance. A daily dose of 60 μg has maintained adults on total parenteral nutrition symptom-free for 6 months in the absence of meaningful intestinal synthesis (Innis and Allardyne, 1983).

Diets supplying 28 to 42 μg of biotin per day were associated with urinary excretion of 20 to 24 μg/day in volunteers. There was no indication of inadequate status in the subjects. In view of the incomplete knowledge of the bioavailability of biotin in foods and of the uncertain contribution of intestinal synthesis to the total intake, a range of 30 to 100 μg is provisionally recommended for adults. This range is lower than that recommended in the previous edition of the RDA, because improved analytical methods for biotin have reduced the estimates of daily intakes compatible with good health.

Pregnancy and Lactation   Blood biotin levels are significantly lower in pregnant than in nonpregnant women and fall progressively throughout gestation. However, low blood biotin levels are not associated with low birth weight infants (Bonjour, 1984). Thus, no increment for pregnancy is recommended. Data are not sufficient for a recommendation to be made for lactation.

Infants and Children   The biotin content of human milk, all in the free, available form, has been variously reported as 3 to 4.7 (Goldsmith et al., 1982), 7 (Paul and Southgate, 1978), and 20 μg/liter (Heard et al., 1987). If a daily milk consumption is assumed to be 750 ml, the intake of infants would range from 2 to 15 μg/day, depending on which analysis is accepted. An intake of 10 and 15 μg/day is tentatively recommended for formula-fed infants during the first and second 6 months, respectively, in agreement with the recommendations of the American Academy of Pediatrics for biotin in infant formulas (AAP, 1976). Recommended intakes for children and adolescents are gradually increased to adult levels above age 11.

Excessive Intakes and Toxicity

There have been no reports of toxicity associated with intakes as high as 10 mg daily (LSRO, 1978).

References

AAP (American Academy of Pediatrics). 1976. Commentary on breast feeding and infant formulas, including proposed standards for formulas. Pediatrics 57:278–285.

Baker, H. 1985. Assessment of biotin status: clinical implications. Ann. N.Y. Acad. Sci. 447:129–132.

Bannister, D.W. 1976. The biochemistry of fatty liver and kidney syndrome. Biochem. J. 156:167–173.

Baugh, C.M., J.W. Malone, and C.E. Butterworth, Jr. 1968. Human biotin deficiency. A case history of biotin deficiency induced by raw egg consumption in a cirrhotic patient. Am. J. Clin. Nutr. 21:173–182.

Bonjour, J.-P. 1984. Biotin. Pp. 403–435 in L.J. Machlin, ed. Handbook of Vitamins: Nutritional, Biochemical and Clinical Aspects. Marcel Dekker, New York.

Bonjour, J.-P. 1985. Biotin in human nutrition. Ann. N.Y. Acad. Sci. 447:97–104.

Goldsmith, S.J., R.R. Eitenmiller, R.M. Feeley, H.M. Barnhart, and F.C. Maddox. 1982. Biotin content of human milk during early lactational states. Nutr. Res. 2:579–583.

Guilarte, T.R. 1985. Analysis of biotin levels in selected foods using a radiometric-microbiological method. Nutr. Rep. Int. 32:837–845.

Heard, G.S., J.B. Redmond, and B. Wolf. 1987. Distribution and bioavailability of biotin in human milk. Fed. Proc. 46:897.

Hoppner, K., and B. Lampi. 1983. The biotin content of breakfast cereals. Nutr. Rep. Int. 28:793–798.

Innis, S.M., and D.B. Allardyce. 1983. Possible biotin deficiency in adults receiving long-term total parenteral nutrition. Am. J. Clin. Nutr. 37:185–187.

LSRO (Life Sciences Research Office). 1978. Evaluation of the Health Aspects of Biotin as a Food Ingredient. SCOGS 92. Federation of American Societies for Experimental Biology, Bethesda, Md. 16 pp.

Marshall, M.W., J.T. Judd, and H. Baker. 1985. Effects of low and high-fat diets varying in ratio of polyunsaturated to saturated fatty acids on biotin intakes and biotin in serum, red cells and urine of adult men. Nutr. Res. 5:801–814.

McClain, C.J. 1983. Biotin deficiency complicating parenteral alimentation. J. Am. Med. Assoc. 250:1028.

Mock, D.M., A.A. deLorimer, W.M. Liebman, L. Sweetman, and H. Baker. 1981. Biotin deficiency: an unusual complication of parenteral alimentation. N. Engl. J. Med. 304:820–823.

Paul, A.A., and D.A.T. Southgate. 1978. The Composition of Foods. Her Majesty's Stationery Office, London.

Sweetman, L. 1981. Two forms of biotin-responsive multiple carboxylase deficiency. J. Inherited Metab. Dis. 4:53–54.

Wolf, B., and G.L. Feldman. 1982. The biotin-dependent carboxylase deficiencies. Am. J. Hum. Genet. 34:699–716.

PANTOTHENIC ACID

Pantothenic acid, a B-complex vitamin, plays its primary physiological roles as a component of the coenzyme A molecule and within the 4'-phosphopantetheine moiety of the acyl carrier protein of fatty acid synthetase, which serves in acyl-group activation and transfer reactions (McCormick, 1988). These reactions are important in the release of energy from carbohydrates; in gluconeogenesis; in the synthesis and degradation of fatty acids; in the synthesis of such vital compounds as sterols and steroid hormones, porphyrins, and acetylcholine; and in acylation reactions in general (Abiko, 1975; Goldman and Vagelos, 1964).

General Signs of Deficiency

Dietary deficiency of pantothenic acid in animals results in a broad spectrum of biochemical defects. These manifest themselves in a variety of abnormalities: retarded growth rates in young animals; infertility, abortion, and frequent neonatal deaths; abnormalities of skin, hair, pigmentation, and feathers; neuromuscular disorder; gastrointestinal malfunction; adrenal cortical failure; and sudden death (Novelli, 1953).

Evidence of dietary deficiency has not been clinically recognized in humans, but deficiency symptoms have been produced by administering a metabolic antagonist, ω-methylpantothenic acid (Hodges et al., 1959), and more recently by feeding subjects a semisynthetic diet virtually free of pantothenic acid for 9 weeks (Fry et al., 1976). The young adult males studied by Fry and colleagues appeared listless and complained of fatigue after 9 weeks on the pantothenic acid-free diet; blood and urinary levels of this nutrient were significantly lower compared to controls. Naturally occurring pantothenic acid deficiencies have not been reliably documented. However, they have been implicated in the "burning feet" syndrome observed among prisoners of war and among malnourished individuals in the Far East, since the symptoms appeared to respond to pantothenic acid preparations and not to other members of the vitamin B complex (Glusman, 1947).

Dietary Sources and Usual Intakes

Pantothenic acid is widely distributed among foods. It is especially abundant in animal tissues, whole grain cereals, and legumes. Smaller amounts are found in milk, vegetables, and fruits. Synthesis of pantothenic acid by intestinal microflora has been suspected, but the amount produced and the availability of the vitamin from this source are unknown. The apparent absence of pantothenic acid deficiency in the human population may therefore be attributed both to its ubiquity in foods and to possible additional contributions from intestinal flora.

The usual intake of pantothenic acid in the United States has been reported to range from 5 to 10 mg/day (Fox and Linkswiler, 1961; Fry et al., 1976). In two more recent studies, investigators reported average intakes of approximately 6 mg/day (Srinivasan et al., 1981; Tarr et al., 1981). Srinivasan and colleagues conducted a study in an elderly population, and showed no difference in intakes between institutionalized and noninstitutionalized subjects. In another study,

Johnson and Nitzke (1975) found that diets consumed by a group of low-income women provided about 4 mg of pantothenic acid per day. In a group of 7- to 9-year-old children, diets that met the recommended allowances for all other nutrients provided 4 to 5 mg of pantothenic acid daily (Pace et al., 1961). In a small group of pregnant, postpartum, and nonpregnant teenagers, the calculated dietary intakes were lower, ranging from 1.1 to 7.2 mg/day (Cohenour and Calloway, 1972).

Estimated Safe and Adequate Daily Dietary Intakes

Adults Urinary excretion generally correlates with dietary intake of pantothenic acid, although individual variation is large. Adults who consume 5 to 7 mg of pantothenic acid daily excrete 2 to 7 mg/day in the urine and 1 to 2 mg/day in the feces (Fox and Linkswiler, 1961). In experimental diets, 10 mg/day has generally been selected for supplementation. At this level, subjects were found to excrete 5 to 7 mg/day in the urine (Fry et al., 1976). This evidence suggests that an intake of 4 to 7 mg/day should be safe and adequate for adults. The subcommittee concluded that there is insufficient evidence to set an RDA for pantothenic acid.

Pregnancy and Lactation The amounts of pantothenic acid secreted in milk can represent a large fraction of the usual dietary intake. Nonetheless, the absence of reports of pantothenic acid deficiency either in pregnant or lactating women indicates that present levels of consumption from the diet (e.g., more than 5 mg/day), possibly supplemented by intestinal microfloral synthesis, is adequate to cover the needs of pregnancy and lactation. Thus, the suggested intake for nonpregnant adults would appear to be adequate for this group.

Infants, Children, and Adolescents Reports of the mean pantothenic acid content of human milk have varied from 1 mg/day (Deodhar and Ramakrishnan, 1960) to 5 mg/day (Johnston et al., 1981), based on an average daily milk production of 750 ml. Song et al. (1984) reported a mean pantothenic acid content at 2 and 12 weeks postpartum of 2.57 mg/liter and 2.55 mg/liter, respectively, for mothers of full-term infants. These values are equivalent to approximately 1.9 mg/day in 750 ml of milk. The differences in the various reports may represent differences in maternal intakes or in analytical techniques. There are no reports of pantothenic acid deficiency in infants, suggesting that intake is adequate. The provisional recommended allowance is set at 2 to 3 mg/day for infants. Recommended intakes for children and adolescents are gradually increased to adult levels by age 11.

Excessive Intakes and Toxicity

Evidence suggests that pantothenic acid is relatively nontoxic. As much as 10 g of calcium pantothenate per day was given to young men for 6 weeks with no toxic symptoms reported (Ralli and Dumm, 1953). Other studies indicate that daily doses of 10 to 20 g may result in occasional diarrhea and water retention (Sebrell and Harris, 1954).

References

Abiko, Y. 1975. Metabolism of coenzyme A. Pp. 1–25 in D.M. Greenberg, ed. Metabolism of Sulfur Compounds, Vol. 7. Metabolic Pathways. Academic Press, New York.

Cohenour, S.H., and D.H. Calloway. 1972. Blood, urine and dietary panthothenic acid levels of pregnant teenagers. Am. J. Clin. Nutr. 25:512–517.

Deodhar, A.D., and C.V. Ramakrishnan. 1960. Studies on human lactation (relation between the dietary intake of lactating women and the chemical composition of milk with regard to vitamin content). J. Trop. Pediatr. 6:44–47.

Fox, H.M., and H. Linkswiler. 1961. Pantothenic acid excretion on three levels of intake. J. Nutr. 75:451–454.

Fry, P.C., H.M. Fox, and H.G. Tao. 1976. Metabolic reponse to a pantothenic acid deficient diet in humans. J. Nutr. Sci. Vitaminol. 22:339–346.

Glusman, M. 1947. Syndrome of "burning feet" (nutritional melalgia) as manifestation of nutritional deficiency. Am. J. Med. 3:211–223.

Goldman, P., and P.R. Vagelos. 1964. Acyl-transfer reactions (CoA-structure, function). Pp. 71–92 in M. Florkin and E. H. Stotz, eds. Comprehensive Biochemistry, Vol. 15. Group-Transfer Reactions. Elsevier, Amsterdam.

Hodges, R.E., W.B. Bean, M.A. Ohlson, and B. Bleiler. 1959. Human pantothenic acid deficiency produced by omega-methylpantothenic acid. J. Clin. Invest. 38:1421–1425.

Johnson, N.E., and S. Nitzke. 1975. Nutritional adequacy of diets of a selected group of low-income women: identification of some related factors. Home Econ. Res. J. 3:241–246.

Johnston, L., L. Vaughan, and H.M. Fox. 1981. Pantothenic acid content of human milk. Am. J. Clin. Nutr. 34:2205–2209.

McCormick, D.B. 1988. Pantothenic acid. Pp. 383–387 in M.E. Shils and V.R. Young, eds. Modern Nutrition in Health and Disease, 7th ed. Lea & Febiger, Philadelphia.

Novelli, G.D. 1953. Metabolic significance of B-vitamins: Symposium; Metabolic functions of pantothenic acid. Physiol. Rev. 33:525–543.

Pace, J.K., L.B. Stier, D.D. Taylor, and P.S. Goodman. 1961. Metabolic patterns in preadolescent children. V. Intake and urinary excretion of pantothenic acid and of folic acid. J. Nutr. 74:345–351.

Ralli, E.P., and M.E. Dumm. 1953. Relation of pantothenic acid to adrenal cortical function. Vitam. Horm. 11:133–158.

Sebrell, W.H., Jr., and R.S. Harris, eds. 1954. Pantothenic acid. Pp. 591–694 in The Vitamins: Chemistry, Physiology, Pathology, Vol. 2. Academic Press, New York.

Srinivasan, V., N. Christensen, B.W. Wyse, and R.G. Hansen. 1981. Pantothenic acid nutritional status in the elderly—institutionalized and noninstitutionalized. Am. J. Clin. Nutr. 34:1736–1742.

Song, W.O., G.M. Chan, B.W. Wyse, and R.G. Hansen. 1984. Effect of pantothenic acid status on the content of the vitamin in human milk. Am. J. Clin. Nutr. 40:317–324.

Tarr, J.B., T. Tamura, and E.L.R. Stokstad. 1981. Availability of vitamin B_6 and pantothenate in an average American diet in man. Am. J. Clin. Nutr. 34:1328–1337.

9
Minerals

CALCIUM

The adult body contains approximately 1,200 g of calcium, approximately 99% of which is present in the skeleton. Bone mineral consists of two chemically and physically distinct calcium phosphate pools—an amorphous phase and a loosely crystallized phase. The skeleton contains two major forms of bone: trabecular (spongy) bone, exemplified by the vertebral bodies, and denser cortical bone, such as the femur. Bone is constantly turning over, a continuous process of resorption and formation. In children and adolescents, the rate of formation of bone mineral predominates over the rate of resorption. In later life, resorption predominates over formation. Therefore, in normal aging, there is a gradual loss of bone (Arnaud, 1988).

The remaining 1% of body calcium is found in extracellular fluids, intracellular structures, and cell membranes. This extraskeletal calcium plays an essential role in such vital functions as nerve conduction, muscle contraction, blood clotting, and membrane permeability. Blood calcium concentration is maintained within very narrow limits by the interplay of several hormones (1,25-dihydroxycholecalciferol, parathyroid hormone, calcitonin, estrogen, testosterone, and possibly others), which control calcium absorption and excretion, as well as bone metabolism.

Levels of soft tissue calcium are maintained at the expense of bone in the face of inadequate calcium intake or absorption. Under such circumstances, there is either inadequate mineralization of bone in the young or mineral is withdrawn from bone with a consequent reduction of bone strength.

174

Calcium is lost from the body in feces, urine, and sweat. The fecal calcium consists of unabsorbed dietary calcium, the amount of which depends on dietary intake and other factors, and a small portion of the endogenously secreted calcium (about 100 to 150 mg/day), which escapes reabsorption. Urinary calcium excretion of adults is about 100 to 250 mg/day, but varies widely among persons consuming self-selected diets (Nordin et al., 1967). Urinary excretion is influenced by hormonal and dietary factors. Among the latter are protein, sodium, and some carbohydrates, which increase calcium excretion, and phosphorus, which decreases it. Except under conditions of extreme sweating, loss of calcium from the skin is small (about 15 mg/day).

Calcium Absorption

Intestinal absorption of calcium is variably influenced by several nutritional and physiological factors (Avioli, 1988). Studies of calcium absorption have frequently been flawed by failure to include the extended period (4 weeks or more) required for adaptation to changes in dietary intake and to control for intervening dietary variables. Nonetheless, the literature is consistent on several points. The efficiency of absorption is increased during periods of high physiologic requirement. Thus, children may absorb up to 75% of ingested calcium as compared to the 20 to 40% typically observed in young adults in the United States. Absorption is impaired in the aged (Heaney et al., 1982). A higher percentage of ingested calcium is absorbed at low intakes than at high intakes. Above an intake of about 800 mg/day in normal adults, absorption is approximately 15% of the amount ingested (Heaney et al., 1975). Vitamin D is a recognized promoter of calcium absorption. The role of protein and phosphorus is less clear. Dietary protein enhances calcium absorption (McCance et al., 1942) in the protein intake range between inadequate and adequate levels, but has little additional effect beyond RDA levels of protein (Chu et al., 1975). The effect of phosphorus differs with the source, but, excluding phytate phosphorus (see below), this element appears to have little if any depressing effect on calcium absorption (Spencer et al., 1978, 1986).

It is uncertain if there are biologically important differences in the absorption of calcium from different foods or diets. In animal models, the presence of lactose tends to enhance paracellular calcium absorption, but this effect has not been consistently demonstrated (Scrimshaw and Murray, 1988). Phytate and oxalate bind calcium, rendering it insoluble, and certain fiber fractions may interfere with calcium absorption. These substances are believed to be of little practical importance at intakes typical for the U.S. diet (Judd et al., 1983; LSRO, 1987; Schwartz et al., 1986).

Dietary Sources and Usual Intakes

Calcium intake varies widely among individuals in the United States but is generally higher in males than in females. The 1977–1978 Nationwide Food Consumption Survey (USDA, 1984) reported an average daily intake of 743 mg for all people, ranging from 530 mg for women 35 to 50 years old to 1,179 mg for 12- to 18-year-old boys. No group of adult females had a calcium intake equal to or greater than the RDA of 800 mg. Black women ingested less dietary calcium than whites (452 compared to 640 mg/day) (USDA, 1987).

Dairy products contribute more than 55% of the calcium intake of the U.S. population (Block et al., 1985). Other contributors to the daily intake of calcium are some leafy green vegetables (such as broccoli, kale, and collards), lime-processed tortillas, calcium-precipitated tofu, and calcium-fortified foods. Bones, especially the soft bones of fish (e.g., sardines, salmon) and tips of poultry leg bones, are rich and often unrecognized sources of calcium. Water is a variable source. Several proprietary antacid preparations are calcium salts that may constitute an underreported calcium source.

Bone Formation and Retention

Although calcium is a major constituent of bone, it is only one of many factors affecting bone health. Genetic influences determine bone mass; sex hormones and physical activity influence bone metabolism. Many dietary constituents are either essential for, or complementary to, the proper utilization of calcium, including vitamin D (Parfitt et al., 1982), copper (Davis and Mertz, 1987), zinc (Hambidge et al., 1986), manganese (Hurley and Keen, 1987), fluorine (Krishnamachari, 1987), silicon (Carlisle, 1986), and boron (Nielsen, 1987).

The growth of the skeleton requires a positive calcium balance until peak bone mass is reached. Mineralization of bone continues for some years after longitudinal bone growth has ceased. Most of the accumulation of bone mineral occurs in humans by about 20 years of age, but some bone mineral is added during the third decade. Bone mass then begins to decline slowly during the fifth decade in both sexes, as evidenced by progressive reduction of bone density. The rate of loss accelerates greatly about the time of menopause in women and remains high for several years. Bone loss accelerates much later in men (by a decade or more). This results in gradually diminishing bone strength and increased risk of fractures. The risk of fracture is less at a given age in people who have achieved larger bone mass during the period of bone mass accretion than in those with lower peak bone mass (Arnaud, 1988; Heaney, 1986).

Peak bone mass appears to be related to intake of calcium during the years of bone mineralization. Investigations have usually involved estimation of past calcium intake from a history of food consumption patterns, in which differing habitual milk consumption is the chief contributor to differences in calcium intake. Thus, intakes of other nutrients (e.g., protein, phosphorus, and, importantly, the vitamin D added to most milk in the United States) are likely to covary with calcium. In a study of two population groups in Yugoslavia with different, long-standing intake patterns (500 and 1,100 mg of calcium per day), greater bone mass was found at all ages and in both sexes in the high calcium community (Matkovic et al., 1979). Since the rate of bone loss was the same in adults of the two communities, the finding of more bone mass in the older age groups of the high-calcium district must reflect higher peak bone mass attainment. In studies conducted in the United States, investigators have reported significant correlations between current bone density and past milk or calcium intake in adult women (Halious and Anderson, 1989; Hurxthal and Vose, 1969; Sandler et al., 1985). In another U.S. study, present calcium intake was compared with bone density of postmenopausal women in two Iowa communities where the water supply contained different levels of calcium over at least a 50–year period (60 compared to 375 mg/liter), resulting in average calcium intakes of 964 compared to 1,326 mg/day, respectively (Sowers et al., 1985). There were no detectable differences in measured bone density between communities. After adjustment for confounding factors, there was a small but significantly higher bone density in the Iowa women who currently consumed *both* 800 mg or more of calcium and 400 IU or more of vitamin D per day. There is, however, no clear evidence that bone density of postmenopausal women is related to concurrent dietary calcium intake within a wide range (Garn, 1970; Garn et al., 1969) except, perhaps, where this reflects a high-calcium food consumption pattern established in childhood.

The postmenopausal rate of decline in bone mineral is strongly dependent on estrogen status. Estrogen replacement slows the rate of bone loss. Evidence that supplementary calcium (1.5 to 2.5 g/day) can retard the rate of postmenopausal bone loss is mixed (NRC, 1989), but the balance of evidence suggests that calcium alone has only a small effect on cortical bone loss and none on trabecular bone (Freudenheim, 1986; Riis et al., 1987). Combined daily treatment with 0.3 mg of conjugated estrogens plus 1 g of calcium supplement has, however, been reported to be as effective as 0.6 mg of conjugated estrogen (widely accepted to be the minimum effective dose for prevention of bone loss) without added calcium (Ettinger et al., 1987). The observed inverse relationship between body weight and risk of hip fracture in older women (heavier women having less risk of fracture) may be due in part to the maintenance of higher levels of estrogen by peripheral conversion of precursor steroids to estrogen in adipose tissue (Kiel et al., 1987).

In the subcommittee's judgment, the most promising nutritional approach to reduce the risk of osteoporosis in later life is to ensure a calcium intake that allows the development of each individual's genetically programmed peak bone mass during the formative years. The importance of meeting recommended allowances at all ages is stressed, but with special attention to intakes throughout childhood to age 25 years.

Relationship to Phosphorus and Protein Intakes

The level of dietary protein and phosphorus can affect the metabolism of, and requirement for, calcium, primarily as a result of their opposing effects on urinary calcium brought about by changes in fractional tubular reabsorption of calcium. The effect on urinary excretion outweighs the small effects on absorption described above. An increase in protein intake reduces fractional tubular reabsorption (Allen et al., 1979; Kim and Linkswiler, 1979) and results in an increase in urinary calcium excretion (Johnson et al., 1970; Margen et al., 1974). In contrast, an increase in phosphorus intake increases fractional reabsorption and causes urinary calcium to decrease (Hegsted et al., 1981; Spencer et al., 1978). Because of the opposing effects of protein and phosphorus on urinary calcium and calcium retention, a simultaneous increase in the intake of both, a pattern characterized by milk, eggs, and meat ingestion, has but little effect on calcium balance at recommended levels of calcium intake (Spencer et al., 1988).

The low ratio of calcium to phosphorus in the U.S. diet was of concern in the past. Animal studies indicated that excessive phosphorus intake led to secondary hyperparathyroidism, resulting in loss of calcium from the skeleton (LSRO, 1981). This effect was not seen in monkeys (Anderson et al., 1977), and studies in humans have failed to demonstrate effects of dietary phosphorus intake on calcium balance at adequate levels of calcium intake (Spencer et al., 1988).

Other Potential Functions

A high intake of calcium has been associated with lower blood pressure in some studies (McCarron et al., 1984), but not in others (Ackley et al., 1983). Animal studies show that high levels of dietary calcium protect against cell proliferation in the colon induced by fat and bile acids (Bird, 1986; Wargovich et al., 1983). The evidence from human studies is, however, insufficient to support an inference that high calcium diets protect against the development of colon tumors. These subjects are reviewed in the Food and Nutrition Board report *Diet and Health* (NRC, 1989).

Recommended Allowances

Adults and Adolescents　An optimal calcium intake is difficult to define, given the substantial adaptive capacity and the long lag period before changes in status can be detected. It is not surprising that recommendations in different countries vary widely, from a low of 400 mg/day for women in Thailand to a high of 1,000 mg for both sexes over 75 years of age in the Netherlands. Concern for the high proportion of postmenopausal women at risk for osteoporosis has led some to suggest that the RDA for calcium should be increased markedly (NIH, 1984). This subcommittee is not persuaded by the evidence in hand that the long-standing RDAs should be revised upward in response to this medical concern. Nor is the subcommittee convinced that levels should be lowered to those recommended by international groups (e.g., FAO, 1962) despite the evidence that many population groups seemingly maintain satisfactory status with much lower intakes of calcium than the RDA.

The age at which peak bone mass is attained is uncertain, but probably is not less than 25 years. The subcommittee thus recommends an extra calcium allowance to permit full mineral deposition through age 24 rather than through age 18 years, as in previous editions of the RDA.

The recommended calcium allowance for adults is based on an estimate of 200 to 250 mg/day of obligatory loss and an estimated absorption rate of 30 to 40%. Calcium accretion during the growing years averages 140 to 165 mg/day and may be as high as 400 to 500 mg/day during the pubertal growth period (Garn, 1970). Intestinal calcium absorption is efficient in youth and adapts in relation to needs. In setting the RDA, however, the absorption rate is conservatively estimated to be 40%.

An intake of 1,200 mg is recommended for both sex groups from ages 11 to 24 years. For older age groups, the previous allowance of 800 mg is retained. These amounts of calcium can easily be obtained if dairy products are included in the diet. A balanced diet furnishes, in addition to calcium, other nutrients necessary for bone health. The subcommittee emphasizes that its recommendations do not address the possible needs of persons who may have osteoporosis and should receive medical attention.

Pregnancy and Lactation The newborn contains approximately 30 g of calcium, most of which is deposited during the third trimester of intrauterine development (Pitkin, 1985). Calcium retention is 200 to 250 mg/day during that period. Human milk contains approximately 320 mg calcium/liter. This concentration corresponds to 240 mg in the average daily milk secretion of 750 ml; 300 mg encompasses the probable upper boundary of production (+2 SDs).

The calcium absorption rate has been reported to increase during pregnancy and lactation in rats (Halloran and DeLuca, 1980) and adolescent girls (Heaney and Skillman, 1971). There is no clear relation between women's bone health and either their number of pregnancies or lactation history in populations that consume currently recommended amounts of calcium (Koetting and Wardlaw, 1988; Lambke et al., 1977). This evidence suggests it is prudent to recommend a calcium intake of 1,200 mg throughout pregnancy and lactation, irrespective of age.

Infants and Children Infants thrive on an average intake of 240 mg of calcium from 750 ml of human milk, of which they retain approximately two-thirds. Allowing 25% for variance, intake would be 300 mg, of which 200 mg is absorbed. The retention of calcium from formulas based on cow's milk is less than one-half. Therefore, the recommendation for formula-fed infants is 400 mg/day for the first 6 months of life. This amount is provided by typical infant formulas now in use in the United States. An allowance of 600 mg/day would suffice for the next 6 months and 800 mg/day at ages 1 to 10 years. These latter allowances are arbitrary, since specific data on requirements of this age group are lacking.

Excessive Intakes and Toxicity

Although no adverse effects have been observed in many healthy adults consuming up to 2,500 mg of calcium per day, high intakes may induce constipation and place up to half of otherwise healthy hypercalciuric males at increased risk of urinary stone formation. A high calcium intake may inhibit the intestinal absorption of iron, zinc, and other essential minerals (Greger, 1988). Ingestion of very large amounts may result in hypercalciuria, hypercalcemia, and deterioration in renal function in both sexes (Avioli, 1988). Supplementation to a total calcium intake much above the RDA is not recommended.

References

Ackley, S., E. Barrett-Connor, and L. Suarez. 1983. Dairy products, calcium and blood pressure. Am. J. Clin. Nutr. 38:457–461.

Allen, L.H., E.A. Oddoye, and S. Margen. 1979. Protein-induced hypercalciuria: a longer term study. Am. J. Clin. Nutr. 32:741–749.

Anderson, M.P., R.D. Hunt, H.J. Griffiths, K.W. McIntyre, and R.E. Zimmerman. 1977. Long-term effect of low dietary calcium:phosphate ratio on the skeleton of *Cebus albifrons* monkeys. J. Nutr. 107:834–839.

Arnaud, C.D. 1988. Mineral and bone homeostasis. Pp. 1469–1479 In J.B. Wyngaarden, L.H. Smith, Jr., and F. Plum, eds. Cecil Textbook of Medicine, 18th ed. W.B. Saunders, Philadelphia.

Avioli, L.V. 1988. Calcium and phosphorus. Pp. 142–158 in M.E. Shils and V.R. Young, eds. Modern Nutrition in Health and Disease, 7th ed. Lea & Febiger, Philadelphia.

Bird, R.P. 1986. Effect of dietary components on the pathobiology of colonic epithelium: possible relationship with colon tumorigenesis. Lipids 21:289–291.

Block, G., C.M. Dresser, A.M. Hartman, and M.D. Carroll. 1985. Nutrient sources in the American diet: quantitative data from the NHANES II survey. I. Vitamins and minerals. Am. J. Epidemiol. 122:13–26.

Carlisle, E.M. 1986. Silicon. Pp. 373–390 in W. Mertz, ed. Trace Elements in Human and Animal Nutrition, 5th ed., Vol. 2. Academic Press, New York.

Chu, J.Y., S. Margen, and F.M. Costa. 1975. Studies on calcium metabolism. II. Effects of low calcium and variable protein intake on human calcium metabolism. Am. J. Clin. Nutr. 28:1028–1035.

Davis, G.K., and W. Mertz. 1987. Copper. Pp. 301–364 in W. Mertz, ed. Trace Elements in Human and Animal Nutrition, 5th ed., Vol. 1. Academic Press, New York.

Ettinger, B., H.K. Genant, and C.E. Cann. 1987. Postmenopausal bone loss is prevented by treatment with low-dosage estrogen with calcium. Ann. Intern. Med. 106:40–45.

FAO (Food and Agricultural Organization). 1962. Calcium Requirements. Report of a Joint FAO/WHO Expert Consultation. FAO Nutrition Meeting Report No. 30. Food and Agriculture Organization, Rome.

Freudenheim, J.L., N.E. Hohnson, and E.L. Smith. 1986. Relationships between usual nutrient intake and bone-mineral content of women 35–65 years of age; longitudinal and cross-sectional analyses. Am. J. Clin. Nutr. 44:863–876.

Garn, S.M. 1970. The earlier gain and the later loss of cortical bone. In Nutritional Perspectives. Charles C Thomas, Springfield, Ill. 146 pp.

Garn, S.M., C.G. Rohmann, B. Wagner, G.H. Davila, and W. Ascoli. 1969. Population similarities in the onset and rate of adult endosteal bone loss. Clin. Orthop. 65:51–60.

Greger, J.L. 1988. Effect of variations in dietary protein, phosphorus, electrolytes and vitamin D on calcium and zinc metabolism. Pp. 205–227 in C.E. Bodwell and J.W. Erdman, Jr., eds. Nutrient Interactions. Marcel Dekker, Inc., New York.

Halious, L., and J.J.B. Anderson. 1989. Lifetime calcium intake and physical activity habits: independent and combined effects on the radial bone of healthy premenopausal Caucasian women. Am. J. Clin. Nutr. 49:534–541.

Halloran, B.P., and H.F. DeLuca. 1980. Calcium transport in small intestine during pregnancy and lactation. Am. J. Physiol. 239:E64-E68.

Hambidge, K.M., C.E. Casey, and N.F. Krebs. 1986. Zinc. Pp. 1–137 in W. Mertz, ed. Trace Elements in Human and Animal Nutrition, 5th ed., Vol. 2. Academic Press, New York.

Heaney, R.P. 1986. Calcium, bone health and osteoporosis. Pp. 255–301 in W.A. Peck, ed. Bone and Mineral Research/4. Elsevier, New York.

Heaney, R.P., and T.G. Skillman. 1971. Calcium metabolism in human pregnancy. J. Clin. Endocrinol. Metab. 33:661–670.

Heaney, R.P., P.D. Sarille, and R.R. Recker. 1975. Calcium absorption as a function of calcium intake. J. Lab. Clin. Med. 85:881–890.

Heaney, R.P., J.C. Gallagher, C.C. Johnston, R. Neer, A.M. Parfitt, and G.D. Whedon. 1982. Calcium nutrition and bone health in the elderly. Am. J. Clin. Nutr. 36:986–1013.

Hegsted, M.S., S.A. Schuette, M.B. Zemel, and H.M. Linkswiler. 1981. Urinary calcium and calcium balance in young men as affected by level of protein and phosphorus intake. J. Nutr. 111:553–562.

Hurley, J.S., and C.L. Keen. 1987. Manganese. Pp. 185–223 in W. Mertz, ed. Trace Elements in Human and Animal Nutrition, 5th ed., Vol. 1. Academic Press, New York.

Hurxthal, L.M., and C.P. Vose. 1969. The relationship of dietary calcium intake to radiographic bone density in normal and osteoporotic persons. Calcif. Tissue Res. 4:245–256.

Johnson, N.E., E.N. Alcantara, and H. Linkswiler. 1970. Effect of level of protein intake on urinary and fecal calcium and calcium retention of young adult males. J. Nutr. 100:1425–1430.

Judd, J.T., J.L. Kelsay, and W. Mertz. 1983. Potential risks from low-fat diets. Semin. Oncol. 10:273–280.

Kiel, D.P., D.T. Felson, J.J. Anderson, P.W.F. Wilson, and M.A. Moskowitz. 1987. Hip fracture and the use of estrogens in postmenopausal women. N. Engl. J. Med. 317:1169–1174.

Kim, Y., and H. Linkswiler. 1979. Effect of level of protein intake on calcium metabolism and on parathyroid and renal function in the adult human male. J. Nutr. 109:1399–1404.

Koetting, C.A., and G.M. Wardlaw. 1988. Wrist, spine and hip bone density in women with variable histories of lactation. Am. J. Clin. Nutr. 48:1479–1481.

Krishnamachari, K.A.V.R. 1987. Pp. 365–415 in W. Mertz, ed. Trace Elements in Human and Animal Nutrition, 5th ed., Vol. 1. Academic Press, New York.

Lambke, B., J. Bruhdin, and P. Moberg. 1977. Changes of bone mineral content during pregnancy and lactation. Acta Obstet. Gynecol. Scand. 56:217–219.

LSRO (Life Sciences Research Office). 1981. Effects of Dietary Factors on Skeletal Integrity in Adults: Calcium, Phosphorus, Vitamin D, and Protein. Federation of American Societies for Experimental Biology, Bethesda, Md.

LSRO (Life Sciences Research Office). 1987. Physiological Effects and Health Consequences of Dietary Fiber. Federation of American Societies for Experimental Biology, Bethesda, Md.

Margen, S., J-Y. Chu, N.A. Kaufmann, and D.H. Calloway. 1974. Studies in calcium metabolism. 1. The calciuretic effect of dietary protein. Am. J. Clin. Nutr. 27:540–549.

Matkovic, V., K. Kostial, I. Simonovic, R. Buzina, A. Brodarec, and B.E.C. Nordin. 1979. Bone status and fracture rates in two regions of Yugoslavia. Am. J. Clin. Nutr. 32:540–549.

McCance, R.A., E.M. Widdowson, and H. Lehmann. 1942. The effect of protein intake on the absorption of calcium and magnesium. Biochem. J. 36:686–691.

McCarron, D.A., C.D. Morris, H.J. Henry, and J.L. Stanton. 1984. Blood pressure and nutrient intake in the United States. Science 224:1392–1397.

Nielsen, F.H. 1987. Effect of dietary boron on mineral, estrogen, and testosterone metabolism in postmenopausal women. FASEB J. 1:394–397.

NIH (National Institutes of Health). 1984. Consensus Conference on Osteoporosis. J. Am. Med. Assoc. 252:799–802.

Nordin, B.E.C., A. Hodgkinson, and M. Peacock. 1967. The measurement and the meaning of urinary calcium. Clin. Orthop. 52:293–322.

NRC (National Research Council). 1989. Diet and Health: Implications for Reducing Chronic Disease Risk. Report of the Committee on Diet and Health, Food and Nutrition Board. National Academy Press, Washington, D.C. 750 pp.

Parfitt, A.M., J.C. Gallagher, R.P. Heaney, C.C. Johnston, R. Neer, and G.D. Whedon. 1982. Vitamin D and bone health in the elderly. Am. J. Clin. Nutr. 36:1014–1031.

Pitkin, R.M. 1985. Calcium metabolism in pregnancy and the perinatal period: a review. Am. J. Obst. Gynecol. 151:99–109.

Riis, B., K. Thomsen, and C. Christiansen. 1987. Does calcium supplementation prevent postmenopausal bone loss? A double-blind controlled clinical study. N. Engl. J. Med. 316:173–177.

Sandler, R.B., C.W. Slemenda, R.E. La Porte, J.A. Cauley, M.M. Schramm, M.L. Baresi, and A.M. Kriska. 1985. Postmenopausal bone density and milk consumption in childhood and adolescence. Am. J. Clin. Nutr. 42:270–274.

Schwartz, R. J. Apgar, and E.M. Wien. 1986. Apparent absorption and retention of Ca, Cu, Mg, Mn, and Zn from a diet containing bran. Am. J. Clin. Nutr. 43:444–455.

Scrimshaw, N.S., and E.A. Murray. 1988. The acceptability of milk and milk products in populations with a high prevalence of lactose intolerance. Am. J. Clin. Nutr. 48:342–390.

Sowers, M.F.R., R.B. Wallace, and J.H. Lemke. 1985. Correlates of midradius bone density among postmenopausal women: a community study. Am. J. Clin. Nutr. 41:1045–1053.

Spencer, H., L. Kramer, D. Osis, and C. Norris. 1978. Effect of phosphorus on the absorption of calcium and on the calcium balance in man. J. Nutr. 108:447–457.

Spencer, H., L. Kramer, N. Rubio, and D. Osis. 1986. The effect of phosphorus on endogenous fecal calcium excretion in man. Am. J. Clin. Nutr. 43:844–851.

Spencer, H., L. Kramer, and D. Osis. 1988. Do protein and phosphorus cause calcium loss? J. Nutr. 118:657–660.

USDA (U.S. Department of Agriculture). 1984. Nationwide Food Consumption Survey. Nutrient Intakes: Individuals in 48 States, Year 1977–78. Report No. I-2. Consumer Nutriton Division, Human Nutrition Information Service. U.S. Department of Agriculture, Hyattsville, Md. 439 pp.

USDA (U.S. Department of Agriculture). 1987. Nationwide Food Consumption Survey. Continuing Survey of Food Intakes of Individuals. Women 19–50 Years

and Their Children 1–5 Years, 4 Days, 1985. Report No. 85-4. Nutrition Monitoring Division, Human Nutrition Information Service, Hyattsville, Md. 182 pp.
Wargovich, M.J., V.W.S. Eng, H.L. Newmark, and W.R. Bruce. 1983. Calcium ameliorates the toxic effect of deoxycholic acid on colonic epithelium. Carcinogenesis 4:1205–1207.

PHOSPHORUS

Phosphorus is an essential component of bone mineral, where it occurs in the mass ratio of 1 phosphorus to 2 calcium. Approximately 85% (700 g) of the phosphorus in the adult body is found in bone. Phosphorus also plays an important role in many and varied chemical reactions in the body. It is present in soft tissues as soluble phosphate ion; in lipids, proteins, carbohydrates, and nucleic acid in an ester or anhydride linkage; and in enzymes as a modulator of their activities. Energy for metabolic processes derives largely from the phosphate bonds of adenosine triphosphate (ATP), creatine phosphate, and similar compounds.

Phosphorus is efficiently absorbed by the small intestine as free phosphate (Avioli, 1988). Phosphorus absorption probably takes place by three different mechanisms: (1) calcium-coupled, vitamin D-dependent; (2) noncalcium-coupled, vitamin D-dependent; and (3) noncalcium coupled, vitamin D-independent (Parfitt and Kleerekoper, 1980).

Infants absorb from 65 to 70% of the phosphorus in cow's milk and 85 to 90% of that in human milk. Children and adults absorb 50 to 70% of the phosphorus in normal diets and as much as 90% when the intake is low (LSRO, 1981).

Polyphosphate (sodium hexametaphosphate), which is used in the processing of food, is efficiently hydrolyzed to orthophosphate in the intestine, where it is well absorbed (Zemel and Linkswiler, 1981). Approximately 50% of phytate phosphorus is absorbed (Parfitt et al., 1964).

Dietary Sources and Usual Intakes

Phosphorus is present in nearly all foods. The amount available in the food supply from unprocessed primary commodities, about 1,430 to 1,520 mg per capita per day, has been relatively constant during the past 75 years, despite marked changes in food consumption patterns (Bunch, 1987). The mean daily phosphorus intake is approximately 1,500 mg/day for adult males (USDA, 1986) and 1,000 mg/day for adult females (USDA, 1987). True intakes may be 15 to 20%

higher, however, since the phosphorus supplied by numerous food additives in processed foods is typically not accounted for in tables of food composition (Oenning et al., 1988).

Major contributors of phosphorus are protein-rich foods and cereal grains. About half the food phosphorus in the U.S. diet comes from milk, meat, poultry, and fish. Cereal products contribute about 12%. Diets based heavily on convenience foods may derive 20 to 30% of phosphorus from food additives (Greger and Krystofiak, 1982).

Meats, poultry, and fish, exclusive of bone, contain 15 to 20 times more phosphorus than calcium. There is twice as much phosphorus as calcium in eggs, grains, nuts, dry beans, peas, and lentils. Only milk, natural cheeses, green leafy vegetables, and bone contain more calcium than phosphorus. Cow's milk contains both more calcium and phophorus than does human milk, and the ratios of the elements differ widely. The ratio of calcium to phosphorus in cow's milk is 1.3 to 1 and that in human milk is 2.3 to 1.

The calcium-to-phosphorus ratio in the U.S. diet varies, depending on food consumption patterns. The calcium-to-phosphorus ratio is higher in diets of infants and children than in diets of adults. The average ratio is 1 to 1.8 for adults between 35 to 50 years of age (USDA, 1984), but may be as low as 1 to 4 for those whose diets are low in dairy products and green vegetables.

General Signs of Deficiency

Because almost all foods contain phosphorus, dietary phosphorus deficiency does not usually occur. An exception is small premature infants fed human milk exclusively. Such infants need more phosphorus than is contained in human milk for the rate of bone mineralization required (Von Sydow, 1946). Without additional phosphorus, hypophosphatemic rickets may develop (Rowe et al., 1979).

Serious phosphorus deficiency has been induced in patients receiving aluminum hydroxide as an antacid for prolonged periods (Bloom and Flinchum, 1960; Lotz et al., 1968). Aluminum hydroxide binds phosphorus, making it unavailable for absorption. Phosphorus deficiency results in bone loss and is characterized by weakness, anorexia, malaise, and pain.

Recommended Allowances

Adults, Children, and Pregnant and Lactating Women   The precise requirement for phosphorus is unknown. Previous editions have set the allowance for phosphorus equal to calcium for all ages except the young infant. Although dietary phosphorus is more abundant than calcium in most U.S. diets with the few exceptions cited, neither inadequate nor excessive intake of phosphorus appears to be a problem. The subcommittee accepts that a 1-to-1 ratio of calcium to phosphorus will provide sufficient phosphorus for most age groups, but if the calcium intake is adequate, the precise ratio of these minerals is unimportant. The RDA for phosphorus is 800 mg for children 1 to 10 years, 1,200 mg for ages 11 to 24 years, and 800 mg for ages beyond 24. A total allowance of 1,200 mg/day is recommended during pregnancy and lactation.

Infants   The phosphorus content of human milk, 14 mg/100 g, is adequate for the full-term infant; the calcium-to-phosphorus ratio is 2.3 to 1. The RDA for calcium in infants is based on the poorer absorption of calcium from formulas than from human milk. Allowances for phosphorus are based on a calcium-to-phosphorus ratio of 1.3 to 1 (the same as in cow's milk) during the first 6 months, and 1.2 to 1 for the second 6 months. This declining ratio is consistent with the gradual addition of supplementary foods to the basic milk diet of the newborn. The RDA of formula-fed infants from birth to 6 months of age is 300 mg/day, and that for infants 6 to 12 months is 500 mg/day.

Excessive Intakes and Toxicity

An excess of phosphorus, i.e., a calcium-to-phosphorus ratio lower than 1 to 2, has been shown in several species of animals to lower the blood calcium level and to cause secondary hyperparathyroidism with resorption and loss of bone. In humans, only the effect on blood calcium level has been observed clinically. High-phosphorus human milk substitutes may contribute to the occurrence of hypocalcemic tetany in early infancy (Mizraki et al., 1968), unless calcium levels are increased commensurately. The phosphorus levels present in normal diets are not likely to be harmful—certainly not in the presence of adequate intakes of calcium and vitamin D.

References

Avioli, L.V. 1988. Calcium and phosphorus. Pp. 142–158 in M.E. Shils and V.R. Young, eds. Modern Nutrition in Health and Disease, 7th ed. Lea & Febiger, Philadelphia.

Bloom, W.L., and D. Flinchum. 1960. Osteomalacia with pseudofractures caused by the ingestion of aluminum hydroxide. J. Am. Med. Assoc. 174:1327–1330.

Bunch, K.L. 1987. Food consumption, prices, and expenditures. 1987. Statistical Bulletin No. 749. U.S. Department of Agriculture, Washington, D.C.

Greger, J.L., and M. Krystofiak. 1982. Phosphorus intake of Americans. Food Technol. 36:78–84.

Lotz, M., E. Zisman, and F.C. Bartter. 1968. Evidence for a phosphorus-depletion syndrome in man. N. Engl. J. Med. 278:409–415.

LSRO (Life Sciences Research Office). 1981. Effects of Dietary Factors on Skeletal Integrity in Adults: Calcium, Phosphorus, Vitamin D and Protein. Federation of American Societies for Experimental Biology, Bethesda, Md.

Mizraki, A., R.D. London, and D. Gribetz. 1968. Neonatal hypocalcemia: its causes and treatment. N. Engl. J. Med. 278:1163–1165.

Oenning, L.L., J. Vogel, and M.S. Calvo. 1988. Accuracy of methods estimating calcium and phosphorus intake in daily diets. J. Am. Diet. Assoc. 88:1076–1078.

Parfitt, A.M., and M. Kleerekoper. 1980. The divalent ion homeostatic system—physiology and metabolism of calcium, phosphorus, magnesium, and bone. Pp. 269–398 in M.H. Maxwell and C.R. Kleeman, eds. Clinical Disorders of Fluid and Electrolyte Metabolism, 3rd ed. McGraw-Hill, New York.

Parfitt, A.M., B.A. Higgins, J.R. Nassim, J.A. Collins, and A. Hilb. 1964. Metabolic studies in patients with hypercalciuria. Clin. Sci. 27:463–482.

Rowe, J.C., D.H. Wood, D.W. Rowe, and L.G. Raisz. 1979. Nutritional hypophosphatemic rickets in a premature fed breast milk. N. Engl. J. Med. 299:293–296.

USDA (U.S. Department of Agriculture). 1984. Table 2A-1: Nutritive value of food intake. Average per individual per day, 1/1977–78. Pp. 154–155 in Nationwide Food Consumption Survey. Nutrient Intakes: Individuals in 48 States, Year 1977–78. Report No. I-2. Consumer Nutrition Division, Human Nutrition Information Service. U.S. Department of Agriculture, Hyattsville, Md.

USDA (U.S. Department of Agriculture). 1986. Nationwide Food Consumption Survey. Continuing Survey of Food Intakes by Individuals. Men 19–50 Years, 1 Day, 1985. Report No. 85-3. Nutrition Monitoring Division, Human Nutrition Information Service. U.S. Department of Agriculture, Hyattsville, Md. 94 pp.

USDA (U.S. Department of Agriculture). 1987. Nationwide Food Consumption Survey. Continuing Survey of Food Intakes by Individuals. Women 19–50 Years and Their Children 1–5 Years, 4 Days, 1985. Report No. 85-4. Nutrition Monitoring Division, Human Nutrition Information Service. U.S. Department of Agriculture, Hyattsville, Md. 182 pp.

Von Sydow, G. 1946. A study of the developments of rickets in premature infants. Acta Paediatr. Scand. 33 Suppl. 2:3.

Zemel, M.B., and H.M. Linkswiler. 1981. Calcium metabolism in the young adult male as affected by level and form of phosphorus intake and level of phosphorus intake. J. Nutr. 111:315–324.

MAGNESIUM

Approximately 40% of the 20 to 28 g of magnesium contained in the adult human body resides in the muscles and soft tissues, about 1% in the extracellular fluid, and the remainder in the skeleton (Aikawa, 1981). Average plasma magnesium concentration is about 0.85 mM (range, 0.65 to 1.0 mM) (Lowenstein and Stanton, 1986). This level is maintained remarkably constant in healthy individuals by poorly understood homeostatic mechanisms.

Numerous biochemical and physiological processes require or are modulated by magnesium. As the complex $Mg-ATP^{2-}$, magnesium is essential for all biosynthetic processes, glycolysis, formation of cyclic-AMP, energy-dependent membrane transport, and transmission of the genetic code (Eichhorn and Marzilli, 1981; Rude and Oldham, 1987; Wacker, 1980; Wester, 1987). More than 300 enzymes are known to be activated by magnesium, either by interaction between substrate and an active site or by induction of conformational change (Garfinkel and Garfinkel, 1985; Mildvan, 1970; Wacker, 1980). Free intracellular magnesium concentrations have been estimated at 0.3 to 1.0 mM (Cittadini and Scarpa, 1983) and are believed to control cellular metabolism by modulating the activity of rate-limiting enzymes (Garfinkel and Garfinkel, 1985; Wacker, 1980). Extracellular magnesium concentrations are critical to the maintenance of electrical potentials of nerve and muscle membranes and for transmission of impulses across neuromuscular junctions (Aikawa, 1981). In these processes, which also depend on calcium, the two cations may act synergistically or antagonistically (Iseri and French, 1984; Livingston and Wacker, 1976).

Magnesium homeostasis does not appear to be regulated by hormonal mechanisms. Plasma magnesium levels are believed to be regulated primarily by the kidney (Heaton, 1969; Quamme, 1986). Approximately 70% of plasma magnesium is not bound to protein and is therefore filterable (Walser, 1967). About 30% of filtered magnesium is reabsorbed in the proximal tubule and another 65% is reabsorbed in the loop of Henle, the site at which major adjustments in response to plasma concentrations appear to take place. A portion of bone magnesium is in passive equilibrium with that in the plasma (Alfrey et al., 1974) and acts as a buffer against fluctuations in extracellular magnesium concentrations.

The rare occurrence of a genetic defect in magnesium absorption in infants (Paunier et al., 1965) suggests that a specific mechanism exists for magnesium absorption (Roth and Werner, 1979), but none has yet been identified. Magnesium secreted into the gut is efficiently reabsorbed. Only 25 to 50 mg of endogenous magnesium are normally excreted in the feces. Fractional magnesium absorption changes inversely with magnesium intake (Graham et al., 1960; Roth and Werner, 1979). Average net magnesium absorption is about 50% (range, 40 to 60%) of intake (Schwartz et al., 1978, 1984; Wilkinson, 1976). The presence of phytate or fiber may reduce magnesium absorption to a minor degree (Kelsay et al., 1979; Reinhold et al., 1976; Schwartz et al., 1984).

General Signs of Deficiency

Magnesium depletion with or without symptoms has been reported in association with numerous disease states (Shils, 1988). Most of these fall into one of four categories: gastrointestinal tract abnormalities associated with malabsorption or excessive fluid and electrolyte losses; renal dysfunction with defects in cation reabsorption; general malnutrition and alcoholism; and iatrogenic causes such as nasogastric suctioning, intravenous or intragastric feeding of mixtures deficient in magnesium, or use of drugs that interfere with magnesium conservation.

Purely dietary magnesium deficiency has not been reported in people consuming natural diets and has been induced experimentally only once (Shils, 1988). In that study, seven patients were fed a formula diet after radical surgery for oral cancer (Shils, 1969). After a month on a formula that supplied adequate magnesium, the formula was changed to supply 12 mg of magnesium. Urinary magnesium fell sharply to levels no longer detectable within a week, demonstrating the efficiency of renal conservation. Fecal magnesium losses were also very low. Nonetheless, plasma magnesium fell continuously. Symptoms were noted at different times after depletion began, the earliest onset occurring in two people after 24 and 26 days. Others remained asymptomatic for more than 100 days, but all eventually showed symptoms. The most prominent and consistent signs were nausea, muscle weakness, irritability, mental derangement, and myographic changes, but not all symptoms were observed in all patients. The signs described by Shils do not coincide entirely with those reported in patients who spontaneously develop symptomatic hypomagnesemia, which is frequently complicated by other deficiencies or diseases (Wacker, 1980). Both hypokalemia and hypocalcemia developed in Shils's patients, although the diet was adequate in potassium and calcium, which led him to conclude that magnesium is important to calcium and potassium homeostasis—a concept still valid today.

Dietary Sources and Usual Intakes

All unprocessed foods contain magnesium, albeit in widely differing amounts. The highest concentrations of magnesium are found in whole seeds such as nuts, legumes, and unmilled grains (Seelig, 1964). More than 80% of the magnesium is lost by removal of the germ and outer layers of cereal grains (Marier, 1986). Green vegetables are another good source of magnesium, much of it in the form of the magnesium-porphyrin complex chlorophyll. Fish, meat, and milk are relatively poor sources of magnesium. So are most commonly eaten fruits, with the exception of bananas. On the whole, diets high in vegetables and unrefined grains are much higher in magnesium than diets that include substantial quantities of refined foods, meat, and dairy products (Abdullah et al., 1981; Marier, 1986).

Average intakes of magnesium have tended to decline in the United States. Per capita magnesium in the U.S. food supply (estimated as food flowing through the food distribution system) was 408 mg/day during the period 1909 to 1913 (Welsh and Marsten, 1982). By 1949, the amount had declined to 368 mg. The amount reported in 1980 was 349 mg of magnesium. These estimates are in close agreement with data reported by Pennington et al. (1984). Chemical analyses of typical diets in the Food and Drug Administration's Total Diet Study showed that the reference adult male, assumed to need 2,850 kcal/day, would have received 354, 328, 326, and 343 mg of magnesium during 1976, 1977, 1980, and 1981–1982, respectively. In 1985, the average magnesium intake of adult men was 329 mg (USDA, 1986), whereas mean intakes for adult women and children 1 to 5 years of age were 207 and 193 mg, respectively (USDA, 1987).

Recommended Allowances

The only practical method for estimating human magnesium requirements is the metabolic balance procedure. Neither the short-lived radioisotope ^{28}Mg nor the stable isotope ^{26}Mg is suitable for whole-body magnesium turnover studies (Schwartz et al., 1978). The other possible alternative for the estimation of requirements (assessment of intake in relation to magnesium status) is unsatisfactory, because there are no reliable noninvasive techniques for determining magnesium status (Elin, 1987; Ryzen et al., 1985).

Adults   Balance data reviewed by Seelig (1964) led her to conclude that an intake of 60 mg/kg per day is needed to ensure adequate magnesium status. Many of the studies she reviewed were conducted before the common use of atomic absorption spectrometry for magnesium analyses. Later studies indicate that magnesium balance can be maintained in healthy men at intakes as low as 3.0 to 4.5 mg/kg (210 to 320 mg/day) (Greger and Baier, 1983; Hunt and Schofield, 1969; Mahalco et al., 1983; Schwartz et al., 1984, 1986).

The subcommittee considered both balance data and the usual intakes of the U.S. population in setting RDAs. Although dietary surveys indicate that magnesium intakes of some segments of the population are lower than current recommendations, there is no unequivocal evidence that magnesium deficiency is a problem among healthy persons in this country. The RDA for adults of both sexes is accepted to be 4.5 mg/kg, the upper range of requirements determined in modern balance studies. This value is approximately the same as the 1980 RDA—280 mg for women and 350 mg for men ages 19 and above.

Pregnancy and Lactation Hathaway (1962) concluded from a compilation of previous data that an intake of 350 mg/day is sufficient to meet the needs of mother and fetus. In a later study, 10 pregnant women on self-selected diets supplying 269 ± 55 mg/day were found, on average, to be in negative magnesium balance (Ashe et al., 1979). Underestimation of intake may have been a contributing factor to negative magnesium (and calcium) balances in this study, since magnesium content of water was not measured.

A healthy full-term fetus is reported to contain approximately 1 g of magnesium (Widdowson and Dickerson, 1964; Ziegler et al., 1976). Most of this is acquired in the last two trimesters of pregnancy at an estimated average rate of about 6 mg/day. An increase of 20 mg of magnesium in the daily recommendation for pregnancy should be enough to meet the needs of the fetus and maternal tissue growth, allowing for individual variation and assuming 50% of dietary magnesium to be absorbed.

Human milk contains about 28 to 40 mg magnesium per liter (Lemons et al., 1982), or about 30 mg in the average volume of 750 ml per day. In the first 6 months of lactation, 60 mg of dietary magnesium per day would replenish average magnesium lost in milk, assuming 50% absorption. To allow for variation, the RDA is 25% higher (+2 SDs), or 75 mg/day in addition to the nonlactating allowance. By the same reasoning, the increase in the RDA for the second 6 months of lactation is 60 mg. These allowances for pregnancy and lactation are far lower than in previous editions. The derivation of previous recommendations was not specified.

Infants and Children There are no data on magnesium requirements of young children. In the first 6 months of life, average magnesium intake of breastfed infants is 30 mg/day. To allow for variability in growth, (2 SDs = 25%), the allowance is 40 mg/day. The allowance for the second 6 months is increased to 60 mg/day. Schwartz et al. (1973) reported that a minimum magnesium intake of 4.6 mg/kg per day was sufficient to support balance in boys aged

13 to 16 years. Greger et al. (1978) found small negative balances in adolescent girls on magnesium intakes of 3.3 to 5.6 mg/kg. The allowance recommended for children of both sexes between 1 and 15 years is 6.0 mg/kg per day, which is substantially lower than the 1980 RDAs for these groups. Allowances for the 15- to 18-year group are maintained at 400 and 300 mg for males and females, respectively, as in the previous edition.

Excessive Intakes and Toxicity

There is no evidence that large oral intakes of magnesium are harmful to people with normal renal function, but impaired renal function resulting in magnesium retention is often associated with hypermagnesemia. Early symptoms of hypermagnesemia include nausea, vomiting, and hypotension. As the condition worsens, bradycardia, cutaneous vasodilatation, electrocardiographic changes, hyporeflexia, and central nervous system depression ensue. At the most severe level of hypermagnesemia, respiratory depression, coma, and asystolic arrest may occur (Mordes and Wacker, 1978).

Most cases of hypermagnesemia occur following the therapeutic use of magnesium-containing drugs. Antacids and laxatives containing relatively low amounts of magnesium generally are regarded as safe.

References

Abdulla, M., I. Andersson, N.G. Asp, K. Berthelsen, D. Birkhed, I. Dencker, C.G. Johansson, M. Jägerstad, K. Kolar, B.M. Nair, P. Nilsson-Ehle, A. Nordén, S. Rassner, B. Åkesson, and P.A. Öckerman. 1981. Nutrient intake and health status of vegans. Chemical analyses of diets using the duplicate portion sampling technique. Am. J. Clin. Nutr. 34:2464–2477.

Aikawa, J.K. 1981. Magnesium: Its Biologic Significance. CRC Press, Boca Raton, Fla.

Alfrey, A.C., N.L. Miller, and D. Butkus. 1974. Evaluation of body magnesium stores. J. Lab. Clin. Med. 84:153–162.

Ashe, J.R., F.A. Schofield, and M.R. Gram. 1979. The retention of calcium, iron, phosphorus, and magnesium during pregnancy: the adequacy of prenatal diets with and without supplementation. Am. J. Clin. Nutr. 32:286–291.

Cittadini, A., and A. Scarpa. 1983. Intracellular Mg^{2+} homeostasis of Ehrlich Ascites tumor cells. Arch. Biochem. Biophys. 227:202–209.

Eichhorn, G.L., and L.G. Marzilli, eds. 1981. Metal Ions in Genetic Information Transfer. Elsevier/North Holland, New York.

Elin, R.J. 1987. Assessment of magnesium status. Clin. Chem. 33:1965–1970.

Garfinkel, L., and D. Garfinkel. 1985. Magnesium regulation of the glycolytic pathway and the enzymes involved. Magnesium 4:60–72.

Graham, L.A., J.J. Caesar, and A.S.V. Burgen. 1960. Gastrointestinal absorption and excretion of Mg^{28} in man. Metabolism 9:646–659.

Greger, J.L., and M.J. Baier. 1983. Effect of dietary aluminum on mineral metabolism of adult males. Am. J. Clin. Nutr. 38:411–419.

Greger, J.L., P. Baligar, R.P. Abernathy, O.A. Bennett, and T. Peterson. 1978. Calcium, magnesium, phosphorus, copper, and manganese balance in adolescent females. Am. J. Clin. Nutr. 31:117–121.

Hathaway, M.L. 1962. Magnesium in human nutrition. Home Economics Research Report No. 19. Agricultural Research Service, U.S. Department of Agriculture, Washington, D.C. 94 pp.

Heaton, F.W. 1969. The kidney and magnesium homeostasis. Ann. NY Acad. Sci. 162:775–785.

Hunt, S.M., and F.A. Schofield. 1969. Magnesium balance and protein intake level in adult human female. Am. J. Clin. Nutr. 22:367–373.

Iseri, L.T., and J.H. French. 1984. Magnesium: nature's physiologic calcium blocker. Am. Heart J. 108:188–193.

Kelsay, J.L., K.M. Behall, and E.S. Prather. 1979. Effect of fiber from fruits and vegetables on metabolic responses of human subjects. II. Calcium, magnesium, iron, and silicon balances. Am. J. Clin. Nutr. 32:1876–1880.

Lemons, J.A., L. Moye, D. Hall, and M. Simmons. 1982. Differences in the composition of preterm and term human milk during early lactation. Pediatr. Res. 16:113–117.

Livingston, D.M., and W.E.C. Wacker. 1976. Magnesium metabolism. Pp. 215–223 in G.D. Aurbach, ed. Handbook of Physiology, Section 7: Endocrinology. Parathyroid Hormone, Vol. VII. American Physiological Society, Washington, D.C.

Lowenstein, F.W., and M.F. Stanton. 1986. Serum magnesium levels in the United States, 1971–1974. J. Am. Coll. Nutr. 5:399–414.

Mahalko, J.R., H.H. Sandstead, L.K. Johnson, and D.B. Milne. 1983. Effect of a moderate increase in dietary protein on the retention and excretion of Ca, Cu, Fe, Mg, P, and Zn by adult males. Am. J. Clin. Nutr. 37:8–14.

Marier, J.R. 1986. Magnesium content of the food supply in the modern-day world. Magnesium 5:1–8.

Mildvan, A.S. 1970. Metals in enzyme catalysis. Pp. 446–536 in P.D. Boyer, ed. The Enzymes, 3rd ed., Vol. 2. Academic Press, New York.

Mordes, J.P., and W.E. Wacker. 1978. Excess magnesium. Pharmacol. Rev. 29:273–300.

Paunier, L., I.C. Radde, S.W. Kooh, P.E. Conen, and D. Fraser. 1965. Primary hypomagnesemia with secondary hypocalcemia in an infant. Pediatrics 41:385–402.

Pennington, J.A.T., D.B. Wilson, R.F. Newell, B.F. Harland, R.D. Johnson, and J.E. Vanderveen. 1984. Selected minerals in foods surveys, 1974 to 1981/82. J. Am. Diet. Assoc. 84:771–780.

Quamme, G.A. 1986. Renal handling of magnesium: drug and hormone interactions. Magnesium 5:248–272.

Reinhold, J.G., B. Faradji, P. Abadi, and F. Ismail-Beigi. 1976. Decreased absorption of calcium, magnesium, zinc and phosphorous by humans due to increased fiber and phosphorus consumption as wheat bread. J. Nutr. 106:493–503.

Roth, P., and E. Werner. 1979. Intestinal absorption of magnesium in man. Int. J. Appl. Radiat. Isot. 30:523–526.

Rude, R.K., and S.B. Oldham. 1987. Hypocalcemia of magnesium deficiency: altered modulation of adenylate cyclase by Mg^{++} and Ca^{++} may result in impaired PTH secretion and PTH end-organ resistance. Pp. 183–195 in B.M. Altura, J. Durlach, and M.S. Seelig, eds. Magnesium in Cellular Processes and Medicine. Karger, Basel.

Ryzen, E., N. Elbaum, F.R. Singer, and R.K. Rude. 1985. Parenteral magnesium tolerance testing in the evaluation of magnesium deficiency. Magnesium 4:137–147.

Schwartz, R., G. Walker, M.D. Linz, and I. MacKellar. 1973. Metabolic responses of adolescent boys to two levels of dietary magnesium and protein. I. Magnesium and nitrogen retention. Am. J. Clin. Nutr. 26:510–518.

Schwartz, R., H. Spencer, and R.A. Wentworth. 1978. Measurement of magnesium absorption in man using stable [26]Mg as a tracer. Clin. Chim. Acta 87:265–273.

Schwartz, R., H. Spencer, and J.J. Welsh. 1984. Magnesium absorption in human subjects from leafy vegetables, intrinsically labeled with stable [26]Mg. Am. J. Clin. Nutr. 39:571–576.

Schwartz, R., B.J. Apgar, and E.M. Wien. 1986. Apparent absorption and retention of Ca, Cu, Mg, Mn, and Zn from a diet containing bran. Am. J. Clin. Nutr. 43:444–455.

Seelig, M.S. 1964. The requirement of magnesium by the normal adult. Am. J. Clin. Nutr. 14:342–390.

Shils, M.E. 1969. Experimental production of magnesium deficiency in man. Ann. NY Acad. Sci. 162:847–855.

Shils, M.E. 1988. Magnesium in health and disease. Annu. Rev. Nutr. 8:429–460.

USDA (U.S. Department of Agriculture). 1986. Nationwide Food Consumption Survey. Continuing Survey of Food Intakes by Individuals. Men 19–50 Years, 1 Day, 1988. Report No. 85-3. Nutrition Monitoring Division, Human Nutrition Information Service. U.S. Department of Agriculture, Hyattsville, Md. 94 pp.

USDA (U.S. Department of Agriculture). 1987. Nationwide Food Consumption Survey. Continuing Survey of Food Intakes by Individuals. Women 19–50 Years and Their Children 1–5 Years, 4 Days, 1985. Report No. 85-4. Nutrition Monitoring Division, Human Nutrition Information Service. U.S. Department of Agriculture, Hyattsville, Md. 182 pp.

Wacker, W.E.C. 1980. Magnesium and Man. Harvard University Press. Cambridge, Mass.

Walser, M. 1967. Magnesium metabolism. Ergebn. Physiol. 59:185–296.

Welsh, S.O., and R.M. Marston. 1982. Review of trends in food use in the United States, 1909 to 1980. J. Am. Diet. Assoc. 81:120–125.

Wester, P.O. 1987. Magnesium. Am. J. Clin. Nutr. 45:1305–1312.

Widdowson, E.M., and J.W.T. Dickerson. 1964. Chemical composition of the body. Pp. 1–247 in C.L. Comar and F. Bronner, eds. Mineral Metabolism, Vol. II. The Elements, Part A. Academic Press, New York.

Wilkinson, R. 1976. Absorption of calcium, phosphorus and magnesium. Pp. 36–112 in B.E.C. Nordin, ed. Calcium, Phosphate and Magnesium Metabolism. Churchill Livingstone, Edinburgh.

Ziegler, E.E., A.M. O'Donnell, S.E. Nelson, and S.J. Fomon. 1976. Body composition of the reference fetus. Growth 40:329–341.

10
Trace Elements

IRON

Iron is a constituent of hemoglobin, myoglobin, and a number of enzymes and, therefore, is an essential nutrient for humans (Bothwell et al., 1979). In addition to these functional forms, as much as 30% of the body iron is found in storage forms such as ferritin and hemosiderin (mainly in the spleen, liver, and bone marrow), and a small amount is associated with the blood transport protein transferrin.

Body iron content is regulated mainly through changes in the amount of iron absorbed by the intestinal mucosa (Finch and Cook, 1984). The absorption of iron is influenced by body stores (Bothwell et al., 1979; Cook et al., 1974), by the amount and chemical nature of iron in the ingested food (Layrisse et al., 1968), and by a variety of dietary factors that increase or decrease the availability of iron for absorption (Gillooly et al., 1983; Hallberg, 1981). When the dietary supply of absorbable iron is sufficient, the intestinal mucosa regulates iron absorption in a manner that tends to keep body iron content constant. In iron deficiency, the efficiency of iron absorption increases (Finch and Cook, 1984). However, this response may not be sufficient to prevent anemia in subjects whose intake of available iron is marginal. Similarly, intestinal regulation is not sufficient to prevent excessive body accumulation of iron in the presence of continued high levels of iron in the diet.

General Signs of Deficiency

Three stages of impaired iron status have been identified. In the first stage, iron depletion, iron stores are diminished, as reflected in a fall in plasma ferritin to levels below 12 μg/liter, but no functional impairment is evident. The second stage is recognized by iron-deficient erythropoiesis, in which the hemoglobin level is within the 95% reference range for age and sex but red cell protoporphyrin levels are elevated, transferrin saturation is reduced to less than 16% in adults, and work capacity performance may be impaired. In the third stage, iron deficiency anemia, total blood hemoglobin levels are reduced below normal values for age and sex of the subject. Severe iron deficiency anemia is characterized by small red blood cells (microcytosis) with low hemoglobin concentrations (hypochromia).

Currently there is no single biochemical indicator available to reliably assess iron inadequacy in the general population. Three approaches for estimating the prevalence of impaired iron status were used by the Life Sciences Research Office (LSRO, 1985). One (the ferritin model) involved the use of three indicators—serum ferritin, transferrin saturation, and erythrocyte protoporphyrin—and required that at least two of these be abnormal. In another, mean cell volume (MCV) was substituted for ferritin, but there was also a requirement that at least two of the three indicators be abnormal. The third approach (hemoglobin percentile shift) was defined as the change in median hemoglobin concentration after exclusion of individuals with one or more abnormal iron status values.

Operational definitions of anemia have been established by a World Health Organization (WHO) Expert Committee (WHO, 1968) in terms of hemoglobin level. For males and females age 14 years and over, anemia is defined as a hemoglobin level below 13 g/dl and 12 g/dl, respectively. For pregnant women, values below 11 g/dl for the first trimester, 10.5 for the second, and 11.0 for the third have recently been proposed by the Centers for Disease Control as levels defining anemia (CDC, 1989). Since the range of normal hemoglobin values is rather broad (13 to 16 g/dl in men and 12 to 16 g/dl in women), the actual deficit in hemoglobin may vary considerably in individuals with a given level of hemoglobin below the cut-off point.

The consequences of iron deficiency are usually ascribed to the resulting anemia, although some effects of deficiency have been found before reduced hemoglobin levels were observed (NRC, 1979). An association between hemoglobin concentration and work capacity is the most clearly identified functional consequence of iron deficiency (Viteri and Torun, 1974). However, there are reports of reduced physical performance in iron deficiency even before anemia is present (Dallman et al., 1978). Iron deficiency also has been associated with decreased immune function as measured by changes in several components of the immune system during iron deficiency. The functional consequences of these immune system changes to actual resistance to infection still remains to be determined. In children, iron deficiency has been associated with apathy, short attention span, irritability, and reduced ability to learn (Lozoff and Brittenham, 1986). The degree to which milder forms of iron deficiency, as opposed to severe anemia, result in impaired school performance by children is uncertain (Pollitt, 1987).

In the United States, iron deficiency may be observed primarily during four periods of life: (1) from about 6 months to 4 years of age, because the iron content of milk is low, the body is growing rapidly, and body reserves of iron are often insufficient to meet needs beyond 6 months; (2) during the rapid growth of early adolescence, because of the needs of an expanding red cell mass and the need to deposit iron in myoglobin; (3) during the female reproductive period, because of menstrual iron losses; and (4) during pregnancy, because of the expanding blood volume of the mother, the demands of the fetus and placenta, and blood losses during childbirth. Analyses of data from the Second National Health and Nutrition Examination Survey (NHANES II) of the U.S. population, 1976–1980, depending on the assessment model used, indicated a prevalence of impaired iron status ranging from 1 to 6% of the total population, including 9% of children aged 1 to 2 years of age, 4 to 12% of males ages 11 to 14 years, and 5 to 14% of females ages 15 to 44 (LSRO, 1985). The frequency of iron depletion as determined by measurement of serum ferritin, and of iron-deficient erythropoiesis as determined by transferrin saturation and protoporphyrin, is substantially greater than the frequency of iron deficiency anemia in the population surveyed in NHANES II (Bothwell et al., 1979; Dallman et al., 1984; Meyers et al., 1983).

Dietary Sources

Iron is widely distributed in the U.S. food supply; meat, eggs, vegetables, and cereals (especially fortified cereal products) are the principal dietary sources. In examining food consumption data for women 18 to 24 years of age from NHANES II, Murphy and Calloway (1986) found that of a daily iron intake of 10.7 mg, 31% came from meat, poultry, and fish and that 25% was provided by iron added to foods, mainly cereals, as fortification or enrichment. Fruits, vegetables, and juices contain varying amounts of iron, but as a group represent another major source of dietary iron. Heme iron, a highly available source, represents from 7 to 10% of the dietary iron of girls and women and from 8 to 12% of dietary iron of boys and men, according to data from the 1977–1978 Nationwide Food Consumption Survey (Raper et al., 1984).

Iron availability may be enhanced by consumption of foods containing ascorbic acid. Ascorbic acid intake is relatively high in U.S. diets, ranging from 86 to 112 mg/day in various groups of men aged 15 years of age and older and from 76 to 92 mg/day for women 15 or more years old and over (Raper et al., 1984).

Absorption of Dietary Iron

Heme and nonheme forms of iron are absorbed by different mechanisms (Bjorn-Rasmussen et al., 1974). Heme iron is highly absorbable. The proportion of heme iron in animal tissues varies, but it averages about 40% of the total iron in all animal tissues, including meat, liver, poultry, and fish. The remaining 60% of the iron in animal tissues and all the iron in vegetable products is present as nonheme compounds.

The absorption of nonheme iron can be enhanced or inhibited by several factors. The two most well-defined enhancers of nonheme iron are some organic acids (especially ascorbic acid) (Gillooly et al., 1983) and the animal tissues present in each meal (Cook and Monsen, 1976). On the other hand, some dietary and medicinal substances such as calcium phosphate, phytates, bran, polyphenols in tea, and antacids may decrease nonheme iron absorption substantially (Gillooly et al., 1983; Monsen et al., 1978). Overall, nonheme iron absorption may vary up to tenfold, depending on the dietary content of such inhibiting and enhancing factors (Hallberg and Rossander, 1984).

The percentage of iron absorbed from a meal decreases as the amount of iron present increases. Bezwoda et al. (1983) reported that mean absorption of nonheme iron decreased from 18 to 6.4% as the nonheme iron content of four meals increased from 1.52 to 5.72 mg, resulting in little variation in the actual amount absorbed from the different meals. This presumably reflects tight control of nonheme iron absorption by the intestinal mucosa. On the other hand, 20% of the heme iron in all four meals was absorbed, despite a heme iron content ranging from 0.28 to 4.48 mg, suggesting that heme iron is less affected by other dietary components and at least partly bypasses intestinal mucosal control. On the basis of results of numerous studies of iron absorption in human subjects, Monsen et al. (1978) have suggested a method for planning and evaluating iron intakes that takes account of the enhancement of nonheme iron absorption by ascorbic acid and the presence of meat in the diet.

Absorption of iron also depends on the iron status of the individual. Mean absorption of dietary iron is relatively low when body stores are high but may be increased when stores are low (Bothwell et al., 1979). Therefore, iron deficiency may not occur to the extent that might be predicted from a given iron intake below recommended allowance levels.

Recommended Allowances

Adults In calculating the RDA, the subcommittee assumed that there are some iron stores, but it concluded that the size of the iron store needed as a reserve against periods of negative iron balance is a value judgment rather than a scientific determination. In U.S. women, average iron stores are approximately 300 mg; in men, they are approximately 1,000 mg (Bothwell et al., 1979). The subcommittee concluded that a dietary intake that achieves a target level of 300 mg of iron stores meets the nutritional needs of all healthy people. This level would be sufficient to provide the iron needs of an individual for several months, even when on a diet nearly devoid of iron.

The average loss of iron in the healthy adult man is estimated to be approximately 1 mg/day (Green et al., 1968). In adult women, there is an additional loss of about 0.5 mg/day, the amount of iron in the average menstrual blood flow averaged over 1 month (Hallberg et al., 1966). In approximately 5% of normal women, however, menstrual losses of more than 1.4 mg/day have been observed. As menstrual losses deplete iron stores, absorption of dietary iron increases. Concordant figures are found using radio-labeled iron loss from circulating erythrocytes. This method gives reliable turnover information for adults and indicates that average requirements to replace daily losses for adults ages 20 to 50 are approximately 14 μg of iron per kilogram of body weight for males (1.10 mg/79 kg) and 22 μg for premenopausal females (1.38 mg/63 kg) (Bothwell and Finch, 1968).

There is little or no population-based information from which to assess variability of iron losses among individuals. A reasonable estimate of the coefficient of variation may be approximately 15% (NRC, 1986), but iron losses are not normally distributed among women. For men, absorbed iron would need to be sufficient to replace a potential loss of 1.3 mg/day (1.03 + 30%) to cover the needs of essentially the entire population. The variability estimate indicates that a replacement of 1.8 mg of iron per day would cover the needs of most women, except for the 5% with the most extreme menstrual losses.

Some impairment of iron status in 9.6 to 14.2% of nonpregnant females 15 to 44 years of age was suggested by population-based data showing two abnormal values among measurements of serum ferritin, erythrocyte protoporphyrin, and transferrin saturation (LSRO, 1985). When hemoglobin was used as an indicator, however, only 2.5 to 4% of the women showed evidence of iron deficiency. The average iron intake of this population group was found to be 10 to 11.0 mg/day in surveys conducted by the U.S. Department of Agriculture (USDA), the National Center for Health Statistics (NCHS), and the Food and Drug Administration (FDA) (Murphy and Calloway, 1986; Pennington et al., 1986; Raper et al., 1984). This suggests that a mean population consumption of about 10 mg/day is associated with adequate iron status in at least 86% of the population of women 15 to 44 years of age. Distribution analysis, considering both the variation in iron losses by menstruating women and in population iron intake, indicate that an iron intake of 14 mg/day is sufficient to meet the needs of all but about 5% of menstruating women (NRC, 1986).

From the available data, it seems reasonable to conclude that a daily intake of 10 to 11 mg of iron from typical U.S. diets is sufficient for most women. Those with high menstrual losses appear to compensate for those losses by improved absorption of dietary iron, since the prevalence of iron deficiency anemia in that group is quite low (Meyers et al., 1983). The most recent WHO recommendations (FAO, 1988) suggest that iron in the diets typical of most populations of industrialized countries is relatively highly available, iron absorption ranging from 10 to 15%. Thus, at an intake of 15 mg/day, approximately 1.5 to 2.2 mg of absorbed iron could be available to replace iron losses in adult women. This level would be expected to replace iron losses of most women.

The subcommittee concluded that an RDA of 15 mg/day would provide a sufficient margin of safety and should cover the needs of essentially all the adult women in the United States except for those with the most extreme menstrual losses, given usual dietary patterns. This is a reduction from the 1980 recommendation of 18 mg/day.

In the United States, very little iron deficiency has been reported for 15- to 60-year-old males (LSRO, 1985), whose average intake is about 15 mg/day. Given usual diets in the United States, an allowance of 10 mg/day for adult males should be sufficient to replace losses of up to 1.5 mg/day—an amount exceeding estimates of usual daily iron loss by men.

There is no evidence of a high prevalence of iron deficiency in the elderly (Lynch et al., 1982). Survey data suggest that inflammatory disease, rather than iron deficiency, is the main cause of anemia in this group (Dallman et al., 1984). In addition, after the menstrual years, the daily iron needs of women approximate those of men. Therefore, the subcommittee recommends the same iron RDA for elderly women and men—10 mg/day.

Pregnancy and Lactation Pregnant women need iron to replace the usual basal losses, to allow expansion of the red cell mass, to provide iron to the fetus and placenta, and to replace blood loss during delivery. Hallberg (1988) estimates that the total iron needed for a pregnancy is approximately 1,040 mg, of which 840 mg are lost from the body permanently and 200 mg are retained and serve as a reservoir of iron when blood volume decreases after delivery. Over the entire period of gestation, the amount of iron absorbed daily averages about 3 mg/day. There is little need for increased iron intake in the first trimester of pregnancy, since the cessation of iron loss from menstruation compensates for any increased needs during this period. In later stages of pregnancy, however, the requirement increases substantially (INACG, 1981). During the later stages of pregnancy, the absorbability of dietary iron also increases (Apte and Iyengar, 1970). To ensure sufficient absorbed iron to satisfy the demands of a normal pregnancy, a daily increment of 15 mg of iron, averaged over the entire pregnancy, should satisfy the needs of most women. However, since the increased pregnancy requirement cannot be met by the iron content of habitual U.S. diets or by the iron stores of at least some women, daily iron supplements are usually recommended.

Loss of iron through lactation is approximately 0.15 to 0.3 mg/day (Lonnerdal et al., 1981). This is less than menstrual loss, which often is absent during lactation (Habicht et al., 1985). Thus, since iron needs for lactating women are not substantially different from those of nonpregnant women, no additional iron allowance for this group is recommended.

Infants Because of stored iron (Dahro et al., 1983), the normal term infant can maintain satisfactory hemoglobin levels from human milk without other iron sources during the first 3 months of life. From birth to age 3 years, infants not breastfed should have an iron intake of approximately 1 mg/kg per day. The RDA for 6 months to 3 years of age is set at 10 mg/day—a level considered adequate for most healthy children during this time. Low birth weight infants (1,000 to 2,500 g) and those with a substantial reduction in total hemoglobin mass require 2 mg/kg per day, starting no later than 2 months of age (AAP, 1976; Dallman et al., 1980). For infants of normal or low birth weight, iron intake should not exceed a maximum of 15 mg/day.

Children and Adolescents   Children and adolescents need iron not only to maintain hemoglobin concentrations but also to increase their total iron mass during the period of growth. Because of the allowance for increases in iron mass related to growth in body size, the iron requirements of children and adolescents are considered to be slightly higher than those of adult men.

To attain a target iron storage level of 300 mg for both sexes by age 20 to 25, an allowance of 10 mg/day is recommended for children. An additional 2 mg/day is recommended for males during the pubertal growth spurt—which occurs between the ages of 10 and 17—and an additional 5 mg for females starting with the pubertal growth spurt and menstruation—which begins at approximately age 10 or shortly thereafter and continues through the menstrual years.

Other Considerations

The RDAs have been established to be adequate for essentially all healthy people who daily consume diets containing 30 to 90 g of meat, poultry, or fish, or foods containing 25 to 75 mg of ascorbate after preparation. People who eat little or no animal protein, such as those whose diets consist largely of beans and rice, and those whose diets are low in ascorbate due to prolonged heating or storage of food (Kies, 1982) may require higher amounts of food iron or a reliable source of ascorbic acid.

Excessive Intakes and Toxicity

In people without genetic defects that increase iron absorption, there are no reports of iron toxicity from foods other than long-term ingestion of home brews made in iron vessels (Walker and Arvidsson, 1953). Deleterious effects of daily intakes between 25 and 75 mg are unlikely in healthy persons (Finch and Monsen, 1972). On the other hand, there are approximately 2,000 cases of iron poisoning each year in the United States, mainly among young children who ingest the medicinal iron supplements formulated for adults. The lethal dose of ferrous sulfate for a 2-year-old child is approximately 3 g; for adults, it ranges from 200 to 250 mg/kg body weight (NRC, 1979).

Some people are genetically at risk from iron overload or hemochromatosis. Idiopathic hemochromatosis, which can result in the failure of multiple organ systems, is the result of an inborn error of metabolism (not yet elucidated), which leads to enhanced iron absorption. The disease is caused by an autosomal recessive gene. Reports suggest that the prevalence of this disease is higher than previously believed (Beaumont et al., 1979; Cartwright et al., 1979; Olsson et al., 1983). The studies by Cartwright et al. (1979) in Utah and Beaumont et al. (1979) in Brittany establish gene frequencies in the relatives of cases identified with the disease and so do not estimate general population prevalence. Olsson et al. (1983) studied a population of males ages 30 to 39 in central Sweden and reported an estimated gene frequency of 6.9%. This would result in a prevalence of heterozygotes in this population of 13.8%. The prevalence of the gene has not been reliably established in the United States. In NHANES II, five of the 3,540 people whose serum ferritin was assessed were diagnosed as having idiopathic hemochromatosis, i.e., they were assumed to be homozygous for the gene. This implies a gene frequency of 3.8% and prevalence of heterozygotes of 7.5% (LSRO, 1985). Further work is needed to determine the prevalence of this gene in the population and to establish the risks of iron fortification of foods to both homozygotes and heterozygotes.

References

AAP (American Academy of Pediatrics). 1976. Iron supplementation for infants. Pediatrics 58:765–768.

Apte, S.V., and L. Iyengar. 1970. Absorption of dietary iron in pregnancy. Am. J. Clin. Nutr. 21:73–77.

Beaumont, C., M. Simon, R. Fauchet, J.-P. Hespel, P. Brissot, B. Genetet, and M. Bourel. 1979. Serum ferritin as a possible marker of the hemochromatosis allele. N. Engl. J. Med. 301:169–174.

Bezwoda, W.R., T.H. Bothwell, R.W. Charlton, J.D. Torrance, A.P. MacPhail, D.P. Derman, and F. Mayet. 1983. The relative dietary importance of haem and non-haem iron. S. Afr. Med. J. 64:552–556.

Bjorn-Rasmussen, E., L. Hallberg, B. Isaksson, and B. Arvidsson. 1974. Food iron absorption in man. Application of the two-pool extrinsic tag method to measure heme and nonheme iron absorption from the whole diet. J. Clin. Invest. 52:247–255.

Bothwell, T.H., and C.A. Finch. 1968. Iron losses in man. Pp. 104–114 in Occurrence, Causes and Prevention of Nutritional Anaemias. Symposia of the Swedish Nutrition Foundation, VI. Almquist and Wiksell, Uppsala.

Bothwell, T.H., R.W. Charlton, J.D. Cook, and C.A. Finch. 1979. Iron Metabolism in Man. Blackwell, Oxford.

Cartwright, G.E., C.Q. Edwards, K. Kravitz, M. Skolnick, D.B. Amos, A. Johnson, and L. Buskjaer. 1979. Hereditary hemochromatosis: phenotypic expression of the disease. N. Engl. J. Med. 301:175–179.

CDC (Centers for Disease Control). 1989. CDC criteria for anemia in children and childbearing-aged women. Morb. Mortal. Week. Rep. 38:400–404.

Cook. J.D., and E.R. Monsen. 1976. Food iron absorption in human subjects. III. Comparison of the effect of animal proteins on honheme iron absorption. Am. J. Clin. Nutr. 29:859–867.

Cook, J.D., D.A. Lipschitz, L.E.M. Miles, and C.A. Finch. 1974. Serum ferritin as a measure of iron stores in normal subjects. Am. J. Clin. Nutr. 27:681–687.

Dahro, M., D. Gunning, and J.A. Olson. 1983. Variations in liver concentrations of iron and vitamin A as a function of age in young American children dying of the sudden infant death syndrome as well as of other causes. Int. J. Vit. Nutr. Res. 53:13–18.

Dallman, P.R., E. Beutler, and C.A. Finch. 1978. Effect of iron deficiency exclusive of anemia. Br. J. Heamatol. 40:179–184.

Dallman, P.R., M.A. Siimes, and A. Stekel. 1980. Iron deficiency in infancy and childhood. Am. J. Clin. Nutr. 33:86–118.

Dallman, P.R., R. Yip, and C. Johnson. 1984. Prevalence and causes of anemia in the United States, 1976 to 1980. Am. J. Clin. Nutr. 39:437–445.

FAO (Food and Agriculture Organization). 1988. Requirements of Vitamin A, Iron, Folate, and Vitamin B12. Report of a Joint FAO/WHO Expert Consultation. FAO Food and Nutrition Series No. 23. Food and Agriculture Organization, Rome. 107 pp.

Finch, C.A., and J.D. Cook. 1984. Iron deficiency. Am. J. Clin. Nutr. 39:471–477.

Finch, C.A., and E.R. Monsen. 1972. Iron nutrition and the fortificaion of food with iron. J. Am. Med. Assoc. 219:1462–1465.

Gillooly, M., T.H. Bothwell, J.D. Torrance, A.P. MacPhail, D.P. Derman, W.R. Bezwoda, W. Mills, and R.W. Charlton. 1983. The effects of organic acids, phytates, and polyphenols on the absorption of iron from vegetables. Br. J. Nutr. 49:331–342.

Green, R., R.W. Charlton, H. Seftel, T.H. Bothwell, F. Mayet, E.B. Adams, C.A. Finch, and M. Layrisse. 1968. Body iron excretion in man: a collaborative study. Am. J. Med. 45:336–353.

Habicht, J.-P., J. DaVanzo, W.P. Butz, and L. Meyers. 1985. The contraceptive role of breastfeeding. Popul. Stud. 39:213–232.

Hallberg, L. 1981. Bioavailability of dietary iron in man. Annu. Rev. Nutr. 1:123–147.

Hallberg, L. 1988. Iron balance in pregnancy. Pp. 115–126 in H. Berger, ed. Vitamins and Minerals in Pregnancy and Lactation. Raven Press, New York.

Hallberg, L., and L. Rossander. 1984. Improvement of iron nutrition in developing countries: comparison of adding meat, soy protein, ascorbic acid, citric acid, and ferrous sulphate on iron absorption from a simple Latin American-type of meal. Am. J. Clin. Nutr. 39:577–583.

Hallberg, L., A.M. Hogdahl, L. Nilsson, and R. Rybo. 1966. Menstrual blood loss— a population study. Variation at different ages and attempts to define normality. Acta Obstet. Gynecol. Scand. 45:320–351.

INACG (International Nutritional Anemia Consultative Group). 1981. Iron Deficiency in Women. A Report for INACG by T.H. Bothwell and R.W. Charlton. University of the Witwatersrand, Johannesburg, South Africa.

Kies, C., ed. 1982. Nutritional Bioavailability of Iron. ACS Symposium Series 203. American Chemical Society, Washington, D.C.

Layrisse, M., C. Martinez-Torres, and M. Roche. 1968. Effect of interaction of various foods on iron absorption. Am. J. Clin. Nutr. 21:1175–1183.

Lönnerdal, B., C.L. Keen, and L.S. Hurley. 1981. Iron, copper, zinc and manganese in milk. Annu. Rev. Nutr. 1:149–174.

Lozoff, B., and G.M. Brittenham. 1986. Behavioral aspects of iron deficiency. Prog. Haematol. 14:23–53.

LSRO (Life Sciences Research Office). 1985. Summary of a report on assessment of the iron nutritional status of the United States population. Am. J. Clin. Nutr. 42:1318–1330.

Lynch, S.R., C.A. Finch, E.R. Monsen, and J.D. Cook. 1982. Iron status of elderly Americans. Am. J. Clin. Nutr. 36:1032–1045.

Meyers, L.D., J.P. Habicht, C.L. Johnson, and C. Brownie. 1983. Prevalences of anemia and iron deficiency anemia in black and white women in the United States estimated by two methods. Am. J. Public Health 73:1042–1049.

Monsen, E.R., L. Hallberg, M. Layrisse, D.M. Hegsted, J.D. Cook, W. Mertz, and C.A. Finch. 1978. Estimation of available dietary iron. Am. J. Clin. Nutr. 31:134–141.

Murphy, S.P., and D.H. Calloway. 1986. Nutrient intakes of women in NHANES II emphasizing trace minerals, fiber, and phytate. J. Am. Diet. Assoc. 86:1366–1372.

NRC (National Research Council). 1979. Iron. A Report of the Subcommittee on Iron, Committee on Medical and Biologic Effects of Environmental Pollutants, Division of Medical Sciences, Assembly of Life Sciences. University Park Press, Baltimore. 248 pp.

NRC (National Research Council). 1986. Nutrient Adequacy: Assessment Using Food Consumption Surveys. Report of the Subcommittee on Criteria for Dietary Evaluation, Coordinating Committee on Evaluation of Food Consumption Surveys, Food and Nutrition Board, Commission on Life Sciences. National Academy Press, Washington, D.C. 146 pp.

Olsson, K.S., B. Ritter, U. Rosen, P.A. Heedman, and F. Staugard. 1983. Prevalence of iron overload in central Sweden. Acta Med. Scand. 213:145–150.

Pennington, J.A.T., B.E. Young, D.B. Wilson, R.D. Johnson, and J.E. Vanderveen. 1986. Mineral content of foods and total diets: the Selected Minerals in Foods Survey, 1982 to 1984. J. Am. Diet. Assoc. 86:876–891.

Pollitt, E. 1987. Effects of iron deficiency on mental development: methodological considerations and substantive findings. Pp. 225–254 in F.E. Johnston, ed. Nutritional Anthropology. Alan R. Liss, New York.

Raper, N.R., J.C. Rosenthal, and C.E. Woteki. 1984. Estimates of available iron in diets of individuals 1 year old and older in the Nationwide Food Consumption Survey. J. Am. Diet. Assoc. 84:783–787.

Viteri, F.E., and B. Torun. 1974. Anaemia and physical work capacity. Clin. Haematol. 3:609–626.

Walker, A.R.P., and U.B. Arvidson. 1953. Iron "overload" in the South African Bantu. Trans. R. Soc. Trop. Med. Hyg. 47:536–548.

WHO (World Health Organization). 1968. Nutritional Anaemias. Report of a WHO Scientific Group. WHO Technical Report Series No. 405. World Health Organization, Geneva.

ZINC

Zinc, a constituent of enzymes involved in most major metabolic pathways, is an essential element for plants, animals, and humans

(Hambidge et al., 1986). Relatively large amounts of zinc are deposited in bone and muscle, but these stores are not in rapid equilibrium with the rest of the organism. The body pool of readily available zinc appears to be small and to have a rapid turnover rate, as shown by the prompt appearance of deficiency signs in laboratory animals. No single enzyme function has yet been identified that could explain the rapid onset of physiological and biochemical changes that follow the induction of zinc deficiency, but the requirement for zinc by many enzymes involved in gene expression (Chesters, 1982) could explain the immediate effect of deficiency on cell growth and repair.

Zinc status is subject to strong homeostatic regulation. Small amounts of zinc are more efficiently absorbed than large amounts, and persons in poor zinc status absorb more efficiently than those in good status. The amount of zinc excreted, predominantly through the intestine, is roughly proportional to dietary intake and to the zinc status of the person. Zinc balance was observed in subjects fed moderately low zinc levels (5.5 mg/day) (King and Turnlund, 1989). Obligatory losses in young men fed a low-zinc diet of 0.3 mg/day were reduced to 0.67 mg/day and resulted in only a small negative balance.

Because of such efficient regulation, a person's zinc requirement, whether determined by balance studies or by factorial calculations of endogenous losses, depends predominantly on that person's zinc status or body pool of mobilizable zinc. The requirement to maintain balance will be high if a high zinc status is to be maintained and low to maintain a low zinc status.

The composition of the diet has important effects on the bioavailability of dietary zinc. Interactions with other dietary components, such as protein, fiber, phytates, and some minerals, have been described. For example, absorption of zinc isotopes added to meals of different composition ranged from 2.4 to 38.2% of the dose supplied (Sandström and Cederblad, 1980; Sandström et al., 1980). The low values were associated with meals containing bran or whole-meal bread, and the higher values, with white bread, meats, milk, and soy products (see below).

General Signs of Deficiency

The signs and symptoms of dietary zinc deficiency in humans include loss of appetite, growth retardation, skin changes, and immunological abnormalities. Studies in laboratory and domestic animals have shown that zinc deficiency during pregnancy may lead to developmental disorders in the offspring (Hurley and Baly, 1982).

Pronounced zinc deficiency in men resulting in hypogonadism and dwarfism has been found in the Middle East (Prasad, 1982). Marginal states of zinc nutrition may exist in segments of the U.S. population, but data are fragmentary. In human patients with low plasma zinc levels, accelerated rates of wound healing have been observed as a result of increased zinc intake, suggesting that the zinc requirement of these subjects was not fully met by their diets (Pories et al., 1976). Marginal zinc deficiency was also described in a survey of apparently healthy children who exhibited low hair zinc levels, suboptimal growth, poor appetite, and impaired taste acuity (Hambidge et al., 1972). Increasing the daily zinc intake by 0.4 to 0.8 mg/kg brought about marked improvement. Supplementation of infant formulas to increase zinc levels from 1.8 to 5.8 mg/liter resulted in increased growth rates in male, but not in female, infants (Walravens and Hambidge, 1976).

Dietary Sources, Bioavailability, and Usual Intakes

Approximately 70% of the zinc consumed by most people in the United States is provided by animal products, especially meat (Welsh and Marston, 1982). Most of the zinc consumed in plant products comes from cereals. Drinking water in the United States generally contains less than 0.1 mg zinc/liter; its contribution to total intake is negligible.

The bioavailability of zinc in different foods varies widely (Inglett, 1983). Meat, liver, eggs, and seafoods (especially oysters) are good sources of available zinc, whereas whole grain products contain the element in a less available form. Of the various factors believed to affect zinc availability adversely, high concentrations of phytate and dietary fiber have great practical importance worldwide, but probably not in the United States, where the phytate content of the average diet is not high enough to impair the utilization of zinc (Erdman et al., 1987; Morris and Ellis, 1983).

For the U.S. population, the interaction of zinc with dietary protein, phosphorus, and iron may have greater practical importance. However, the data are not consistent. Sandstead (1985) observed that increasing dietary intake of phosphorus greatly increased zinc requirements of humans in balance studies. Others have observed that the ingestion of additional phosphorus, as polyphosphates but not generally as orthophosphates, tended to depress zinc absorption slightly (Greger, 1988).

Several investigators have observed that alterations in dietary protein levels and composition affected zinc utilization. Although Sandstead (1985) noted that zinc requirements were increased somewhat when protein intake was increased, others observed improved zinc utilization when protein levels were increased (Greger, 1988; Lönnerdal, 1987).

The simultaneous ingestion of equal amounts of ferrous iron and zinc (as sulfates) depressed zinc absorption in volunteers, but no such effects occurred with heme iron or when a food source of zinc was used (Solomons and Jacob, 1981). Thus, it is unlikely that the iron-zinc interaction has a major influence on zinc requirements under most dietary conditions (Solomons and Cousins, 1984).

The zinc content of typical mixed diets of North American adults has been reported to furnish between 10 and 15 mg/day. Pennington et al. (1984), in a survey of U.S. foods, found 13.2 mg of zinc in a 2,850 kcal diet. Infant and toddler diets containing 880 and 1,300 kcal contained 5.5 and 8.5 mg zinc, respectively. Elderly people generally have been found to consume 7 to 10 mg zinc daily (Greger, 1989).

Recommended Allowances

Adults   Because of the lack of sensitive indicators of zinc status, the estimation of a zinc requirement for adults and the setting of a recommended allowance is beset with several uncertainties. As discussed above, strong homeostatic control of absorption and excretion can maintain persons in zinc balance with intakes lower than those furnished by typical U.S. diets. The long-term health effects of such intakes for adults are not known, but it has been postulated that marginal zinc status is responsible for delayed wound healing, disturbances of taste and smell acuity, and declining immune functions sometimes observed in older populations (Greger, 1989). Such conditions are usually treated with massive zinc supplements; therefore, these therapeutic trials provide no quantitative information on which to base the zinc requirement to maintain optimal health.

To estimate zinc requirements, the subcommittee assumed that the zinc status of healthy young adult men and women consuming mixed U.S. diets was adequate for all zinc-dependent functions. The zinc requirements to maintain that status can be determined either by balance studies or by determining endogenous zinc losses and translating the requirement for *absorbed* zinc into a dietary requirement, taking into account that zinc is incompletely absorbed to an extent that varies with the nature of the diet.

An evaluation of the most reliable balance studies indicates that at least 12 mg of zinc in a mixed U.S. diet is required to maintain the existing zinc status of healthy young men (Sandstead, 1985). This is a conservative estimate, valid for diets of moderate phytate and fiber content, and it does not include dermal and seminal losses. Another long-term study in 28 men and women eating self-selected diets with approximately 10 mg of zinc per day resulted in an average negative balance of 1 to 2 mg/day (Patterson et al., 1984). Endogenous losses estimated by regression analysis in adequately nourished, healthy young men were 2.2 mg/day (Baer and King, 1984), including 0.8 mg through dermal losses. Seminal emissions contained an average of 0.6 mg of zinc per ejaculum. Thus, the daily loss can be estimated to be between 2.2 and 2.8 mg, similar to the average of 2.7 mg determined by turnover measurements of metastable zinc in men and women (Foster et al., 1979).

Taking into account the uncertainties in determining dermal and seminal zinc excretion, the subcommittee assumed an average requirement for absorbed zinc of 2.5 mg/day and an absorption efficiency of 20%. This assumption is arbitrary and includes a generous safety factor. Although zinc is absorbed with a higher efficiency from meat-containing meals, the factor of 20% was used to take into account the lower absorption of zinc from fiber-rich diets.

The resulting dietary requirement of 12.5 mg/day agrees with the 12.7 mg/day estimated from balance studies in men (Sandstead, 1985). To meet the needs of practically all healthy persons, including those who habitually consume diets with low zinc bioavailability, the recommended allowance for adult men is set at 15 mg/day. The allowance for adult women, because of their lower body weight, is set at 12 mg/day.

Pregnancy and Lactation Sandstead (1973) estimated the additional average need for absorbed zinc due to the products of conception as less than 0.1, approximately 0.4, and 0.75 mg/day during the first 10, the second 10, and the last 20 weeks of gestation, respectively, as compared to more recent estimates of 0.1, 0.2, and 0.6 mg/day (Swanson and King, 1987). Hambidge et al. (1986) pointed out that the actual zinc concentrations in the fetus may be higher than those on which the above calculations were based. Thus, in the absence of evidence for increased absorption efficiency in pregnant women (Swanson et al., 1983), a dietary zinc intake of 15 mg/day is recommended during pregnancy.

The increased zinc requirement of lactating women can be calculated from the amount of zinc lost each day in the different phases of lactation. The mean zinc content of human milk in the United States is approximately 1.5 and 1.0 mg/liter during the first and second half year, respectively (Krebs et al., 1985; Moser and Reynolds, 1983), the highest concentrations occurring during the first month of lactation. Average milk productions of 750 ml/day and 600 ml/day during the first and second 6 month periods, respectively, uses an extra 1.2 and 0.6 mg of absorbed zinc. Assuming an absorption efficiency of 20% and a coefficient of variation of 12.5% in milk production, the subcommittee recommends extra dietary intakes of 7 and 4 mg/day for the first and second 6 months of lactation.

Infants and Children   Full-term infants consuming only human milk do not show any signs of zinc depletion (Hambidge et al., 1979). Therefore, their zinc requirement must be satisfied by the zinc in their mother's milk plus liver stores. During the first month of life, breastfed infants consume an average of 2 mg of zinc per day (Casey et al., 1985). Beyond the age of 6 months, infants would receive from 600 ml of breast milk only 0.6 mg of zinc per day—an amount that is usually augmented by the zinc in solid foods. The dietary zinc requirement of infants consuming formula is higher than that of breastfed infants because of lower zinc availability of the formulae (Casey et al., 1981; Lönnerdal et al., 1984). Walravens and Hambidge (1976) demonstrated that male infants consuming formula supplemented with zinc to a total of 5.8 mg/liter grew better than those on an unsupplemented formula containing 1.8 mg/liter. Assuming a consumption of 750 ml/day, plus two standard deviations, the subcommittee recommends 5 mg/day of zinc as the intake for formula-fed infants.

Although earlier balance studies suggested a zinc requirement of 6 to 7 mg/day for preadolescent children (Engel et al., 1966), Walravens et al. (1983) found low hair and plasma zinc levels suggestive of marginal deficiency in Spanish-American children 2 to 6 years old whose intake was 5 to 6 mg/day. Their height-for-age was below the tenth percentile, and their rate of linear growth improved as a result of supplementation to a total zinc intake of approximately 10 mg/day. That intake is recommended for preadolescent children.

Excessive Intakes and Toxicity

Acute toxicity, resulting in gastrointestinal irritation and vomiting, has been observed following the ingestion of 2 g or more of zinc in the form of sulfate (Prasad, 1976). The more subtle effects of moderately elevated intakes, not uncommon in the U.S. population, are of greater concern, because they are not easily detected. Impairment of the copper status of volunteers by dietary zinc intakes of 18.5 mg

(Festa et al., 1985) or 25 mg/day (Fischer et al., 1984) has been reported. Patients given zinc in quantities 10 to 30 times the RDA for several months developed hypocupremia, microcytosis, and neutropenia (Prasad et al., 1978). Zinc supplementation of healthy adults with amounts 20 times the RDA for 6 weeks resulted in the impairment of various immune responses (Chandra, 1984). Daily supplements of 80 to 150 mg caused a decline of high-density lipoproteins in serum after several weeks (Hooper et al., 1980). For these reasons, chronic ingestion of zinc supplements exceeding 15 mg/day is not recommended without adequate medical supervision.

References

Baer, M.T., and J.C. King. 1984. Tissue zinc levels and zinc excretion during experimental zinc depletion in young men. Am. J. Clin. Nutr. 39:556–570.

Casey, C.E., P.A. Walravens, and K.M. Hambidge. 1981. Availability of zinc: loading tests with human milk, cow's milk, and infant formulas. Pediatrics 68:394–396.

Casey, C.E., K.M. Hambidge, and M.C. Neville. 1985. Studies in human lactation: zinc, copper, manganese, and chromium in human milk in the first month of lactation. Am. J. Clin. Nutr. 41:1193–1200.

Chandra, R.K. 1984. Excessive intake of zinc impairs immune responses. J. Am. Med. Assoc. 252:1443–1446.

Chesters, J.K. 1982. Metabolism and biochemistry of zinc. Pp. 221–238 in A.S. Prasad, ed. Clinical, Biochemical, and Nutritional Aspects of Trace Elements. Current Topics in Nutrition and Disease, Vol. 6. Alan R. Liss, New York.

Engel, R.W., R.F. Miller, and N.O. Price. 1966. Metabolic patterns in preadolescent children. XIII. Zinc balance. Pp. 326–338 in A.S. Prasad, ed. Zinc Metabolism. Charles C Thomas, Springfield, Ill.

Erdman, J.W., Jr., S. Garcia-Lopez, and A.R. Sherman. 1987. Processing and fortification: How do they affect mineral interactions? Pp. 23–26 in O.A. Levander, ed. Nutrition 1987. American Institute of Nutrition, Bethesda, Md.

Festa, M.D., H.L. Anderson, R.P. Dowdy, and M.R. Ellersieck. 1985. Effect of zinc intake on copper excretion and retention in men. Am. J. Clin. Nutr. 41:285–292.

Fischer, P.W.F., A. Giroux, and M.R. L'Abbé. 1984. Effect of zinc supplementation on copper status in adult man. Am. J. Clin. Nutr. 40:743–746.

Foster, D.M., R.L. Aamodt, R.I. Henkin, and M. Berman. 1979. Zinc metabolism in humans: a kinetic model Am. J. Physiol. 237:R340–R349.

Greger, J.L. 1988. Effect of variations in dietary protein, phosphorus, electrolytes and vitamin D on calcium and zinc utilization. Pp. 205–227 in C.E. Bodwell and J.W. Erdman, Jr., eds. Nutrient Interactions. Marcel Dekker, New York.

Greger, J.L. 1989. Potential for trace mineral deficiencies and toxicities in the elderly. Pp. 171–200 in C.W. Bales, ed. Mineral Homeostasis in the Elderly. Current Topics in Nutrition and Disease, Vol. 21. Alan R. Liss, New York.

Hambidge, K.M., C. Hambidge, M. Jacobs, and J.D. Baum. 1972. Low levels of zinc in hair, anorexia, poor growth, and hypogensia in children. Pediatr. Res. 6:868–874.

Hambidge, K.M., P.A. Walravens, C.E. Casey, R.M. Brown, and C. Bender. 1979. Plasma zinc concentrations of breast-fed infants. J. Pediatr. 94:607–608.

Hambidge, K.M., C.E. Casey, and N.F. Krebs. 1986. Zinc. Pp. 1–137 in W. Mertz, ed. Trace Elements in Human and Animal Nutrition, Vol. 2. 5th ed. Academic Press, Orlando, Fla.

Hooper, P.L., L. Visconti, P.J. Garry, and G.E. Johnson. 1980. Zinc lowers high-density lipoprotein-cholesterol levels. J. Am. Med. Assoc. 244:1960–1961.

Hurley, L.S., and D.L. Baly. 1982. The effects of zinc deficiency during pregnancy. Pp. 145–159 in A.S. Prasad, ed. Clinical, Biochemical, and Nutritional Aspects of Trace Elements. Current Topics in Nutrition and Disease, Vol. 6. Alan R. Liss, New York.

Inglett, G.E., ed. 1983. Nutritional Bioavailability of Zinc. ACS Symposium Series No. 210. American Chemical Society, Washington, D.C.

King, J.C., and J.R. Turnlund. In press. Human zinc requirements. C.F. Mills, ed. Zinc in Human Biology. International Life Sciences Institute. London.

Krebs, N.F., K.M. Hambidge, M.A. Jacobs, and J.O. Rasbach. 1985. The effects of a dietary zinc supplement during lactation on longitudinal changes in maternal zinc status and milk zinc concentrations. Am. J. Clin. Nutr. 41:560–570.

Lönnerdal, B. 1987. Protein-mineral interactions. Pp. 32–36 in O.A. Levander, ed. Nutrition 1987. American Institute of Nutrition, Bethesda, Md.

Lönnerdal, B., A. Cederblad, L. Davidsson, and B. Sandström. 1984. The effect of individual components of soy formula and cows' milk formula on zinc bioavailability. Am. J. Clin. Nutr. 40:1064–1070.

Morris, E.R., and R. Ellis. 1983. Dietary phytate/zinc molar ratio and zinc balance in humans. Pp. 159–172 in G.E. Inglett, ed. Nutritional Bioavailability of Zinc. ACS Symposium Series No. 210. American Chemical Society, Washington, D.C.

Moser, P.B., and R.D. Reynolds. 1983. Dietary zinc intake and zinc concentrations of plasma erythrocytes, and breast milk in antepartum and postpartum lactating and nonlactating women: a longitudinal study. Am. J. Clin. Nutr. 38:101–108.

Patterson, K.Y., J.T. Holbrook, J.E. Bodner, J.L. Kelsay, J.C. Smith, Jr., and C. Veillon. 1984. Zinc, copper, and manganese intake and balance for adults consuming self-selected diets. Am. J. Clin. Nutr. 40:1397–1403.

Pennington, J.A.T., D.B. Wilson, R.F. Newell, B.F. Harland, R.D. Johnson, and J.E. Vanderveen. 1984. Selected minerals in foods surveys, 1974 to 1981/82. J. Am. Diet. Assoc. 84:771–780.

Pories, W.J., E.G. Mansour, F.R. Plecha, A. Flynn, and W.H. Strain. 1976. Metabolic factors affecting zinc metabolism in the surgical patient. Pp. 115–141 in A.S. Prasad, ed. Trace Elements in Health and Disease. Vol. I, Zinc and Copper. Academic Press, New York.

Prasad, A.S. 1976. Deficiency of zinc in man and its toxicity. Pp. 1–20 in A.S. Prasad, ed. Trace Elements in Health and Disease. Vol. I, Zinc and Copper. Academic Press, New York.

Prasad, A.S. 1982. Clinical and biochemical spectrum of zinc deficiency in human subjects. Pp. 3–62 in A.S. Prasad, ed. Clinical, Biochemical, and Nutritional Aspects of Trace Elements. Current Topics in Nutrition and Disease, Vol. 6. Alan R. Liss, New York.

Prasad, A.S., G.J. Brewer, E.B. Schoomaker, and P. Rabbani. 1978. Hypocupremia induced by zinc therapy in adults. J. Am. Med. Assoc. 240:2166–2168.

Sandstead, H.H. 1973. Zinc nutrition in the United States. Am. J. Clin. Nutr. 26:1251–1260.

Sandstead, H.H. 1985. Are estimates of trace element requirements meeting the needs of the user? Pp. 875–878 in C.F. Mills, I. Bremner, and J.K. Chesters, eds. Trace Elements in Man and Animals, TEMA-5. Commonwealth Agricultural Bureaux, Farnham Royal, United Kingdom.

Sandström, B., and Å. Cederblad. 1980. Zinc absorption from composite meals. II. Influence of the main protein source. Am. J. Clin. Nutr. 33:1778–1783.

Sandström, B., B. Arvidsson, Å. Cederblad, and E. Björn-Rasmussen. 1980. Zinc absorption from composite meals. I. The significance of wheat extraction rate, zinc, calcium, and protein content in meals based on bread. Am. J. Clin. Nutr. 33:739–745.

Solomons, N.W., and R. J. Cousins. 1984. Zinc. Pp. 125–197 in N.W. Solomons and I.H. Rosenberg, eds. Absorption and Malabsorption of Mineral Nutrients. Alan R. Liss, New York.

Solomons, N.W., and R.A. Jacob. 1981. Studies on the bioavailability of zinc in humans: effects of heme and non-heme iron on the absorption of zinc. Am. J. Clin. Nutr. 34:475–482.

Swanson, C.A., and J.C. King. 1987. Zinc and pregnancy outcome. Am. J. Clin. Nutr. 46:763–771.

Swanson, C.A., J.R. Turnlund, and J.C. King. 1983. Effect of dietary zinc sources and pregnancy on zinc utilization in adult women fed controlled diets. J. Nutr. 113:2557–2567.

Walravens, P.A., and K.M. Hambidge. 1976. Growth of infants fed a zinc supplemented formula. Am. J. Clin. Nutr. 29:1114–1121.

Walravens, P.A., N.F. Krebs, and K.M. Hambidge. 1983. Linear growth of low income preschool children receiving a zinc supplement. Am. J. Clin. Nutr. 38:195–201.

Welsh, S.O., and R.M. Marston. 1982. Zinc levels of the U.S. food supply: 1909–1980. Food Technol. 36:70–76.

IODINE

Iodine, an integral part of the thyroid hormones thyroxine and triiodothyronine, is an essential micronutrient for all animal species, including humans (Hetzel and Maberly, 1986). It is present in food and water predominantly as iodide and, to a lesser degree, organically bound to amino acids. Iodide is rapidly and almost completely absorbed and transported to the thyroid gland for synthesis into the thyroid hormones, to salivary and gastric glands, and to the kidneys for excretion into the gastrointestinal tract and urine. Organically bound iodine is less well absorbed, and part of it is excreted in the feces. Since all the iodide secreted into the gastrointestinal tract is reabsorbed, the main excretory route for the inorganic form of iodine is the urine. Although losses in the milk of lactating women and losses in sweat in hot climates can be considerable, urinary excretion is a reliable indicator of iodine status under most circumstances.

Iodine is unevenly distributed in the environment. In large areas, often mountainous, environmental levels are inadequate for humans and animals. Deficiency can lead to a wide spectrum of diseases, ranging from severe cretinism with mental retardation to barely visible enlargement of the thyroid. Endemic goiter and the more severe forms of iodine deficiency disorders continue to be a worldwide problem. In 1983 there were an estimated 400 million iodine-deficient persons in the less developed regions of the world (Hetzel and Maberly, 1986), an an estimated 112 million in the more developed areas (Matovinovic, 1983).

Iodine deficiency disorders, including goiter, can be prevented but not cured by providing an adequate iodine intake. The incidence of endemic goiter in the United States fell sharply after the introduction of iodized salt in 1924 (Brush and Atland, 1952). There are, however, residual cases of goiter remaining, mainly in women and children living in certain areas of the United States (California, Texas, Kentucky, Louisiana, and South Carolina) (Matovinovic, 1970; McGanity, 1970) and in the prairie regions of Canada (Nutrition Canada National Survey, 1973). These are most probably not caused by iodine deficiency, since they bear no relation to urinary iodine excretion, which is accepted as a reliable indicator of iodine status. Natural goitrogens, such as those found in cabbage or cassava, have been implicated in the pathogenesis of goiter in some parts of the world. It is not known if they pose a problem in the United States (Matovinovic, 1983).

Dietary Sources and Usual Intakes

The environmental levels of iodine and their contribution to the daily intake of animals and humans vary widely in the United States. In the coastal areas, seafoods, water, and iodine-containing mist from the ocean are important sources, whereas further inland, the iodine content of plant and animal products is variable, depending on the geochemical environment and on fertilizing, feeding practices, and food processing. In these areas, iodized table salt is a reliable source, providing 76 μg of iodine per gram of salt.

In addition, several adventitious sources of iodine find their way into the U.S. diet. Iodates are still used as dough oxidizers in the continuous bread making process, adding about 500 μg/100 g of bread. Dairy products accumulate iodine because of the use of iodine-containing disinfectants on cows, milking machines, and storage tanks, and by iodine-containing additives to the animals' feeds. All this can raise iodine concentrations severalfold over natural levels (Hemken, 1979).

The U.S. Food and Drug Administration in its Total Diet Study has found a tendency toward steadily declining iodine levels since 1982. In 1985–1986, the typical intake for men and women was 250 μg and 170 μg/day, respectively, excluding intakes from iodized salt (Pennington et al., 1989).

Recommended Allowances

Adults   Because of the high contribution by adventitious sources to the daily iodine intake in the United States, maintenance of the existing nutritional status is not a valid criterion for determining iodine requirements. It is customary to relate urinary iodine excretion, a reliable indicator of iodine intake and status, to the risk for goiter and other iodine deficiency disorders. An expert group of the Pan American Health Organization considered an excretion of more than 50 μg of iodine per gram of creatinine as adequate for normal function, excretion of 25 to 50 μg/g as associated with increased risk for hypothyroidism, and excretion of less than 25 μg/g as indicative of serious risk for endemic cretinism (Querido et al., 1974). Since dietary iodine is well absorbed, albeit not completely, a minimum intake of 50 to 75 μg/day is needed to maintain the higher level of iodine excretion in a population (NRC, 1970).

Although the levels of goitrogens in the U.S. diet and their effects on the iodine requirement have not been quantified, the recommended allowance for adults of both sexes is set at 150 μg/day to provide an extra margin of safety. This amount is close to the 160 μg calculated to maintain plasma inorganic iodide levels within the normal range in most of the U.S. population (Wayne et al., 1964).

Pregnancy and Lactation   An increment of 25 μg/day in the dietary allowance is recommended during pregnancy to cover the extra demands of the fetus. The additional allowance for lactating women, 50 μg/day, is based on the estimated need of the infant, not on the iodine loss via breast milk (Fomon, 1984; Man and Benotti, 1964).

Infants and Children   The amounts of iodine in the milk of North American women are much greater than the needs of their infants. They reflect the elevated dietary iodine intakes of the mothers (Gushurst et al., 1984). In the absence of a better basis, the relative energy requirements of adults has been used to set the iodine allowance for infants and children.

Excessive Intakes and Toxicity

The acute toxicity of iodides and iodates has been thoroughly studied (LSRO, 1975). Amounts between 200 and 500 mg/kg per day produced death in different species of laboratory animals.

The potential chronic toxic effects of dietary iodine are less clear. In an attempt to reduce the high incidence of goiter in Tasmania, bread was fortified with iodine to yield a concentration of 2 to 4 μg/ g (dry) bread. Once the iodinated bread was available to the islanders, the incidence of thyrotoxicosis more than doubled. Most patients were in the older age groups and had been exposed to decades of iodine deficiency (Connolly, 1973). Goiter induced by high iodine intake has also been documented in Japan, where seaweeds rich in iodine (up to 4.5 mg/g dry weight) are consumed (Nagataki, 1974).

Generally, iodine intakes of up to 2 mg/day have caused no adverse physiological reactions in healthy adults, and 1 mg/day produced no indications of physiological abnormalities in children (Crocco and White, 1981). There is no evidence of adverse reactions, such as chronic toxicity or hypersensitivity, to the much lower iodine intakes in the United States, and the present iodine intake by the majority of the U.S. population is considered to be adequate and safe (LSRO, 1975).

Other Considerations

The public health value of iodized salt in the prevention of iodine deficiency disorders is well established. The use of iodized salt in all noncoastal regions where environmental and dietary levels are low is recommended.

The present iodine intake in the United States is safe and decreasing toward recommended levels. The subcommittee notes that the use of iodine-containing compounds has declined and recommends that no additional sources of iodine be introduced into the U.S. diet.

References

Brush, B.E., and J.K. Altland. 1952. Goiter prevention with iodized salt: results of a thirty-year study. J. Clin. Endocrin. Metab. 12:1380–1388.

Connally, R.J. 1973. The changing age incidence of iodbasedow in Tasmania. Med. J. Austr. 2:171–174.

Crocco, S.C., and P.L. White. 1981. Iodine: Fifty Years After Goiter. Proceedings of the Stokely-Van Camp Annual Symposium, Food in Contemporary Society: Emerging Patterns, May 27–29, 1981. University of Tennessee, Knoxville. 16 pp.

Fomon, S.J. 1974. Infant Nutrition, 2nd ed. Saunders, Philadelphia. 575 pp.

Gushurst, C.A., J.A. Mueller, J.A. Green, and F. Sedor. 1984. Breast milk iodide: reassessment in the 1980s. Pediatrics 73:354–357.

Hemken, R.W. 1979. Factors that influence the iodine content of milk and meat: a review. J. Anim. Sci. 48:981–985.

Hetzel, B.S., and G.F. Maberly. 1986. Iodine. Pp. 139-208 in W. Mertz, ed. Trace Elements in Human and Animal Nutrition, 5th ed. Academic Press, New York.

LSRO (Life Sciences Research Office). 1975. Evaluation of the Health Aspects of Potassium Iodide, Potassium Iodate, and Calcium Iodate as Food Ingredients. Federation of American Societies for Experimental Biology, Bethesda, Md.

Man, E.B., and J. Benotti. 1969. Butanol-extractable iodine in human and bovine colostrum and milk. Clin. Chem. 15:1141–1146.

Matovinovic, J. 1970. Extent of iodine insufficiency in the United States. Pp. 1–5 in Iodine Nutriture in the United States. Report of the Committee on Food Protection, Food and Nutrition Board, National Academy of Sciences, Washington, D.C.

Matovinovic, J. 1983. Endemic goiter and cretinism at the dawn of the third millennium. Annu. Rev. Nutr. 3:341–412.

McGanity, W. 1970. Extent of iodine insufficiency in the United States. Pp. 5–8 in Iodine Nutriture in the United States. Food and Nutrition Board, National Research Council. National Academy of Sciences, Washington, D.C.

Nagataki, S. 1974. Effect of excess quantities of iodide. Pp. 329–344 in Handbook of Physiology, III, Endocrinology. American Physiological Society, Washington, D.C.

NRC (National Research Council). 1970. Iodine Nutriture in the United States. Summary of a Conference, October 31, 1970. Report of the Committee on Food Protection, Food and Nutrition Board, National Academy of Sciences. Washington, D.C. 53 pp.

Nutrition Canada National Survey. 1973. Nutrition Problems in Perspective. Information Canada, Ottawa. 115 pp.

Pennington, J.A.T., B.E. Young, and D.B. Wilson. 1989. Nutritional elements in U.S. diets: results from the Total Diet Study, 1982 to 1986. J. Am. Diet. Assoc. 89:659–664.

Querido, A., F. Delange, J.T. Dunn, R. Fierro-Benítez, H.K. Ibbertson, D.A. Koutras, and H. Perinetti. 1974. Definitions of endemic goiter and cretinism, classification of goiter size and severity of endemias, and survey techniques. Pp. 267–272 in J.T. Dunn and G.A. Medeiros-Neto, eds. Endemic Goiter and Cretinism: Continuing Threats to World Health. Scientific Publ. No. 292. Pan American Health Organization, Washington, D.C.

Wayne, E.J., D.A. Koutras, and W.D. Alexander. 1964. Clinical Aspects of Iodine Metabolism. Blackwell, Oxford. 303 pp.

SELENIUM

The biochemical basis for the essentiality of selenium is its presence at the active site of glutathione peroxidase, an enzyme that catalyzes the breakdown of hydroperoxides (Hoekstra, 1975). Although the role of selenium in hydroperoxide destruction helps explain its close metabolic interrelationship with the antioxidant vitamin E, evidence for other possible functions is accumulating (Burk, 1983).

Direct evidence of a requirement for selenium in human nutrition was lacking until 1979, when Chinese scientists reported an association between low selenium status and Keshan disease, a cardiomyopathy that affects primarily young children and women of childbearing age (Keshan Disease Research Group, 1979a). A large-scale intervention trial involving several thousand Chinese children demonstrated the value of selenium in preventing the disease (Keshan Disease Research Group, 1979b). Selenium deficiency cannot account for all aspects of Keshan disease, and the possible involvement of a cardiotoxic virus has been suggested (Yang et al., 1988), but it seems clear that selenium deficiency is the underlying condition predisposing people to the development of the disease.

General Signs of Deficiency

In animals, many diseases are caused by simultaneous deficiencies of selenium and vitamin E, and they can be prevented or cured by supplementation with either nutrient alone (NRC, 1983). Pure selenium deficiency in the presence of adequate levels of vitamin E has been demonstrated conclusively only in rats fed a selenium-deficient diet for two generations (McCoy and Weswig, 1969). Signs of selenium deficiency observed in squirrel monkeys (Muth et al., 1971) have not been seen in more recent studies of rhesus monkeys (Butler et al., 1988). Nutritional pancreatic atrophy in chicks, long believed to be a selenium-specific deficiency syndrome, has now been shown to respond to high dietary levels of vitamin E and certain other antioxidants (Whitacre et al., 1987).

Intravenous feeding solutions used in total parenteral nutrition (TPN) are practically devoid of selenium, and patients undergoing TPN have low erythrocyte glutathione peroxidase activities and low levels of selenium in plasma and red cells (Levander and Burk, 1986). In three such patients, muscular discomfort or weakness responded to selenium therapy (Brown et al., 1986; Kien and Ganther, 1983; van Rij et al., 1979), thereby providing additional evidence of a selenium requirement for humans. Some cases of cardiomyopathy have also occurred in TPN patients with low selenium status (Fleming et al., 1982; Johnson et al., 1981).

Dietary Sources and Usual Intakes

Seafoods, kidney, and liver, and to a lesser extent other meats, are consistently good sources of selenium, whereas grains and other seeds are more variable, depending on the selenium content of the soils in which they are grown (WHO, 1987). Fruits and vegetables generally contain little selenium. Drinking water usually makes only a small contribution to selenium intake (WHO, 1987).

Studies in animals have shown that the bioavailability of selenium in certain fish is less than that in other foods (Mutanen, 1986). Few data exist on the bioavailability of selenium in foods consumed by humans. However, bioavailability trials conducted in subjects with poor selenium status indicated that organically bound forms of selenium are retained better than inorganic selenium, but all forms tested caused similar increases in glutathione peroxidase activity (Levander et al., 1983; Thomson et al., 1982).

Analyses of national food composites in the United States indicate that the overall adult mean dietary selenium intake was 108 μg/day between 1974 and 1982. The daily means for each year ranged from 83 to 129 μg (Pennington et al., 1984).

Assessment of Selenium Status

Selenium status in humans is commonly assessed by estimating dietary selenium intakes, measuring selenium levels in various tissues and excreta, or determining glutathione peroxidase activity in certain blood components (for a review, see Levander, 1985). Dietary selenium intakes are difficult to estimate because of the variation in the selenium content of locally produced and consumed foods, which is determined by the selenium content of the soil in which the food is grown. Selenium levels in erythrocytes are an index of longer term selenium status than levels in plasma, and animal studies indicate that the latter may not always reflect other body selenium pools, especially when sudden shifts in selenium intake occur. It is easier to measure glutathione peroxidase activity than to perform the chemical analysis for selenium. Moreover, the enzymatic method has the advantage of measuring only biologically active selenium. However, glutathione peroxidase activity is a valid index of human selenium status only in populations with low selenium intakes, since the activity of the enzyme plateaus at higher intakes (Whanger et al., 1988).

Recommended Allowances

Adults   Several balance studies have been conducted to investigate selenium requirements of humans. However, humans apparently can adjust their selenium homeostatic mechanisms to remain in balance over rather wide ranges of dietary intakes. Therefore, the balance technique is of little help in delineating the selenium requirements of humans (Levander, 1987).

Another approach to estimating human selenium requirements is to examine dietary intakes in areas with and without selenium deficiency. In China, for example, dietary surveys of selenium intake in endemic and nearby nonendemic Keshan disease areas indicated that the minimum daily selenium requirements for adult Chinese men and women are 19 and 13 μg, respectively (Yang et al., 1988). In New Zealand, however, daily selenium intakes of 33 μg by men and

23 μg by women were not associated with any selenium deficiency symptoms (Thomson and Robinson, 1980).

A so-called physiological human selenium requirement was estimated by following increases in plasma glutathione peroxidase activity in adult Chinese men with low selenium status (i.e., a daily dietary intake of approximately 10 μg), who were supplemented with graded doses of selenomethionine (Yang et al., 1987). After 5 months, the plasma glutathione peroxidase activity plateaued at similar levels for groups receiving 30 μg or more of supplemental selenium per day. On this basis, the authors suggested a physiological selenium requirement of approximately 40 μg/day (diet plus supplement) for their adult Chinese male subjects. Since the Chinese men in this study weighed approximately 60 kg and the selenium requirement of adults appears to be related to body weight, the estimated requirements for the reference North American adult male and female must be adjusted for differences in body weight, i.e., 79 kg for males and 63 kg for females. Individual variation in selenium requirements was accounted for by using a safety factor of 1.3, which was based on an arbitrarily assumed coefficient of variation of 15%. Multiplying the Chinese estimate of the physiological human selenium requirement by these two factors (adjustments for body weight and individual variation) results in a recommended dietary selenium allowance of 0.87 μg/kg or, with rounding, 70 and 55 μg/day for the reference adult North American male and female, respectively. In the absence of specific data on requirements of the elderly, the figures for younger adults are used.

Pregnancy and Lactation   A metabolic balance study demonstrated that the amounts of selenium retained during the second and fourth quarters of pregnancy were 10 and 23 μg/day, respectively (Swanson et al., 1983). However, these retention values were believed to be high because the levels of dietary selenium fed during that study (150 μg/day) were elevated, compared to the usual intake of the subjects, and resulted in positive selenium balances, even in the nonpregnant subjects. If a factorial technique is used to estimate the human selenium requirement for pregnancy, and it is assumed that 5 kg of lean tissue containing an average selenium concentration of 0.25 mg/kg (Schroeder et al., 1970) is deposited during pregnancy, a total of 1.25 mg of selenium would have to be retained. Thus, an average selenium accretion of 5 μg/day, or 6.5 μg/day allowing for variability, would be needed. If an absorption rate of 80% is assumed (Levander, 1983), the average increase in dietary selenium during pregnancy would be 10 μg/day.

Milk from North American women contains an average selenium concentration of 15 to 20 μg/liter (Mannon and Picciano, 1987). During lactation, a daily selenium loss of 13 μg may occur in a secretion of 750 ml of milk. If a population variance is allowed and a dietary absorption of 80% is assumed, an additional selenium allowance of 20 μg/day is recommended for lactation to maintain a satisfactory level of the mineral in milk and to prevent depletion in the mother.

Infants and Children The maintenance selenium requirements for infants, extrapolated from adult values, would be 5 μg/day from birth to 6 months of age. To allow for growth, this figure was increased to 10 μg/day. The North American breastfed infant would receive ample selenium, since consumption of 750 ml of breast milk per day would result in an intake of about 13 μg of selenium per day. The allowance during the second 6 months, calculated similarly, is 15 μg/day. Moreover, these recommendations provide a substantial margin of safety, since infants in Finland and New Zealand suffer no observable ill effects of low selenium intake even though the average selenium content of human milk in those countries ranges from only 6 to 8 μg/liter (Kumpulainen et al., 1983; Williams, 1983), in contrast to 15 to 20 μg/liter in the United States.

Because little is known about the selenium requirements of children, recommendations for them have been extrapolated from adult values on the basis of body weight, and a factor arbitrarily allowed for growth.

Excessive Intakes and Toxicity

The level of dietary selenium exposure needed to cause chronic poisoning in humans is not known with certainty, but approximately 5 mg/day from foods resulted in fingernail changes and hair loss in a seleniferous zone of China (Yang et al., 1983). The Chinese investigators also reported that a person who had consumed 1 mg of selenium daily as sodium selenite for more than 2 years had thickened but fragile nails and a garlic odor in dermal excretions. In the United States, 13 people developed selenium intoxication after taking an improperly manufactured dietary supplement that contained 27.3 mg of selenium per tablet. Symptoms included nausea, abdominal pain, diarrhea, nail and hair changes, peripheral neuropathy, fatigue, and irritability (Helzlsouer et al., 1985). The woman who consumed the most selenium (2,387 mg over a 2.5-month period) experienced hair loss, fingernail tenderness and loss, nausea and vomiting, a sour-milk breath odor, and increasing fatigue (Jensen et al., 1984). The molecular mechanism of selenium toxicity has not been clearly established (Levander, 1982), and sensitive biochemical indicators of selenium poisoning are not known.

References

Brown, M.R., H.J. Cohen, J.M. Lyons, T.W. Curtis, B. Thunberg, W.J. Cochran, and W.J. Klish. 1986. Proximal muscle weakness and selenium deficiency associated with long term parenteral nutrition. Am. J. Clin. Nutr. 43:549–554.

Burk, R.F. 1983. Biological activity of selenium. Annu. Rev. Nutr. 3:53–70.

Butler, J.A., P.D. Whanger, and N.M. Patton. 1988. Effect of feeding selenium-deficient diets to rhesus monkeys (*Macaca mulatta*). J. Am. Coll. Nutr. 7:43–56.

Fleming, C.R., J.T. Lie, J.T. McCall, J.F. O'Brien, E.E. Baillie, and J.L. Thistle. 1982. Selenium deficiency and fatal cardiomyopathy in a patient on home parenteral nutrition. Gastroenterology 83:689–693.

Helzlsouer, K., R. Jacobs, and S. Morris. 1985. Acute selenium intoxication in the United States. Fed. Proc. 44:1670.

Hoekstra, W.G. 1975. Biochemical function of selenium and its relation to vitamin E. Fed. Proc. 34:2083–2089.

Jensen, R., W. Closson, and R. Rothenberg. 1984. Selenium intoxication—New York. Morb. Mortal. Week. Rep. 33:157–158.

Johnson, R.A., S.S. Baker, J.T. Fallon, E.P. Maynard, J.N. Ruskin, Z. Wen, K. Ge, and H.J. Cohen. 1981. An accidental case of cardiomyopathy and selenium deficiency. N. Engl. J. Med. 304:1210–1212.

Keshan Disease Research Group. 1979a. Epidemiologic studies on the etiologic relationship of selenium and Keshan disease. Chin. Med. J. 92:477–482.

Keshan Disease Research Group. 1979b. Observations on effect of sodium selenite in prevention of Keshan disease. Chin. Med. J. 92:471–476.

Kien, C.L., and H.E. Ganther. 1983. Manifestations of chronic selenium deficiency in a child receiving total parenteral nutrition. Am. J. Clin. Nutr. 37:319–328.

Kumpulainen, J., E. Vuori, P. Kuitunen, S. Mäkinen, and R. Kara. 1983. Longitudinal study on the dietary selenium intake of exclusively breast-fed infants and their mothers in Finland. Int. J. Vit. Nutr. Res. 53:420–426.

Levander, O.A. 1982. Selenium: biochemical actions, interactions and some human health implications. Pp. 345–368 in A.S. Prasad, ed. Clinical, Biochemical, and Nutritional Aspects of Trace Elements. Current Topics in Nutrition and Disease, Vol. 6. Alan R. Liss, New York.

Levander, O.A. 1983. Considerations in the design of selenium bioavailability studies. Fed. Proc. 42:1721–1725.

Levander, O.A. 1985. Considerations on the assessment of selenium status. Fed. Proc. 44:2579–2583.

Levander, O.A. 1987. A global view of selenium nutrition. Annu. Rev. Nutr. 7:227–250.

Levander, O.A., and R.F. Burk. 1986. Report on the 1986 A.S.P.E.N. Research Workshop on Selenium in Clinical Nutrition. J. Parenter. Enteral. Nutr. 10:545–549.

Levander, O.A., G. Alfthan, H. Arvilommi, C.G. Gref, J.K. Huttunen, M. Kataja, P. Koivistoinen, and J. Pikkarainen. 1983. Bioavailability of selenium to Finnish men as assessed by platelet glutathione peroxidase activity and other blood parameters. Am. J. Clin. Nutr. 37:887–897.

Mannan, S., and M.F. Picciano. 1987. Influence of maternal selenium status on human milk selenium concentration and glutathione peroxidase activity. Am. J. Clin. Nutr. 46:95–100.

McCoy, K.E.M., and P.H. Weswig. 1969. Some selenium responses in the rat not related to vitamin E. J. Nutr. 98:383–389.

Mutanen, M. 1986. Bioavailability of selenium. Ann. Clin. Res. 18:48–54.

Muth, O.H., P.H. Weswig, P.D. Whanger, and J.E. Oldfield. 1971. Effect of feeding selenium-deficient ration to the subhuman primate (*Saimiri sciureus*). Am. J. Vet. Res. 32:1603–1605.

NRC (National Research Council). 1983. Selenium in Nutrition, rev. ed. Report of the Subcommittee on Selenium, Committee on Animal Nutrition, Board on Agriculture. National Academy Press, Washington, D.C. 174 pp.

Pennington, J.A.T., D.B. Wilson, R.F. Newell, B.F. Harland, R.D. Johnson, and J.E. Vanderveen. 1984. Selected minerals in foods surveys, 1974 to 1981/82. J. Am. Diet. Assoc. 84:771–780.

Schroeder, H.A., D.V. Frost, and J.J. Balassa. 1970. Essential trace metals in man: selenium. J. Chronic Dis. 23:227–243.

Swanson, C.A., D.C. Reamer, C. Veillon, J.C. King, and O.A. Levander. 1983. Quantitative and qualitative aspects of selenium utilization in pregnant and nonpregnant women: an application of stable isotope methodology. Am. J. Clin. Nutr. 38:169–180.

Thomson, C.D., and M.F. Robinson. 1980. Selenium in human health and disease with emphasis on those aspects peculiar to New Zealand. Am. J. Clin. Nutr. 33:303–323.

Thomson, C.D., M.F. Robinson, D.R. Campbell, and H.M. Rea. 1982. Effect of prolonged supplementation with daily supplements of selenomethionine and sodium selenite on glutathione peroxidase activity in blood of New Zealand residents. Am. J. Clin. Nutr. 36:24–31.

van Rij, A.M., C.D. Thomson, J.M. McKenzie, and M.F. Robinson. 1979. Selenium deficiency in total parenteral nutrition. Am. J. Clin. Nutr. 32:2076–2085.

Whanger, P.D., M.A. Beilstein, C.D. Thomson, M.F. Robinson, and M. Howe. 1988. Blood selenium and glutathione peroxidase activity of populations in New Zealand, Oregon, and South Dakota. FASEB J. 2:2996–3002.

Whitacre, M.E., G.F. Combs, Jr., S.B. Combs, and R.S. Parker. 1987. Influence of dietary vitamin E on nutritional pancreatic atrophy in selenium-deficient chicks. J. Nutr. 117:460–467.

WHO (World Health Organization). 1987. Selenium. Environmental Health Criteria 58: A Report of the International Programme on Chemical Safety. World Health Organization, Geneva.

Williams, M. 1983. Selenium and glutathione peroxidase in mature human milk. Proc. Univ. Otago Med. Sch. 61:20–21.

Yang, G., S. Wang, R. Zhou, and S. Sun. 1983. Endemic selenium intoxication of humans in China. Am. J. Clin. Nutr. 37:872–881.

Yang, G., L.Z. Zhu, S.J. Liu, L.Z. Gu, P.C. Qian, J.H. Huang, and M.O. Lu. 1987. Human selenium requirements in China. Pp. 589–607 in G.F. Combs, Jr., J.E. Spallholz, O.A. Levander, and J.E. Oldfield, eds. Proceedings of the Third International Symposium on Selenium in Biology and Medicine. AVI Publishing, Westport, Conn.

Yang, G., K. Ge, J. Chen, and X. Chen. 1988. Selenium-related endemic diseases and the daily selenium requirement of humans. World Rev. Nutr. Diet. 55:98–152.

COPPER

Copper is an essential nutrient for all vertebrates and some lower animal species (Davis and Mertz, 1987). Several abnormalities have been observed in copper-deficient animals, including anemia, skeletal defects, demyelination and degeneration of the nervous system, defects in pigmentation and structure of hair or wool, reproductive failure, myocardial degeneration, and decreased arterial elasticity. There are a number of important copper-containing proteins and enzymes, some of which are essential for the proper utilization of iron (Davis and Mertz, 1987).

Assessment of Copper Status

Although hypocupremia is readily produced in animals during experimental copper deficiency, circulating copper concentration is not necessarily a valid index of copper nutriture in humans (Solomons, 1979). Ceruloplasmin, a protein-copper complex, is strongly influenced by hormonal changes or inflammation, thus limiting its usefulness as an indicator (Mason, 1979). Determination of erythrocyte superoxide dismutase (SOD) activity appears to be a promising technique for assessing copper status in humans (Uauy et al., 1985).

Evidence for Human Requirement

Severe copper deficiency is rare in human beings (Cartwright and Wintrobe, 1964; Danks, 1988). Copper depletion sufficient to cause hypocupremia has been observed during total parenteral nutrition (Shike, 1984) and in cases of Menkes' steely hair disease—a rare, inherited disease resulting in impaired copper utilization (Menkes et al., 1962). The hypocupremia reported in protein-calorie malnutrition, sprue, nephrotic syndrome, and certain other diseases is probably unrelated to dietary copper intake and is believed to be secondary to a state of hypoproteinemia and inability to provide adequate amounts of the aproprotein for ceruloplasmin synthesis (Mason, 1979). Under normal circumstances, dietary copper deficiency is not known to occur in adults, but it has been observed in malnourished children in Peru; its manifestations are anemia, neutropenia, and severe bone demineralization (Cordano et al., 1964). In the early 1970s in the United States, similar findings were recognized in a few very small premature infants who were hospitalized for long periods and exclusively fed modified cow's milk formula or received prolonged parenteral alimentation. Presumably, these aberrations reflected a deficient dietary intake of copper (Cordano, 1974). More recently, copper deficiency has been shown to impair the growth of Chilean infants recovering from malnutrition (Castillo-Duran and Uauy, 1988).

The concentration of copper in the human fetus increases substantially during gestation, about half of the total fetal copper accumulating in the liver (Widdowson et al., 1974). These hepatic reserves are believed to protect the full-term infant against copper deficiency during the first few months of life. In the United States, tissue copper concentrations remain remarkably steady throughout adult life (Schroeder et al., 1966). The relatively constant copper concentrations in most tissues indicate sufficient dietary intake and effective homeostatic control of copper.

Epidemiological and experimental animal studies suggest a positive correlation between the zinc-to-copper ratio in the diet and the incidence of cardiovascular disease (Klevay, 1984). Elevated plasma cholesterol levels, impaired glucose tolerance, and heart-related abnormalities have been observed in some human subjects consuming only 0.8 to 1.0 mg copper per day (Klevay et al., 1984; Reiser et al., 1985), but not in others (Turnlund et al., 1989).

Dietary Sources and Usual Intakes

Organ meats, especially liver, are the richest sources of copper in the diet, followed by seafoods, nuts, and seeds. The concentration of copper in drinking water is highly variable; it is much influenced by the interaction of the water's acidity with the piping system. Additional contributions to intake may come from adventitious sources, such as copper-containing fungicides sprayed on agricultural products. Human milk contains approximately 0.3 mg/liter; cow's milk only about 0.09 mg/liter (Varo et al., 1980)

Older analytical data indicating that most U.S. diets provide a daily copper intake between 2 and 5 mg are now being reexamined and questioned (Klevay, 1984). The Total Diet Study, based on the extensive dietary analyses performed by the U.S. Food and Drug Administration, showed that the daily intake of copper for adult males and females averaged about 1.2 and 0.9 mg, respectively, from 1982 to 1986 (Pennington et al., 1989). The intakes for infants 6 to 11 months old and toddlers 2 years old were 0.45 and 0.57 mg daily.

Bioavailability

Several different factors may affect the bioavailability of dietary copper. Jacob et al. (1987) observed that high intakes of vitamin C (605 mg/day) decreased serum ceruloplasmin but had no effect on overall body copper status. Zinc intakes slightly above RDA levels reduced apparent copper retention in young men and adolescent females (Festa et al., 1985; Greger et al., 1978). The degree of copper deficiency may be influenced by the type of carbohydrate consumed, since rats fed a diet containing fructose developed more severe signs of copper deficiency than did rats fed a diet containing either glucose or starch (Fields et al., 1984). Although it may be assumed that the interaction between copper and ascorbic acid involves reduction and chelation of the metal in the intestine, the nature of the interaction of copper with zinc or carbohydrates is not yet known.

Estimated Safe and Adequate Daily Dietary Intakes

Adults In the past, estimates of the copper requirement for humans were derived from metabolic balance studies. However, the balance technique can lead to false estimates of nutritional requirements because the efficiency of copper absorption is increased or decreased in response to low or high copper intakes, respectively (Turnlund et al., 1989). Older balance studies suggested that the adult requirement for copper ranged from 2.0 to 2.6 mg/day, whereas later studies indicated that intakes less than 2.0 mg/day, and often not much more than 1.0 mg/day, could maintain positive copper balance (Mason, 1979). In a recent metabolic ward study, 13 men consuming a variety of typical U.S. diets were found to need 1.30 mg/day to replace fecal and urinary losses (Klevay et al., 1980).

Whole-body surface losses of copper are highly variable. Such variability makes it difficult to select an appropriate value for the losses incurred through this pathway, but recent estimates indicate that copper losses from the body's surface are less than 0.1 mg/day (Turnlund et al., 1989). If the true gastrointestinal absorption of copper at intakes of 1.7 to 2.0 mg is 36% ($\pm$ 1.3 SEM) (Turnlund et al., 1989), then a dietary intake of 0.3 mg/day is required to replace body surface losses. Adding this figure to the average dietary intake of 1.3 mg/day needed to replace urinary and fecal losses indicates that a total dietary copper intake of approximately 1.6 mg/day is required to maintain balance in adult men.

Many U.S. diets provide less than 1.6 mg of copper daily (Klevay, 1984). Since anemia or neutropenia ascribable to copper deficiency has not been observed in adults consuming typical U.S. diets, there is an obvious discrepancy between the experimentally derived copper requirement as defined by balance studies and currently estimated dietary copper intakes. This suggests either a long-term homeostatic adaptation to low copper intakes, or an incorrect estimate of dietary copper intake due to the underreporting of certain foods and water that are sources of the element. Because of the uncertainty about the quantitative human requirement for copper, it is not possible to establish an RDA for this trace element. Rather, the subcommittee recommends 1.5 to 3 mg/day as a safe and adequate range of dietary copper intake for adults.

Infants and Children   The average daily intake of copper by exclusively breastfed North American infants was 0.23 ± .07 mg over the first 4 months of lactation (Butte et al., 1987), or approximately 40 ± 16 μg/kg per day. This intake is substantially less than the 80 μg/kg per day recommended by a World Health Organization Expert Committee (WHO, 1973), but approaches the lower limit of the estimated requirement range of 45 to 135 μg/kg per day suggested by Cordano (1974) for rapidly growing infants with poor stores. Positive copper balance has been observed in normal children ages 3 months to 8 years with intakes as low as 35 ± 22 μg/kg per day (Alexander et al., 1974).

Studies in animals have shown high bioavailability of copper from human milk (Lönnerdal et al., 1985). Furthermore, the sizeable hepatic copper reserve built up during fetal development appears to contribute to the early needs of the growing full-term infant (Widdowson et al., 1974). After 3 months of age, the recommended copper intake of 75 μg/kg/day translates into dietary ranges of 0.4 to 0.6 and 0.6 to 0.7 mg/day for reference infants from birth to 6 months and from 6 to 12 months old, respectively. The introduction of solid foods at 4 to 6 months of age should enable the older infant fed a mixed diet to meet the copper recommendations (Gibson and De Wolfe, 1980), but the exclusively breastfed infant will have difficulty in achieving those levels because copper levels in human milk decline from 0.6 to 0.2 mg/liter during the first 6 months of lactation (Vuori and Kuitunen, 1979). These recommended intakes may be inadequate for the premature infant, who is always born with low copper stores (Shaw, 1973).

The American Academy of Pediatrics has recently recommended that infant formulas provide 60 μg of copper per 100 kcal (AAP, 1985). By following this recommendation, a typical formula-fed infant from birth to 6 months of age receiving 700 kcal per day would consume approximately 0.4 mg of copper per day.

In preadolescent and adolescent girls, fecal and urinary losses were at or near equilibrium with a dietary copper intake of 1 to 1.3 mg/day (35 to 45 µg/kg body weight per day) (Engel et al., 1967; Greger et al., 1978; Price and Bunce, 1972). The recommended copper range of 1.0 to 2.0 mg/day for 7- to 10-year-old children provides at least 40 µg/kg body weight/day.

Excessive Intakes and Toxicity

An FAO/WHO Expert Committee concluded that no deleterious effects can be expected in humans whose copper intake is 0.5 mg/kg body weight per day (FAO/WHO, 1971). Usual diets in the United States rarely supply more than 5 mg/day, and an occasional intake of up to 10 mg/day is probably safe for human adults. Although storing or processing acidic foods or fluids in copper vessels can add to the daily intake, overt toxicity from dietary sources is extremely rare in the U.S. population (NRC, 1977)

References

AAP (American Academy of Pediatrics). 1985. Recommended ranges of nutrients in formulas. Appendix I. Pp. 356–357 in Pediatric Nutrition Handbook, 2nd ed. American Academy of Pediatrics, Elk Grove Village, Ill.

Alexander, F.W., B.E. Clayton, and H.T. Delves. 1974. Mineral and trace-metal balances in children receiving normal and synthetic diets. Q.J. Med. 43:89–111.

Butte, N.F., C. Garza, E.O. Smith, C. Wills, and B.L. Nichols. 1987. Macro- and trace-mineral intakes of exclusively breast-fed infants. Am. J. Clin. Nutr. 45:42–48.

Cartwright, G.E., and M.M. Wintrobe. 1964. The question of copper deficiency in man. Am. J. Clin. Nutr. 15:94–110.

Castillo-Duran, C., and R. Uauy. 1988. Copper deficiency impairs growth of infants recovering from malnutrition. Am. J. Clin. Nutr. 47:710–714.

Cordano, A. 1974. The role played by copper in the physiopathology and nutrition of the infant and the child. Ann. Nestle 33:1–16.

Cordano, A., J.M. Baertl, and G.G. Graham. 1964. Copper deficiency in infancy. Pediatrics 34:324–336.

Danks, D.M. 1988. Copper deficiency in humans. Annu. Rev. Nutr. 8:235–257.

Davis, G.K., and W. Mertz. 1987. Copper. Pp. 301–364 in W. Mertz, ed. Trace Elements in Human and Animal Nutrition, 5th ed., Vol. 2. Academic Press, Orlando, Fla.

Engel, R.W., N.O. Price, and R.F. Miller. 1967. Copper, manganese, cobalt, and molybdenum balance in pre-adolescent girls. J. Nutr. 92:197–204.

FAO/WHO (Food and Agriculture Organization/World Health Organization). 1971. Evaluation of Food Additives. WHO Technical Report Series No. 462. World Health Organization, Geneva.

Festa, M.D., H.L. Anderson, R.P. Dowdy, and M.R. Ellersieck. 1985. Effect of zinc intake on copper excretion and retention in men. Am. J. Clin. Nutr. 41:285–292.

Fields, M., R.J. Ferretti, J.C. Smith, and R. Reiser. 1984. The interaction of type of dietary carbohydrates with copper deficiency. Am. J. Clin. Nutr. 39:289–295.

Gibson, R.S., and M.S. DeWolfe. 1980. The dietary trace metal intake of some Canadian full-term and low birthweight infants during the first twelve months of infancy. J. Can. Diet. Assoc. 41:206–215.

Greger, J.L., S.C. Zaikis, R.P. Abernathy, O.A. Bennett, and J. Huffman. 1978. Zinc, nitrogen, copper, iron and manganese balance in adolescent females fed two levels of zinc. J. Nutr. 108:1449–1456.

Jacob, R.A., J.H. Skala, S.T. Omaye, and J.R. Turnlund. 1987. Effect of varying ascorbic acid intakes on copper absorption and ceruloplasmin levels of young men. J. Nutr. 117:2109–2115.

Klevay, L.M. 1984. The role of copper, zinc, and other chemical elements in ischemic heart disease. Pp. 129–157 in O.M. Rennert and W.-Y. Chan, eds. Metabolism of Trace Metals in Man, Vol. 1. Developmental Aspects. CRC Press, Boca Raton, Fla.

Klevay, L.M., S.J. Reck, R.A. Jacob, G.M. Logan, Jr., J.M. Munoz, and H.H. Sandstead. 1980. The human requirement for copper. I. Healthy men fed conventional American diets. Am. J. Clin. Nutr. 33:45–50.

Klevay, L.M., L. Inman, K. Johnson, M. Lawler, J.R. Mahalko, D.B. Milne, H.C. Lukaski, W. Bolonchuk, and H.H. Sandstead. 1984. Increased cholesterol in plasma in a young man during experimental copper depletion. Metabolism 33:1112–1118.

Lönnerdal, B., J.G. Bell, and C.L. Keen. 1985. Copper absorption from human milk, cow's milk, and infant formulas using a suckling rat model. Am. J. Clin. Nutr. 42:836–844.

Mason, K.E. 1979. A conspectus of research on copper metabolism and requirements of man. J. Nutr. 109:1979–2066.

Menkes, J.H., M. Alter, G.K. Steigledger, D.R. Weakley, and J.H. Sung. 1962. A sexlinked recessive disorder with retardation of growth, peculiar hair, and focal cerebral and cerebellar degeneration. Pediatrics 29:764–779.

NRC (National Research Council). 1977. Medical and Biological Effects of Environmental Pollutants: Copper. Report of the Committee on Medical and Biologic Effects of Environmental Pollutants, Division of Medical Sciences, Assembly of Life Sciences, National Academy of Sciences, Washington, D.C. 115 pp.

Pennington, J.A.T., B.E. Young, and D.B. Wilson. 1989. Nutritional elements in U.S. diets: results from the Total Diet Study, 1982–86. J. Am. Diet. Assoc. 89:659–664.

Price, N.O., and G.E. Bunce, 1972. Effect of nitrogen and calcium on balance of copper, manganese, and zinc in preadolescent girls. Nutr. Rep. Int. 5:275–280.

Reiser, S., J.C. Smith, Jr., W. Mertz, J.T. Holbrook, D.J. Scholfield, A.S. Powell, W.K. Canfield, and J.J. Canary. 1985. Indices of copper status in humans consuming a typical American diet containing either fructose or starch. Am. J. Clin. Nutr. 42:242–251.

Schroeder, H.A., A.P. Nason, I.H. Tipton, and J.J. Balassa. 1966. Essential trace elements in man: copper. J. Chronic Dis. 19:1007–1034.

Shaw, J.C.L. 1973. Parenteral nutrition in the management of sick low birthweight infants. Pediatr. Clin. North Am. 20:333–358.

Shike, M. 1984. Copper in parenteral nutrition. Bull. N.Y. Acad. Med. 60:132–143.

Solomons, N.W. 1979. On the assessment of zinc and copper nutriture in man. Am. J. Clin. Nutr. 32:856–871.

Turnlund, J.R., W.R. Keyes, H.L. Anderson, and L.L. Acord. 1989. Copper absorption and retention in young men at three levels of dietary copper using the stable isotope, [65]Cu. Am. J. Clin. Nutr. 49:870–878.

Uauy, R., C. Castillo-Duran, M. Fisberg, N. Fernandez, and A. Valenzuela. 1985. Red cell superoxide dismutase activity as an index of human copper nutrition. J. Nutr. 115:1650–1655.

Varo, P., M. Nuurtamo, E. Saari, and P. Koivistoinen. 1980. Mineral element composition of Finnish foods. VIII. Dairy products, eggs and margarine. Acta Agric. Scand. Suppl. 22:115–126.

Vuori, E., and P. Kuitunen. 1979. The concentrations of copper and zinc in human milk. A longitudinal study. Acta Paediatr. Scand. 68:33–37.

WHO (World Health Organization). 1973. Trace Elements in Human Nutrition. Report of a WHO Expert Committee. WHO Technical Report Series No. 532. World Health Organization, Geneva.

Widdowson, E.M., J. Dauncey, and J.C.L. Shaw. 1974. Trace elements in foetal and early postnatal development. Proc. Nutr. Soc. 33:275–284.

MANGANESE

Manganese has been shown to be an essential element in every animal species studied. Signs of deficiency include poor reproductive performance, growth retardation, congenital malformations in the offspring, abnormal formation of bone and cartilage, and impaired glucose tolerance (Hurley and Keen, 1987). Several enzymes, such as decarboxylases, hydrolases, kinases, and transferases, are nonspecifically activated by manganese *in vitro*. There are two known manganese metalloenzymes: pyruvate carboxylase and superoxide dismutase, both localized in mitochondria.

Manganese deficiency has never been observed in noninstitutionalized human populations because of the abundant supply of manganese in edible plant materials compared to the relatively low requirements of mammals (Underwood, 1981). Analyses of a variety of tissues taken from humans of various ages have indicated that there is no tendency for either a decrease or an increase in manganese accumulation throughout most of the life cycle (Schroeder et al., 1966). This constancy of manganese concentration in the tissues suggests adequate dietary intake coupled with strong homeostatic control. There has been only one recorded case of a possible manganese deficiency in a human—a male subject in a vitamin K deficiency study who was fed a purified diet from which manganese was inadvertently omitted (Doisy, 1973). His total diet (food and water) furnished only about 0.35 mg of manganese per day. Retrospective analyses revealed that there were 55 and 85% declines in his serum and stool manganese levels, respectively, over a 17-week period (Doisy, 1974).

Progress in the field of manganese nutrition has been hampered because of the lack of a practical method for assessing manganese status. Blood manganese levels appear to reflect body manganese status of rats fed deficient or adequate amounts of manganese (Keen et al., 1983), but consistent changes in blood or plasma manganese levels have not been observed in depleted or repleted human subjects (Freeland-Graves et al., 1988; Friedman et al., 1987). Animal studies have shown that the activity of mitochondrial superoxide dismutase is a function of dietary manganese intake, but practical usefulness of this enzyme as an indicator is uncertain since tissues containing mitochondria are generally not readily available for nutritional status assessment purposes.

Dietary Sources and Usual Intakes

Whole grains and cereal products are the richest dietary sources of manganese, and fruits and vegetables are somewhat less so. Dairy products, meat, fish, and poultry are poor sources. Tea is a rich source of manganese, but typical drinking water consumed at the rate of 2 liters daily contributes only about 40 to 64 μg, or about 2 to 3% of the amount furnished by diet (NRC, 1980).

Although there is now a body of data concerning the levels of manganese in the diet, little is known about the chemical form or nutritional bioavailability of the manganese in foods (Kies, 1987). Extreme dietary habits can result in manganese intake outside the provisionally recommended limits; consumption of a varied and balanced diet will reliably furnish safe and adequate amounts.

The Total Diet Study conducted in the United States between 1982 and 1986 indicated that the mean daily dietary manganese intake was 2.7 and 2.2 mg for adult men and women, respectively (Pennington et al., 1989). Teenage boys consumed an average of 2.8 mg/day, whereas girls consumed only 1.8 mg/day. Mean manganese intakes were 1.1 and 1.5 mg/day for 6- to 11-month-old babies and 2-year-old toddlers, respectively.

Estimated Safe and Adequate Daily Dietary Intakes

Adults   Several short-term balance studies in adult humans fed different amounts of manganese have been conducted in an attempt to define the requirement for this trace element (reviewed by Freeland-Graves et al., 1987). However, there are many problems with using the balance method to estimate trace element requirements (Freeland-Graves et al., 1988). At best, such studies determine the intake needed to maintain a given pool size of a nutrient in test subjects (Mertz, 1987). Factorial methods have also been used to estimate manganese requirements (Freeland-Graves et al., 1988; Friedman et al., 1987), but as with zinc, endogenous manganese loss is likely to be a function of manganese status. Therefore, the validity of this approach is also doubtful. Given the apparent lack of manganese deficiency as a practical nutritional problem in adults, it would seem that current dietary intakes satisfy needs for the element. Therefore, a provisional daily dietary manganese intake for adults of 2.0 to 5.0 mg is recommended.

Infants and Children   Little is known about the manganese requirement of human infants. McLeod and Robinson (1972) reported the manganese content of human milk to average 15 ng/ml (range, 12 to 20.2 ng/ml). Casey et al. (1985) calculated that the average daily intake of manganese from human milk from North American mothers during the first month after birth was only 2 μg. Such low intakes are associated with negative manganese balances (Widdowson, 1969), which are reflected in the decreases in tissue manganese levels that occur during the first weeks of life (Schroeder et al., 1966). Nonetheless, no cases of manganese deficiency in human infants have been documented (Lönnerdal et al., 1983). This suggests utilization of tissue reserves built up in the infant during gestation, but the site of such reserves, if any, is not clear, since manganese, unlike copper, is not stored in the fetal liver (Widdowson et al., 1972). In the absence of reports on manganese deficiency in human infants, no supplementation of the breastfed infant is recommended.

With the introduction of other foods at an assumed age of 4 months, manganese consumption increases accordingly and intakes of 71 and 80 μg/kg have been reported for infants 6 and 12 months old, respectively (Gibson and De Wolfe, 1980). For reference infants at birth to 0.5 year old and at 0.5 to 1 year of age, this would be equivalent to intakes of 0.4 and 0.7 mg/day, respectively. Therefore, the provisional recommended ranges for daily dietary intakes of manganese for these age groups are 0.3 to 0.6 and 0.6 to 1.0 mg/day, respectively. The ranges for children and adolescents are derived through extrapolation on the basis of body weight and expected food intake.

Pregnancy and Lactation   The requirement for manganese during pregnancy is not known, since the manganese content of the fetus has not been determined (Shaw, 1980). If an increased need exists, however, it may be met largely by enhanced absorption. Studies in isolated rat intestinal sacs have shown that manganese absorption during the third trimester is triple that of nonpregnant, nonlactating controls (Kirchgessner et al., 1982). Because the manganese content of human milk is so low (Casey et al., 1985), lactation is not likely to result in any appreciable additional demand for dietary manganese.

Excessive Intakes and Toxicity

In animals, the toxicity of ingested manganese is low and signs of a toxic response generally appear only after concentrations higher than 1,000 μg/g diet are fed (Hurley and Keen, 1987). In contrast, when the element was injected or inhaled as dust, adverse effects on the central nervous system became apparent at much smaller doses. The biochemical mechanism of manganese neurotoxicity has not been established, but studies in rats suggest that higher valency forms of the element might potentiate the autooxidation of catecholamines (Donaldson et al., 1982).

In humans, toxicity has been observed only in workers exposed to high concentrations of manganese dust or fumes in air, but not as a consequence of dietary intake by people consuming 8 to 9 mg of manganese per day in their food (WHO, 1973). In view of the remarkably steady tissue concentrations of manganese in the U.S. population (Schroeder et al., 1966) and the low toxicity of dietary manganese, an occasional intake of 10 mg/day by adults can be considered safe. To include an extra margin of safety, however, the subcommittee recommends a range of manganese intake from 2 to 5 mg/day for adults.

In the young of certain animal species, the homeostatic mechanism for manganese is relatively undeveloped (Cotzias et al., 1976). There have also been reports that learning disabilities in children might be associated with increased manganese levels in hair (Collipp et al., 1983); however, more evidence is required before this association can be substantiated.

References

Casey, C.E., K.M. Hambidge, and M.C. Neville. 1985. Studies in human lactation: zinc, copper, manganese, and chromium in human milk in the first month of lactation. Am. J. Clin. Nutr. 41:1193–1200.

Collipp, P.J., S.Y. Chen, and S. Maitinsky. 1983. Manganese in infant formulas and learning disability. Ann. Nutr. Metab. 27:488–494.

Cotzias, G.C., S.T. Miller, P.S. Papavasiliou, and L.C. Tang. 1976. Interactions between manganese and brain dopamine. Med. Clin. N. Am. 60:729–738.

Doisy, E.A., Jr. 1973. Micronutrient controls on biosynthesis of clotting proteins and cholesterol. Pp. 193–199 in D.D. Hemphill, ed. Trace Substances in Environmental Health—VI. University of Missouri, Columbia, Mo.

Doisy, E.A., Jr. 1974. Effects of deficiency in manganese upon plasma levels of clotting proteins and cholesterol in man. Pp. 668–670 in W.G. Hoekstra, J.W. Suttie, H.E. Ganther, and W. Mertz, eds. Trace Element Metabolism in Animals—2. University Park Press, Baltimore.

Donaldson, J., D. McGregor, and F. La Bella. 1982. Manganese neurotoxicity: a model for free radical mediated neurodegeneration. Can. J. Physiol. Pharmacol. 60:1398–1405.

Freeland-Graves, J.H., C.W. Bales, and F. Behmardi. 1987. Manganese requirements of humans. Pp. 90–104 in C. Kies, ed. Nutritional Bioavailability of Manganese. American Chemical Society, Washington, D.C.

Freeland-Graves, J.H., F. Behmardi, C.W. Bales, V. Dougherty, P.-H. Lin, J.B. Crosby, and P.C. Trickett. 1988. Metabolic balance of manganese in young men consuming diets containing five levels of dietary manganese. J. Nutr. 118:764–773.

Friedman, B.J., J.H. Freeland-Graves, C.W. Bales, F. Behmardi, R.L. Shorey-Kutschke, R.A. Willis, J.B. Crosby, P.C. Trickett, and S.D. Houston. 1987. Manganese balance and clinical observations in young men fed a manganese-deficient diet. J. Nutr. 117:133–143.

Gibson, R.S., and M.S. De Wolfe. 1980. The dietary trace metal intake of some Canadian full-term and low birthweight infants during the first twelve months of infancy. J. Can. Diet. Assoc. 41:206–215.

Hurley, L.S., and C.L. Keen. 1987. Manganese. Pp. 185-223 in W. Mertz, ed. Trace Elements in Human and Animal Nutrition, Vol. 1. Academic Press, Orlando, Fla.

Keen, C.L., M.S. Clegg, B. Lönnerdal, and L.S. Hurley. 1983. Whole-blood manganese as an indicator of body manganese. N. Engl. J. Med. 308:1230.

Kies, C., ed. 1987. Nutritional Bioavailability of Manganese. American Chemical Society, Washington, D.C.

Kirchgessner, M., Y.S. Sherif, and F.J. Schwarz. 1982. Changes in absorption of manganese during pregnancy and lactation. Ann. Nutr. Metab. 26:83–89.

Lönnerdal, B., C.L. Keen, M. Ohtake, and T. Tamura. 1983. Iron, zinc, copper, and manganese in infant formulas. Am. J. Dis. Child. 137:433–437.

McLeod, B.E., and Robinson, M.F. 1972. Dietary intake of manganese by New Zealand infants during the first six months of life. Br. J. Nutr. 27:229–232.

Mertz, W. 1987. Use and misuse of balance studies. J. Nutr. 117:1811–1813.

NRC (National Research Council). 1980. The contribution of drinking water to mineral nutrition in humans. Pp. 265–403 in Drinking Water and Health, Vol. 3. Report of the Safe Drinking Water Committee, Board on Toxicology and Environmental Health Hazards, Assembly of Life Sciences. National Academy Press, Washington, D.C. 415 pp.

Pennington, J.A.T., B.E. Young, and D.B. Wilson. 1989. Nutritional elements in U.S. diets: results from the Total Diet Study, 1982–86. J. Am. Diet. Assoc. 89:659–664.

Schroeder, H.A., J.J. Balassa, and I.H. Tipton. 1966. Essential trace elements in man: manganese. J. Chronic Dis. 19:545–571.

Shaw, J.C.L. 1980. Trace elements in the fetus and young infant. II. Copper, manganese, selenium, and chromium. Am. J. Dis. Child. 134:74–81.

Underwood, E.J. 1981. The incidence of trace element deficiency diseases. Phil. Trans. R. Soc. Lond. B 294:3–8.

WHO (World Health Organization). 1973. Trace elements in human nutrition. Report of a WHO Expert Committee. WHO Technical Report Series No. 532. World Health Organization, Geneva.

Widdowson, E.M. 1969. Trace elements in human development. Pp. 85–98 in D. Barltrop, ed. Mineral Metabolism in Paediatrics. Blackwell, Oxford.

Widdowson, E.M., H. Chan, G.E. Harrison, and R.D.G. Milner. 1972. Accumulation of Cu, Zn, Mn, Cr and Co in the human liver before birth. Biol. Neonate 20:360–367.

FLUORIDE

Fluorine[a] is present in small but widely varying concentrations in practically all soils, water supplies, plants, and animals, and is a constituent of all diets. The major tissues known to incorporate fluoride are bones and tooth enamel, the incorporation being proportional to the total intake (Hodge and Smith, 1970). The primary route of fluoride excretion is the kidney, and urine generally accounts for approximately 90% of the total fluoride excreted (Maheshwari et al., 1981; Spencer et al., 1981). There is a direct linear relationship between plasma fluoride level and the concentration of fluoride in the community water supply up to 6 mg/liter (Taves and Guy, 1979), but there can be substantial diurnal variations of these levels (Ekstrand, 1978).

The status of fluorine as an essential nutrient has been debated. Several studies in rodents have provided conflicting results. Addition of 2.5 mg of fluoride per kilogram of basal diet, the content of which varied but occasionally dropped below 0.04 mg/kg, stimulated the growth of rats housed in a trace element-controlled environment (Milne and Schwarz, 1974; Schwarz and Milne, 1972). In contrast, no effect of fluoride was seen in mice fed another low-fluorine diet (0.2 mg/kg) containing ingredients grown hydroponically, even when the diet was fed over six generations (Weber and Reid, 1974). An earlier report that fluoride added to the drinking water at 50 mg/liter protected pregnant mice against impaired reproduction and severe anemia (Messer et al., 1973) was not confirmed (Tao and Suttie, 1976). These contradictory results do not justify a classification of fluorine as an essential element, according to accepted standards. Nonetheless, because of its valuable effects on dental health, fluorine is a beneficial element for humans.

[a]Fluoride is the term for the ionized form of the element fluorine, as it occurs in drinking water. The two terms are used interchangeably.

Effects on Dental Caries

The negative correlation between tooth decay in children and fluoride concentrations in their drinking water was first demonstrated in a large study in the United States almost 50 years ago (Dean et al., 1942). Subsequently, many studies (see review by Burt, 1982) proved that fluoridation of public water supplies, wherever natural fluoride concentrations are low, is an effective and practical means of reducing dental caries (Council on Dental Therapeutics, 1982). Recommendations approved by virtually all national and international health organizations call for fluoride concentrations between 0.7 and 1.2 mg/liter, depending on average local temperature (as a predictor of water intake).

There is evidence that dental health has been improving, even in communities with low water fluoride concentrations, presumably because of increased fluoride intake from other sources (e.g., from foods processed with fluoridated water, topical fluoride applications by dentists, fluoride supplementation, and unintentional ingestion of fluoride dentifrices).

Although no one theory explains completely the exact role of fluoride in reducing caries (Council on Dental Therapeutics, 1982), it is known that fluoride replaces hydroxyl ions in developing enamel prior to tooth eruption, thereby forming an apatite crystal that is less susceptible to solubilization by acid and, hence, more resistant to caries formation. Some topically applied fluoride is also taken up by the enamel. The protective effect against caries is greatest during maximal tooth formation, i.e., during the first 8 years of childhood, but there is evidence to suggest that adults as well as children continue to benefit from the consumption of fluoridated water (Council on Dental Therapeutics, 1982).

Effects on Bone Disease

Although it has been suggested that fluoride intakes greater than those recommended for caries control may have some benefit in protecting adult bone, definitive evidence for such an effect is lacking. Bernstein et al. (1966) found a higher prevalence of reduced bone density and of collapsed vertebrae in an area with low-fluoride water (0.15 to 0.30 mg/liter) compared to that in an area with naturally high-fluoride water (4 to 5.8 mg/liter); these findings have not yet been confirmed.

Dietary Sources and Usual Intakes

A recent estimate of fluoride intake in the United States from food, beverages, and water ranged from approximately 0.9 mg/day in an area with unfluoridated water to 1.7 mg/day in an area with fluoridation (Singer et al., 1980). Daily fluoride intake was reported to be approximately 1.8 mg from a hospital diet in a fluoridated area of the United States (Taves, 1983), but drinking water was not taken into account. Most of the difference in fluoride intake between the fluoridated and unfluoridated areas was due to beverages, since foods marketed in different parts of the country contributed only 0.3 to 0.6 mg/day. This suggests that any effect of locally grown foods is largely negated by the supraregional distribution of the majority of foods in the United States.

Food processing has a strong influence on the fluoride content of foods. The fluoride content of various foods can be increased severalfold by cooking them in fluoridated water (Marier and Rose, 1966; Martin, 1951). Even the type of cooking vessel can be important. Cooking in utensils treated with Teflon, a fluoride-containing polymer, can increase the fluoride content, whereas an aluminum surface can reduce it (Full and Parkins, 1975).

The richest dietary sources of fluoride are tea and marine fish that are consumed with their bones (Kumpulainen and Koivistoinen, 1977). The bones of some land-based animals also contain high levels of fluoride. In countries where tea drinking is common, this beverage can make a substantial contribution to the total fluoride intake. In the United Kingdom Total Diet Study, tea was the main source of dietary fluoride for adults, accounting for 1.3 mg of the total daily intake of 1.8 mg (Walters et al., 1983).

Current intake estimates for 6-month-old infants range from 0.23 to 0.42 mg/day in different regions of the United States (Ophaug et al., 1985). This small range is due to the agreement among the producers of infant formulas to use only water low in fluoride for all their products (Barness, 1981; Horowitz and Horowitz, 1983).

The fluoride content of cow's milk is approximately 20 μg/liter (Taves, 1983). Mean reported values of human milk range from 5 to 25 μg/liter (Esala et al., 1982; Krishnamachari, 1987; Spak et al., 1983), reflecting maternal intake. The low and high concentrations in human milk were found in samples from mothers drinking water with fluoride concentrations of 0.2 and 1.7 mg/liter, respectively.

The quantitative estimates of fluoride intake discussed above give no indication about the relative absorption of dietary fluoride (see review by Subba Rao, 1984). In general, free fluoride as it exists in water is more available than the protein-bound fluorine in foods, and the absorption of fluoride from sodium fluoride in aqueous solution is estimated to be 100%. In young adults, the absorption of fluoride from sodium fluoride added to milk or baby formula was only 72 and 65%, respectively, of that added to water in a study by Spak et al. (1982). An even poorer absorption, from 37 to 54%, has been reported for the fluorine in bone meal (Krishnamachari, 1987). These differences in fluoride absorption indicate the difficulties in establishing dietary recommendations for fluoride based solely on quantitative data about the fluoride content of foods and drinking water.

Excessive Intakes and Toxicity

Fluorine, like other trace elements, is toxic when consumed in excessive amounts. Chronic toxicity—fluorosis—affects bone health, kidney function, and possibly muscle and nerve function (Krishnamachari, 1987). The condition occurs after years of daily exposures of 20 to 80 mg of fluorine, far in excess of the average intake in the United States. Mottling of the teeth in children has been observed at 2 to 8 mg/kg concentrations of fluoride in diet and drinking water (NRC, 1971). Many detailed epidemiological studies in the United States and abroad have failed to find any indication for an increased cancer risk associated with fluoride in the water supply (IARC, 1982).

The acute toxicity of fluoride resulting in death has been described in a 70-kg adult who ingested one dose of 5 to 10 g of sodium fluoride (Heifetz and Horowitz, 1984). Recently, investigators have suggested that the use of pharmacological doses of fluoride (50 mg/day) for 3 months was helpful in the treatment of women with osteoporosis (Pak et al., 1989). At these doses there is a potential for toxicity, and these patients should be monitored carefully.

Estimated Safe and Adequate Daily Dietary Intakes

The estimated range of safe and adequate intakes of fluoride for adults is 1.5 to 4.0 mg/day. This takes into account the widely varying fluoride concentrations of diets consumed in the United States and includes both food sources and drinking water. For younger age groups, the range is reduced to a maximal level of 2.5 mg in order to avoid mottling of the teeth. Ranges of 0.1 to 1 mg during the first year of life and 0.5 to 1.5 mg during the subsequent 2 years are suggested as adequate and safe.

Infants receiving human milk, ready-to-use formula, or concentrated formulas prepared with nonfluoridated water are all ingesting low levels of fluoride. In such cases, the American Academy of Pediatrics Committee on Nutrition advises the use of a fluoride supplement of 0.25 mg/day for children from 2 weeks to 2 years of age (Barness, 1981).

In view of fluoride's beneficial effects on dental health and its safety at the prescribed intakes, the Food and Nutrition Board recommends fluoridation of public water supplies if natural fluoride levels are substantially below 0.7 mg/liter.

References

Barness, L.A. 1981. Fluoride in infant formulas and fluoride supplementation. Pediatrics 67:582–583.

Bernstein, D.S., N. Sadowsky, D.M. Hegsted, C.D. Guri, and F.J. Stare. 1966. Prevalence of osteoporosis in high- and low-fluoride areas in North Dakota. J. Am. Med. Assoc. 198:499–504.

Burt, B.A. 1982. The epidemiological basis for water fluoridation in the prevention of dental caries. J. Public Health Policy 3:391–407.

Council on Dental Therapeutics. 1982. Fluoride compounds. Pp. 344–368 in Accepted Dental Therapeutics, 39th ed. American Dental Association, Chicago, Ill.

Dean, H.T., F.A. Arnold, Jr., and E. Elvove. 1942. Domestic water and dental caries: additional studies of relation of fluoride domestic waters to dental caries experience in 4,425 white children aged 12 to 14 years, of 13 cities in 4 states. Public Health Rep. 57:1155–1179.

Ekstrand, J. 1978. Relationship between fluoride in the drinking water and the plasma fluoride concentration in man. Caries Res. 12:123–127.

Esala, S., E. Vuori, and A. Helle. 1982. Effect of maternal fluorine intake on breast milk fluorine content. Br. J. Nutr. 48:201–204.

Full, C.A., and F.M. Parkins. 1975. Effect of cooking vessel composition on fluoride. J. Dent. Res. 54:192.

Heifetz, S.B., and H.S. Horowitz. 1984. The amounts of fluoride in current fluoride therapies: safety considerations for children. J. Dent. Child. 51:257–269.

Hodge, H.C., and F.A. Smith. 1970. Minerals: fluorine and dental caries. Pp. 93–115 in R.F. Gould, ed. Dietary Chemicals vs. Dental Caries. Advances in Chemistry Series No. 94. American Chemical Society, Washington, D.C.

Horowitz, A.M., and H.S. Horowitz. 1983. Fluorides and dental caries. Science 220:142–144.

IARC (International Agency for Research on Cancer). 1982. Inorganic fluorides used in drinking-water and dental preparations. Pp. 237–303 in IARC Monographs on the Evaluation of the Carcinogenic Risk of Chemicals to Humans, Vol. 27. Some Aromatic Amines, Anthraquinones and Nitroso Compounds, and Inorganic Fluorides Used in Drinking-Water and Dental Preparations. IARC, Lyon, France.

Krishnamachari, K.A.V.R. 1987. Fluorine. Pp. 365–415 in W. Mertz, ed. Trace Elements in Human and Animal Nutrition, Vol. 1. Academic Press, San Diego, Calif.

Kumpulainen, J., and P. Koivistoinen. 1977. Fluorine in foods. Residue Rev. 68:37–57.

Maheshwari, U.R., J.T. McDonald, V.S. Schneider, A.J. Brunetti, L. Leybin, E. New-brun, and H.C. Hodge. 1981. Fluoride balance studies in ambulatory healthy men with and without fluoride supplements. Am. J. Clin. Nutr. 34:2679–2684.

Marier, J.R., and D. Rose. 1966. The fluoride content of some food and beverages—A brief survey using a modified Zr-SPADNS method. J. Food Sci. 31:941–946.

Martin, D.J. 1951. The Evanston Dental Caries Study. VIII. Fluorine content of vegetables cooked in fluorine containing waters. J. Dent. Res. 30:676–681.

Messer, H.H., W.D. Armstrong, and L. Singer. 1973. Influence of fluoride intake on reproduction in mice. J. Nutr. 103:1319–1326.

Milne, D.B., and K. Schwarz. 1974. Effect of different fluorine compounds on growth and bone fluoride levels in rats. Pp. 710-714 in W. G. Hoekstra, J. W. Suttie, H. E. Ganther, and W. Mertz, eds. Trace Element Metabolism in Animals, 2. University Park Press, Baltimore.

NRC (National Research Council). 1971. Fluorides. Report of the Committee on Biologic Effects of Atmospheric Pollutants. National Academy of Sciences, Washington, D.C. 295 pp.

Ophaug, R.H., L. Singer, and B.F. Harland. 1985. Dietary fluoride intake of 6-month and 2-year-old children in four dietary regions of the United States. Am. J. Clin. Nutr. 42:701–707.

Pak, C.Y.C., K. Sakhafe, J.E. Zerwekh, C. Parcel, R. Peterson, and K. Johnson. 1989. Safe and effective treatment of osteoporosis with intermittent slow release sodium fluoride: augmentation of vertebral bone. J. Clin. Endocrinol. Metab. 68:150–159.

Schwarz, K., and D.B. Milne. 1972. Fluorine requirement for growth in the rat. Bioinorg. Chem. 1:331–338.

Singer, L., R.H. Ophaug, and B.F. Harland. 1980. Fluoride intake of young male adults in the United States. Am. J. Clin. Nutr. 33:328–332.

Spak, C.J., J. Ekstrand, and D. Zylberstein. 1982. Bioavailability of fluoride added to baby formula and milk. Caries Res. 16:249–256.

Spak, C.J., L.I. Hardell, and P. deChateau. 1983. Fluoride in human milk. Acta Paediatr. Scand. 72:699–701.

Spencer, H., D. Osis, and M. Lender. 1981. Studies of fluoride metabolism in man: a review and report of original data. Sci. Total Environ. 17:1–12.

Subba Rao, G. 1984. Dietary intake and bioavailability of fluoride. Annu. Rev. Nutr. 4:115–136.

Tao, S., and J.W. Suttie. 1976. Evidence for a lack of an effect of dietary fluoride level on reproduction in mice. J. Nutr. 106:1115–1122.

Taves, D.R. 1983. Dietary intake of fluoride ashed (total fluoride) v. unashed (inorganic fluoride) analysis of individual foods. Br. J. Nutr. 49:295–301.

Taves, D.R., and W.S. Guy. 1979. Distribution of fluoride among body compartments. Pp. 159–185 in E. Johansen, D.R. Taves, and T.O. Olsen, eds. Continuing Evaluation of the Use of Fluorides. Westview Press, Boulder, Colo.

Walters, C.B., J.C. Sherlock, W.H. Evans, and J.I. Read. 1983. Dietary intake of fluoride in the United Kingdom and fluoride content of some foodstuffs. J. Sci. Food Agric. 34:523–528.

Weber, C.W., and B.L. Reid. 1974. Effect of low-fluoride diets fed to mice for six generations. Pp. 707–709 in W.G. Hoekstra, J.W. Suttie, H.E. Ganther, and W. Mertz, eds. Trace Element Metabolism in Animals, 2. University Park Press, Baltimore.

CHROMIUM

Trivalent chromium is required for maintaining normal glucose metabolism in laboratory animals; it acts as a cofactor for insulin (Mertz, 1969). Experimental chromium deficiency has been induced in several animal species, resulting in impaired glucose tolerance in the presence of normal concentrations of circulating insulin and, in severe cases, in a diabetes-like syndrome (Schroeder, 1966). Three cases of pronounced chromium deficiency have been reported in patients on long-term total parenteral alimentation (Brown et al., 1986; Freund et al., 1979; Jeejeebhoy et al., 1977); all three had in common a relative insulin resistance and peripheral or central neuropathy. Chromium-responsive impairment of glucose tolerance has been reported in malnourished children, in some but not all studies of mild diabetics, and in middle-aged subjects with impaired glucose tolerance. (For a review, see IPCS, 1988.)

Chromium concentrations in human tissues decline with age, except for the lungs in which chromium accumulates. Parity, juvenile diabetes, and coronary artery disease are associated with low-chromium concentrations in hair or serum (IPCS, 1988).

The intestinal absorption of dietary chromium at daily intakes of 40 µg and more is approximately 0.5% of the total amount present; intakes of less than 40 µg/day are absorbed with an increasing efficiency, up to about 2% of the total (Anderson and Kozlovsky, 1985). Absorbed chromium is excreted almost completely through the urine.

Usual Intakes

Chromium intake from typical Western diets varies widely between a low of 25 µg/day in elderly persons in England to approximately 200 µg in Belgian and Swedish diets, but in the most recent international studies (IPCS, 1988), intakes below 100 µg/day were reported. Two experimental diets prepared to meet the RDAs for all nutrients and furnishing 2,800 calories contained 62 and 89 µg of chromium at a fat content of 43 and 25% of the energy, respectively (Kumpulainen et al., 1979). This is in contrast to the average chromium intake of 33 and 25 µg/day from self-selected diets of adults in Beltsville, Maryland, in diets containing 2,300 and 1,600 kcal, respectively (Anderson and Kozlovsky, 1985).

Estimated Safe and Adequate Daily Dietary Intakes

Because of the lack of methods to diagnose chromium status, it is difficult to estimate a chromium requirement. In the majority of all chromium supplementation studies in the United States, at least half the subjects with impaired glucose tolerance improved upon chromium supplementation, suggesting that the lower ranges of chromium intakes from typical U.S. diets are not optimal with regard to chromium nutriture (Anderson et al., 1983).

Experiments *in vitro* and in animals have demonstrated substantial differences in the biological activity of different chromium compounds. Although the chemical forms of chromium in foods are not known with certainty, a chromium-dinicotinic acid-glutathione complex with high bioavailability has been identified in brewer's yeast. The bioavailability of chromium in calf's liver, American cheese, and wheat germ is also relatively high. More precise data on the nutritional value of chromium in various foods are not yet available. Thus, the best assurance of an adequate and safe chromium intake is the consumption of a varied diet balanced with regard to other essential nutrients. A range of chromium intakes between 50 and 200 µg/day is tentatively recommended for adults. This range is based on the absence of signs of chromium deficiency in the major part of the U.S. population consuming an average of 50 µg/day. The safety of an intake of 200 µg has been established in long-term supplementation trials in human subjects receiving 150 µg/day in addition to the dietary intake (Glinsmann and Mertz, 1966). Habitual dietary intakes of around 200 µg/day have been reported in several studies; no adverse effects of such intakes are known. The suggested range of chromium intake is predicated on the assumption that a varied diet providing an adequate intake of other essential micronutrients will furnish chromium with an average absorbability of 0.5%.

The tentative recommendations for younger age groups are derived by extrapolation on the basis of expected food intake. Until more precise recommendations can be made, the consumption of a varied diet, balanced with regard to other essential nutrients, remains the best assurance of an adequate and safe chromium intake.

Excessive Intakes and Toxicity

The toxicity of trivalent chromium, the chemical form that occurs in diets, is so low that there is a substantial margin of safety between the amounts normally consumed and those considered to have harmful effects. No adverse effects were seen in rats and mice consuming 5 mg/liter in drinking water throughout their lifetimes, and no toxicity was observed in rats exposed to 100 mg/kg in the diet (IPCS, 1988).

An increased incidence of bronchial cancer has been correlated with chronic occupational exposure of workers to dusts containing chromate, the hexavalent form of chromium (IPCS, 1988). Humans cannot oxidize the nontoxic trivalent food chromium to the potentially carcinogenic hexavalent chromate compounds. Therefore, the carcinogenicity of certain chromates bears no relevance to the nutritional role of trivalent chromium.

References

Anderson, R.A., and A.S. Kozlovsky. 1985. Chromium intake, absorption, and excretion of subjects consuming self-selected diets. Am. J. Clin. Nutr. 41:1177–1183.

Anderson, R.A., M.M. Polansky, N.A. Bryden, E.E. Roginski, W. Mertz, and W.H. Glinsmann. 1983. Chromium supplementation of human subjects: effects on glucose, insulin, and lipid variables. Metabolism 32:894–899.

Brown, R.O., S. Forloines-Lynn, R.E. Cross, and W.D. Heizer. 1986. Chromium deficiency after long-term total parenteral nutrition. Dig. Dis. Sci. 31:661–664.

Freund, H., S. Atamian, and J.E. Fischer. 1979. Chromium deficiency during total parenteral nutrition. J. Am. Med. Assoc. 241:496–498.

Glinsmann, W.H., and W. Mertz. 1966. Effect of trivalent chromium on glucose tolerance. Metabolism 15:510–520.

IPCS (International Programme on Chemical Safety). 1988. Chromium. Environmental Health Criteria 61. World Health Organization, Geneva.

Jeejeebhoy, K.N., R.C. Chu, E.B. Marliss, G.R. Greenberg, and A. Bruce-Robertson. 1977. Chromium deficiency, glucose intolerance and neuropathy reversed by chromium supplementation in a patient receiving long-term total parenteral nutrition. Am. J. Clin. Nutr. 30:531–538.

Kumpulainen, J.T., W.R. Wolf, C. Veillon, and W. Mertz. 1979. Determination of chromium in selected United States diets. J. Agric. Food Chem. 27:490–494.

Mertz, W. 1969. Chromium occurrence and function in biological systems. Physiol. Rev. 49:163–239.

Schroeder, H.A. 1966. Chromium deficiency in rats: a syndrome simulating diabetes mellitus with retarded growth. J. Nutr. 88:439–445.

MOLYBDENUM

Molybdenum plays a biochemical role as a constituent of several mammalian enzymes, such as aldehyde oxidase, xanthine oxidase, and sulfite oxidase (Rajagopalan, 1988); however, production of characteristic pathological lesions in animals due to nutritional molybdenum deficiency has been difficult (Mills and Bremner, 1980). Although naturally occurring deficiency, uncomplicated by antagonists, is not known with certainty, molybdenum deficiency has been produced experimentally in goats by feeding them purified rations containing less than 0.07 μg of molybdenum per gram of diet. The consequences are retarded weight gain, decreased food consumption, impaired reproduction, and shortened life expectancy (Anke et al., 1985). On the basis of these studies, Anke et al. (1985) suggested that the minimum molybdenum requirement of goats was approximately 100 μg/kg of ration dry matter. However, the molybdenum requirement of monogastric species may be less than that of ruminants because of the molybdenum needs of rumen microflora (Anke et al., 1985).

Two recent lines of investigation have suggested a role for molybdenum in human nutrition. The first involved a patient on long-term total parenteral nutrition who developed a variety of symptoms, including amino acid intolerance, irritability, and, ultimately, coma (Abumrad et al., 1981). This person also displayed hypermethioninemia, increased urinary excretion of xanthine and sulfite, and decreased urinary excretion of uric acid and sulfate. Treatment with 300 μg of ammonium molybdate (equivalent to about 163 μg of molybdenum) per day resulted in clinical improvement and normalization of sulfur metabolism and uric acid production. The authors concluded that this may be the first report of a feeding-induced molybdenum deficiency in humans.

The second line of evidence concerns a rare inborn error of metabolism that leads to a combined deficiency of sulfite oxidase and xanthine dehydrogenase (Rajagopalan, 1988). This metabolic disease is due to a lack of the molybdenum cofactor (molybdopterin), which is an essential constituent of these enzymes. Patients with this defect display severe neurological dysfunction, dislocated ocular lenses, and mental retardation. Biochemical abnormalities are similar to those observed in the intravenously fed patient cited above. Structural characterization of molybdopterin indicates the presence of a reduced pterin ring, a 4-carbon side chain containing an enedithiol, and a terminal phosphate ester (Rajagopalan, 1988).

Dietary Sources and Usual Intakes

The concentration of molybdenum in food varies considerably, depending on the environment in which the food was grown (Mills and Davis, 1987). Therefore, tabulations of expected molybdenum concentrations in various foods are of limited value (Chappell, 1977). Tsongas et al. (1980) calculated that the dietary intake of molybdenum in the United States ranged from 120 to 240 μg/day, depending on age and sex, and averaged about 180 μg/day. The foods that contributed the most to the molybdenum intake were milk, beans, breads, and cereals. Pennington and Jones (1987) found a lower molybdenum content in the 1984 collection of the Food and Drug

Administration's Total Diet Study ranging from 76 to 109 μg/day for adult females and males, respectively. Human milk contains very low levels of molybdenum, and after the first month of lactation, furnishes only approximately 1.5 μg/day (Casey and Neville, 1987). Little is known about the chemical form or nutritional bioavailability of molybdenum in foods. Most public water supplies would be expected to contribute between 2 to 8 μg of molybdenum per day (NRC, 1980), which would constitute 10% or less of the lower limit of the provisional recommended intake. Since most diets should meet the molybdenum requirements of humans, supplements of additional molybdenum are not recommended.

Estimated Safe and Adequate Daily Dietary Intakes

Aside from the exceptions discussed above, no disturbances in uric acid or sulfate production have ever been related to molybdenum deficiency in humans. The human requirement apparently is so low that it is easily furnished by common U.S. diets. Therefore, the provisional recommended range for the dietary intake of molybdenum, based on average reported intakes, is set at 75 to 250 μg/day for adults and older children. The range for other age groups is derived through extrapolation on the basis of body weight.

Excessive Intakes and Toxicity

The toxicity of molybdenum presents a substantial problem for animal nutrition because molybdenum is antagonistic to the essential element copper (Mills and Davis, 1987). Adverse effects of high environmental concentrations of molybdenum were observed in humans living in a province of the USSR (Koval'skiy and Yarovaya, 1966). The authors suggested that the excessive dietary intake of 10 to 15 mg/day may be the cause of a high incidence of a goutlike syndrome associated with elevated blood levels of molybdenum, uric acid, and xanthine oxidase. Even a moderate dietary exposure of 0.54 mg/day has been associated with loss of copper in the urine (Deosthale and Gopalan, 1974).

References

Abumrad, N.N., A.J. Schneider, D. Steel, and L.S. Rogers. 1981. Amino acid intolerance during prolonged total parenteral nutrition reversed by molybdate therapy. Am. J. Clin. Nutr. 34:2551–2559.

Anke, M., B. Groppel, and M. Grun. 1985. Essentiality, toxicity, requirement and supply of molybdenum in humans and animals. Pp. 154–157 in C.F. Mills, I. Bremner, and J.K. Chesters, eds. Trace Elements in Man and Animals—TEMA 5. Commonwealth Agricultural Bureaux, Slough, United Kingdom.

Casey, C.E., and M.C. Neville. 1987. Studies in human lactation 3: molybdenum and nickel in human milk during the first month of lactation. Am. J. Clin. Nutr. 45:921–926.

Chappell, W.R., ed. 1977. Proceedings: Symposium on Molybdenum in the Environment, Vol. 2. Marcel Dekker, New York. 812 pp.

Deosthale, Y.G., and C. Gopalan. 1974. The effect of molybdenum levels in sorghum (*Sorghum vulgare Pers.*) on uric acid and copper excretion in man. Br. J. Nutr. 31:351–355.

Koval'skiy, V.V., and G.A. Yarovaya. 1966. Molybdenum-infiltrated biogeochemical provinces. Agrokhimiya 8:68–91.

Mills, C.F., and I. Bremner. 1980. Nutritional aspects of molybdenum in animals. Pp. 517–542 in M.P. Coughlan, ed. Molybdenum and Molybdenum-Containing Enzymes. Pergamon Press, Oxford.

Mills, C.F., and G.K. Davis. 1987. Molybdenum. Pp. 429–463 in W. Mertz, ed. Trace Elements in Human and Animal Nutrition, 5th ed, Vol. 1. Academic Press, Orlando, Fla.

NRC (National Research Council). 1980. The contribution of drinking water to mineral nutrition in humans. Pp. 265–404 in Drinking Water and Health, Vol. 3. Safe Drinking Water Committee, Board on Toxicology and Environmental Health Hazards, Assembly of Life Sciences. National Academy Press, Washington, D.C.

Pennington, J.A.T., and J.W. Jones. 1987. Molybdenum, nickel, cobalt, vanadium, and strontium in total diets. J. Am. Diet. Assoc. 87:1644–1650.

Rajagopalan, K.V. 1988. Molybdenum: an essential trace element in human nutrition. Annu. Rev. Nutr. 8:401–427.

Tsongas, T.A., R.R. Meglen, P.A. Walravens, and W.R. Chappell. 1980. Molybdenum in the diet: an estimate of average daily intake in the United States. Am. J. Clin. Nutr. 33:1103–1107.

11

Water and Electrolytes

Although water and the principal electrolytes (sodium, potassium, and chloride) are often excluded from lists of nutrients, these substances are essential dietary components, in that they must be acquired from the diet either exclusively or—in the case of water—in amounts well in excess of that produced by metabolism in the body. Concerns about possible overconsumption (sodium and chloride) or underconsumption (potassium) of these substances in the United States are comparatively recent (NRC, 1989; Tobian, 1979).

WATER

Water is the most abundant constituent of the human body, accounting for one-half to four-fifths of body weight, depending mainly on body fat content. Accordingly, body water, as a percentage of body mass, is higher in men than in women and tends to fall with age in both.

Figure 11-1 shows the routes and approximate magnitudes of water intake and loss in an environment cool enough to prevent sweating. The normal daily turnover of water via these routes is approximately 4% of total body weight in adults and much higher, 15% of total body weight, in infants. As Figure 11-1 shows, even in the absence of visible perspiration, approximately one-half of the turnover occurs through what is called insensible water loss, i.e., water lost from the lungs and skin. These insensible losses can all be increased under certain conditions, including high temperatures, high altitude, and dry air. Exertion under any of these conditions can cause up to a 10-

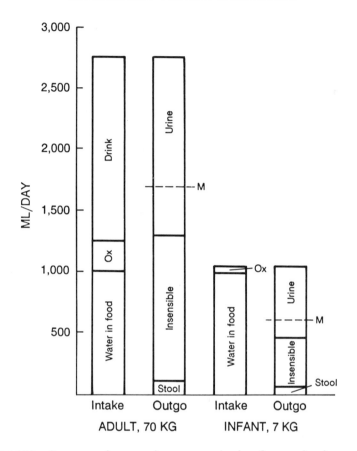

FIGURE 11-1 Routes and approximate magnitude of water intake and outgo without sweating. From NRC, 1980b. M is minimal urine volume at maximal solute concentration. Ox is water of oxidation.

fold increase in water loss from skin and lungs. Diarrhea can increase intestinal loss dramatically.

Figure 11-1 includes an estimate of minimal urine volume required when urinary solute concentration is maximal (about 1,400 mosmol/liter in the healthy adult and 700 mosmol/liter in the infant). Because the kidney must excrete waste products, the solute load—composed of the nitrogen-containing breakdown products of protein metabolism (principally urea), sulfates, phosphates, and other electrolytes—determines the minimal volume of water required for urine formation. Normally functioning kidneys can adjust urine osmolarity from 40 to 1,400 mosmol/liter, depending both on water intake and on dietary solute load. Despite the kidney's ability to compensate, its limitations require the effective use of the thirst sensation to maintain water balance. If the sensation of thirst is not met by water consumption, or if the thirst mechanism is inoperative because of intense, sustained exertion, especially at a high altitude (Buskirk and Mendez, 1967), dehydration will eventually result. This can become life threatening when more than 10% of body weight is lost.

Sources

Although water, consumed as water, is a major source of liquid in some parts of the world, much of the water consumed in the United States is taken in the form of other beverages. Median daily intake of water as such among respondents in the 1977–1978 Nationwide Food Consumption Survey was 2.8 cups (USDA, 1984). In 1981, daily per capita milk consumption was approximately one and one-third cups, per capita coffee and tea consumption was about one and one-half cups, and soft drink consumption was one and three-fourths cups per capita. In addition, many solid foods, especially fruits and vegetables, contain from 85 to 95% water.

Estimate of Requirements

The primary determinant of maintenance water requirement appears to be metabolic (Holliday and Segar, 1957), but the actual estimation of water requirement is highly variable and quite complex. Because the water requirement is the amount necessary to balance the insensible losses (which can vary markedly) and maintain a tolerable solute load for the kidneys (which may vary with dietary composition and other factors), it is impossible to set a general water requirement.

Adults For practical purposes, 1 ml/kcal of energy expenditure can be recommended as the water requirement for adults under average conditions of energy expenditure and environmental exposure. However, there is so seldom a risk of water intoxication that the specified requirement for water is often increased to 1.5 ml/kcal to cover variations in activity level, sweating, and solute load.

Special attention must be given to the water needs of the elderly whose thirst sensation may be blunted. Even though these people may be less physically active, they may still have a high water requirement, especially during the summer. If uncorrected, water depletion with heat exhaustion, resulting from inadequate replacement of fluid losses, can eventually cause a loss of consciousness and heat stroke (NRC, 1980b).

Pregnancy and Lactation   Pregnancy is associated with an increased need for water because of the expanded extracellular fluid space, the needs of the fetus, and the amniotic fluid. However, calculations indicate that the increment amounts to only about 30 ml/day. A lactating woman, on the other hand, requires an increased volume of water to match that secreted in the milk. Since milk is 87% water and average milk secretion is 750 ml/day for the first 6 months, the extra fluid required would be less than 1,000 ml/day.

Infants and Children   Infants must be treated as a separate category for several reasons: their large surface area per unit of body weight, their higher percentage of body water and its high rate of turnover, the limited capacity of their kidneys for handling the solute load from high protein intakes required for growth, and their susceptibility to severe dehydration due in part to their inability to express thirst. It is prudent, therefore, to recommend an average water intake of 1.5 ml/kcal of energy expenditure for infants. This figure corresponds to the water-to-energy ratio in human milk and common formulas and has been well established as a satisfactory level for the growing infant.

Excessive Intakes and Toxicity

Toxicity results from the ingestion of water at a rate beyond the capacity of the kidneys to excrete the extra load, resulting in hyposmolarity. Such a condition is rarely observed in a normal healthy adult. The manifestations usually include a gradual mental dulling, confusion, coma, convulsion, and even death.

SODIUM

Sodium, the principal cation of extracellular fluid, is the primary regulator of extracellular fluid volume. Both the body content of sodium and its concentration in body fluids are under homeostatic control, and the volume of extracellular fluid is thus normally determined by its sodium content. In addition to its role in regulating extracellular fluid volume, sodium is important in the regulation of osmolarity, acid-base balance, and the membrane potential of cells. Sodium is also involved in active transport across cell membranes and must be pumped out in exchange for potassium in order to maintain an appropriate intracellular milieu—a process that requires an appreciable fraction of the energy required in the basal metabolic state.

Sodium homeostasis is maintained over a wide range of environmental and dietary circumstances, primarily through the action of the hormone aldosterone on the renal tubules of the kidney. When sodium intake is high, the aldosterone level decreases and urinary sodium increases. When dietary sodium intake is low, the aldosterone level increases and urinary excretion of sodium rapidly falls almost to zero. Although the kidney can thus conserve sodium, there is some obligatory loss via feces and sweat. Sodium deficiency resulting from low dietary intake thus does not normally occur, even among those existing on very low sodium diets (Page, 1976, 1979). Even relatively heavy sweating does not normally create a need to provide salt supplements (Conn, 1949). The body may be depleted of sodium under extreme conditions of heavy and persistent sweating, or where trauma, chronic diarrhea, or renal disease produce an inability to retain sodium (Gothberg et al., 1983). These latter conditions require medical attention.

Dietary Sources and Usual Intakes

Foods and beverages containing sodium chloride (39% sodium by weight) are the primary sources of sodium. Sources other than table salt—e.g., sodium bicarbonate and monosodium glutamate—are believed to account for less than 10% of total dietary sodium intake (Sanchez-Castillo, 1987a). Water from community systems usually contains less than 20 mg of sodium per liter, and it has been estimated that water contributes less than 10% of daily sodium intake (NRC, 1977). By using a lithium chloride marker to trace the use of salt in cooking and at the table, Sanchez-Castillo et al. (1987a, 1987b) found that only 10% of the salt came from the natural salt content of foods, 15% from salt added during cooking and at the table, and fully 75% from salt added during processing and manufacturing.

Because of the high proportion of dietary sodium accounted for by processing, the highest salt intakes are normally associated with a diet high in processed foods and the lowest intakes are associated with diets emphasizing fresh fruits, vegetables, and legumes. In the first National Health and Nutrition Examination Survey (Abraham and Carroll, 1981), 32% of the sodium chloride consumed came from baked goods and cereals, approximately 21% came from meats, and 14% from dairy products. The FDA's Total Diet Study, in which a very different methodology was used, showed similar results (Pennington et al., 1984).

Usual levels of sodium consumption have been estimated in dietary surveys by assessing salt intake and by measuring urinary sodium. Reported dietary intakes of sodium range from 1.8 g/day to 5 g/day in various studies, depending on the methods of assessment used (Abraham and Carroll, 1981; Dahl, 1960; Pennington et al., 1984) and on whether or not discretionary sodium use is assessed. The discretionary intake of sodium is quite variable and can be quite large. In one 28-day study, males were found to add about 5.5 g of sodium chloride (2.2 g of sodium) to their food per day (Mickelson et al., 1977).

Because of the difficulty of assessing sodium use from dietary recall, dietary surveys probably underestimate total sodium intake, even when contributions of water and other marginal sources are included. From data on daily urinary sodium excretion over 24 hours, Dahl and Love (1957) calculated the average daily adult intake of salt to be 10 g/day (4 g of sodium per day). Dahl subsequently reported a mean sodium chloride intake of 10.3 g (range, 4 to 24 g) for 71 working men in New York. Coatney et al. (1958) reported that a 5-month sodium excretion in a military population corresponded to an intake of 11 g of salt per day. Sanchez-Castillo et al. (1987a, b) found sodium chloride excretion over a 12-day period to be 10.6 ± 0.55 g in men and 7.4 ± 2.9 g in women.

Estimate of Requirements

Calculations of sodium requirements (shown in Table 11-1) are based on estimates of what is needed for growth and for replacement of obligatory losses. The amount needed to support growth depends on the rate at which extracellular fluid volume is expanded, a rate that varies with age and reproductive status.

Adults In a temperate climate, the healthy adult can maintain sodium balance with a very low intake of sodium (Kempner, 1948). Dole et al. (1950) have estimated obligatory urinary and fecal losses by adults to be 23 mg (1 mEq)[a] per day. The other source of loss is sweat, which normally averages a sodium concentration of 25 mEq/liter (Consolazio et al., 1963). Sanchez-Castillo et al. (1987a) found that sweat and fecal excretion contributed only 2 to 5% of the sodium lost by British men and women. Obligatory dermal losses have been assumed to range from 46 to 92 mg (2 to 4 mEq) per day (Fregley,

---

[a] 1 mEq of sodium is 23 mg, and 1 mmol of sodium chloride is 58.5 mg.

TABLE 11-1 Estimated Sodium, Chloride, and Potassium
Minimum Requirements of Healthy Persons[a]

Age	Weight (kg)[a]	Sodium (mg)[a,b]	Chloride (mg)[a,b]	Potassium (mg)[c]
Months				
0–5	4.5	120	180	500
6–11	8.9	200	300	700
Years				
1	11.0	225	350	1,000
2–5	16.0	300	500	1,400
6–9	25.0	400	600	1,600
10–18	50.0	500	750	2,000
>18[d]	70.0	500	750	2,000

[a] No allowance has been included for large, prolonged losses from the skin through sweat.
[b] There is no evidence that higher intakes confer any health benefit.
[c] Desirable intakes of potassium may considerably exceed these values (~3,500 mg for adults—see text).
[d] No allowance included for growth. Values for those below 18 years assume a growth rate at the 50th percentile reported by the National Center for Health Statistics (Hamill et al., 1979) and averaged for males and females. See text for information on pregnancy and lactation.

1984). Thus, a minimum average requirement for adults can be estimated under conditions of maximal adaptation and without active sweating as no more than 5 mEq/day, which corresponds to 115 mg of sodium or approximately 300 mg of sodium chloride per day. In consideration of the wide variation of patterns of physical activity and climatic exposure, a safe minimum intake might be set at 500 mg/day. Such an intake is substantially exceeded by usual diets in the United States, even in the absence of added sodium chloride. Although no optimal range of salt intake has been established, there is no known advantage in consuming large amounts of sodium, and clear disadvantages for those susceptible to hypertension. From this and other considerations, a Food and Nutrition Board committee recently recommended that daily intakes of sodium chloride be limited to 6 g (2.4 g of sodium) or less (NRC, 1989).

Pregnancy and Lactation   During pregnancy, there is an increased need for sodium because of the increased extracellular fluid volume in the mother, the requirements of the fetus, and the level of sodium in the amniotic fluid. This need is normally met in part by physiological responses of the renin-angiotensin-aldosterone systems (Pike and Smiciklas, 1972). Given a pregnancy weight gain of 11 kg (70% of which is extracellular water containing 150 mEq of sodium per liter), the average total sodium requirement for the duration of pregnancy is 3 mEq (69 mg) per day in addition to the normal requirement. Since the average intake is, as has been noted, considerably above that, the sodium requirement for pregnancy is met by usual salt intake.

Lactation increases sodium requirements considerably. Since human milk contains about 7.8 mEq of sodium (180 mg) per liter (AAP, 1985), and the average milk secretion when established is about 750 ml, lactation would add about 6 mEq (135 mg) per day to the usual adult requirement. This increase is easily met by the usual dietary sodium intake.

Infants and Children   The sodium requirement is obviously highest in infants and young children in whom extracellular fluid volume is rapidly expanding. Forbes (1952) calculated that from birth to 3 months of age, 0.5 mEq/kg (11.5 mg/kg) daily is needed for growth, or approximately 2 mEq (46 mg) per day for the reference infant. At 6 months of age, the daily requirement for growth is approximately 0.2 mEq (4.6 mg)/kg. According to calculations by Cooke et al. (1950), daily losses of sodium from the skin range from 0.4 to 0.7 mEq/kg (9 to 16 mg/kg). Because sodium losses from the kidney can be regulated precisely when intakes are not excessive, the convenient value of 1 mEq/kg (23 mg/kg) daily is considered more than satisfactory for the healthy infant and young child residing in a temperate climate. Human milk contains 7 mEq of sodium per liter (range, 3 to 19 mEq/liter) (Gross, 1983; Macy, 1949). Consumed at a rate of 750 ml/day, this provides the reference infant with an average of 120 mg/day, which corresponds to 1.16 mEq/kg (27 mg/kg) daily from birth through 2 months of age and 0.8 mEq/kg (18 mg/kg) daily from 3 through 5 months of age. Except for the premature infant, in whom hyponatremia can occur (Roy et al., 1976), human milk certainly provides adequate sodium for the growing infant.

Formula-fed infants consuming 750 ml/day now receive a minimum of 100 mg/day and a maximum of 300 mg/day (AAP, 1985). The American Academy of Pediatrics has estimated that there is a threefold increase in dietary sodium between 2 and 12 months of age (AAP, 1981).

Excessive Intakes and Toxicity

Acute excessive intake of sodium chloride leads to an increase in the extracellular space as water is pulled from cells to maintain sodium concentration. The end result is edema and hypertension. Such acute toxicity from dietary sodium is not a concern, however, since as long as water needs can be met, the kidney can excrete the excess sodium. Sustained overconsumption of sodium, particularly as salt, has been related to development of hypertension in sensitive individuals (NRC, 1989; Tobian, 1979).

POTASSIUM

Potassium is the principal intracellular cation, occurring in cell water at a concentration of 145 mEq/liter,[b] more than 30 times the concentration at which it is found in plasma and interstitial fluid (3.8 to 5.0 mEq/liter). This small percentage of extracellular potassium is, however, of great physiological importance, contributing to the transmission of nerve impulses, to the control of skeletal muscle contractility, and to the maintenance of normal blood pressure.

More than 90% of ingested potassium is absorbed from the gastrointestinal tract, but higher or lower intakes are not reflected in fluctuations in plasma potassium concentrations because the kidney can regulate potassium balance. Potassium is lost from the body in the urine and, to a lesser extent, in gastrointestinal secretions, whereas only minimal amounts are excreted in sweat.

Under normal circumstances, dietary deficiency of potassium does not occur. The most important cause of potassium deficiency is excessive losses, usually through the alimentary tract or the kidneys. Large alimentary potassium losses may occur through prolonged vomiting, chronic diarrhea, or laxative abuse. The most common cause of excessive renal loss is the use of diuretic agents, especially for the treatment of hypertension. Some forms of chronic renal disease and metabolic disturbances (e.g., diabetic acidosis) can also lead to severe potassium loss. Deficiency symptoms include weakness, anorexia, nausea, listlessness, apprehension, drowsiness, and irrational behavior. Severe hypokalemia may result in cardiac dysrhythmias that can be fatal.

Dietary Sources and Usual Intakes

Potassium is widely distributed in foods, since it is an essential constituent of all living cells. Animal tissue concentration of potassium is fairly constant, but varies inversely with the amount of fat. Some potassium is also added in food processing, but the overall effect of

---

[b]1 mEq of potassium is 39 mg.

processing on the food supply has been to increase the sodium and decrease the potassium (NRC, 1989). Thus, the richest dietary sources are unprocessed foods, especially fruits, many vegetables, and fresh meats. The contribution of drinking water to potassium intake is negligible. The mean concentration in household tap water was reported to be 2.15 mg/liter (range, 0.72 to 8.3 mg/liter) (Greathouse and Crown, 1979; NRC, 1980a).

Potassium intakes vary considerably, depending on food selection. People who eat large amounts of fruits and vegetables have a high potassium intake, on the order of 8 to 11 g/day (NRC, 1989). In the FDA's Total Diet Study, mean potassium intake in the United States during 1981–1982 was found to be 1,500 mg/day for 6-month-old infants, 1,800 mg/day for 2-year-old children, and 3,400 mg/day for 15- to 20-year olds (Pennington et al., 1984). Urban whites eat about 2,500 mg/day (Khaw and Barrett-Connor, 1987); low intakes of about 1,000 mg/day have been reported in blacks (Grim et al., 1980; Langford, 1985).

Human milk contains about 500 mg (12.8 mEq) of potassium per liter, and therefore provides the reference infant consuming 750 ml daily with 375 mg/day. Infant formulas contain slightly more potassium than human milk on the average, and cow's milk contains almost 3 times as much, 1,365 mg (35 mEq) per liter.

Estimate of Requirements

Adults Potassium requirements have been evaluated in only a few studies. Although losses on a low or "minimum" potassium diet are small, potassium is less well conserved than sodium (see Table 11-1). Fecal losses are less than 400 mg (10 mEq) per day, and renal losses may approach 200 to 400 mg (5 to 10 mEq) per day (Squires and Huth, 1959). Other losses (e.g., in sweat) are negligible. On intakes of about 20 mEq/day, metabolic balance is achieved at the expense of reduced body potassium stores (up to 250 mEq) and in some cases with reduced plasma levels (<4 mEq/liter). To maintain normal body stores and a normal concentration in plasma and interstitial fluid, an intake of about 40 mEq/day may be needed (Sebastian et al., 1971). Therefore, it would appear that the minimum requirement is approximately 1,600 to 2,000 mg (40 to 50 mEq) per day. There is considerable evidence that dietary potassium exerts a beneficial effect in hypertension, and recommendations for increased intake of fruits and vegetables (NRC, 1989) would raise potassium intake of adults to about 3,500 mg (90 mEq) per day.

Pregnancy and Lactation   There is no evidence that potassium requirements are appreciably increased during pregnancy, except for the increment needed to build new tissue, which is easily satisfied by the usual ingestion of potassium. Since maternal milk contains about 500 mg (12.8 mEq) per liter, this increased loss must be considered during lactation, but is supplied by usual intakes.

Infants and Children   Since potassium is a necessary constituent of each body cell, an increase in lean body mass is a major determinant of potassium needs. From 60 to 80 mEq are required for each kilogram of weight gained. Using growth rates for infants and children calculated from the reference weight data reported by Hammill et al. (1979), and assuming that 70 mEq of potassium are required for each kg of body weight, one may estimate that the potassium requirement for growth averages 65 mg/day for infants, 15 to 20 mg/day for 1- to 10-year-old children, and 35 mg/day for adolescents.

To allow for obligatory urinary, cutaneous, and fecal losses, dietary intake must, of course, be higher than the amount required at the tissue level. Holliday and Segar (1957) have estimated that in general, 78 mg (2 mEq) per 100 kcal should maintain potassium balance in children of all ages as long as there is no preexisting potassium deficit or ongoing excessive loss. This is in keeping with data on potassium intake in infants and children showing that average potassium intake (from milk and solid foods) ranges from about 780 mg/day at 2 months of age to about 1,600 mg/day at the end of the first year of life (AAP, 1981).

Excessive Intakes and Toxicity

In the absence of markedly increased losses of potassium from the body, acute intoxication (hyperkalemia) will result from sudden enteral or parenteral increases in potassium intake to levels about 12.0 g/m^2 (250 to 300 mEq/m^2) of surface area per day—about 18 g for an adult (NRC, 1980b). Although urinary excretion provides some protection, acute hyperkalemia can prove fatal because it can cause cardiac arrest.

CHLORIDE

Chloride, the principal inorganic anion in the extracellular fluid compartment, is essential in maintaining fluid and electrolyte balance, and is a necessary component of gastric juice. It occurs in plasma in concentrations of 96 to 106 mEq/liter,[c] and in a more concentrated form in cerebrospinal fluid and gastrointestinal secretions. Its concentration in most cells is low.

Under normal circumstances, dietary deficiency of chloride does not occur. The only known instance of diet-related chloride depletion occurred in healthy infants inadvertently fed diets containing 1 to 2 mEq/liter (Grossman et al., 1980; Rodriguez-Soriano et al., 1983; Roy and Arant, 1981) rather than the minimum of 10.4 mEq/liter now recommended (AAP, 1985). Chloride loss tends to parallel losses of sodium; hence, conditions associated with sodium depletion (e.g., heavy, persistent sweating, chronic diarrhea or vomiting, trauma, or renal disease) will also cause chloride loss, resulting in hypochloremic metabolic alkalosis.

Dietary Sources and Usual Intakes

Dietary chloride comes almost entirely from sodium chloride. Much smaller amounts are supplied from potassium chloride. Therefore, dietary sources of chloride are essentially the same as those described for sodium, and processed foods are the major source. Although chloride is also found in almost all natural waters, estimates by the Environmental Protection Agency (EPA, 1975) suggest a daily contribution of 42 mg/day. This is insignificant compared to the roughly 6 g of chloride a day contributed by added salt.

Estimate of Requirements

Because both the intake of chloride from food and its losses from the body under normal conditions parallel those of sodium, the requirements specified for all age and sex groups except infants parallel those of sodium on a mEq basis (see Table 11-1).

Human milk contains 11 mEq of chloride per liter, which makes the chloride level higher than the sodium level on a mEq basis. The American Academy of Pediatrics has suggested a similar level (10.4 mEq/liter) for infant formulas on the grounds that a 1.5–2.0 ratio of sodium plus potassium to chloride maintained good acid-base regulation in infants (AAP, 1985).

Excessive Intakes and Toxicity

The toxicity of salts containing the chloride ion depends mainly on the characteristics of the cation. The only known dietary cause of

---

[c] 1 mEq of chloride is 35.5 mg.

hyperchloremia is water-deficiency dehydration. Sustained ingestion of high levels of chloride (as salt) has been associated with elevated blood pressure in sensitive individuals and animal models (Kurtz et al., 1987; Whitescarver et al., 1986).

REFERENCES

AAP (American Academy of Pediatrics). 1981. Sodium intake of infants in the United States. Pediatrics 68:444–445.

AAP (American Academy of Pediatrics). 1985. Pediatric Nutrition Handbook, 2nd Ed. American Academy of Pediatrics, Elk Grove Village, Ill.

Abraham, S., and M.D. Carroll. 1981. Fats, Cholesterol and Sodium Intake in the Diet of Persons 1–74 Years: United States. Advance Data No. 54. U.S. Department of Health, Education, and Welfare, Washington, D.C.

Buskirk, E.R., and J. Mendez. 1967. Nutrition, environment and work performance with special reference to altitude. Fed. Proc. 26:1760–1767.

Coatney, G.R., O. Nickelson, R.W. Burgess, M.D. Young, and C.I. Pirkle. 1958. Chloroquin or pyrimethamine in salt as a suppressive against sporozoite-induced vivax malaria (Chesson strain). Bull. W.H.O. 19:56–67.

Conn, J.W. 1949. The mechanisms of acclimitization to heat. Adv. Intern. Med. 3:373–393.

Consolazio, C.F., L.O. Matoush, R.A. Nelson, R.S. Harding, and J.E. Canham. 1963. Excretion of sodium, potassium, magnesium and iron in human sweat and the relation of each to balance and requirements. J. Nutr. 79:407–415.

Cooke, R.E., E.L. Pratt, and D.C. Darrow. 1950. Metabolic response to heat stress. Yale J. Biol. Med. 22:227.

Dahl, L.K. 1960. Possible role of salt intake in the development of essential hypertension. Pp. 53–65 in P. Cottier and K.D. Bock, eds. Essential Hypertension: An International Symposium. Springer-Verlag, Heidelberg, Federal Republic of Germany.

Dahl, L.K., and R.A. Love. 1957. Etiological role of sodium chloride intake in essential hypertension in humans. J. Am. Med. Assoc. 164:397.

Dole, V.P., L.K. Dahl, G.C. Cotzias, H.A. Eder, and M.E. Krebs. 1950. Dietary treatment of hypertension. Clinical metabolic studies of patients on the rice-fruit diet. J. Clin. Invest. 39:1189.

EPA (U.S. Environmental Protection Agency). 1975. Region V. Federal/State Survey of Organics and Inorganics in Selected Drinking Water Supplies. U.S. Environmental Protection Agency, Chicago. 317 pp.

Forbes, G.B. 1952. Chemical growth in man. Pediatrics 9:58.

Fregley, M.J. 1984. Sodium and potassium. Pp. 439–458 in Nutrition Reviews' Present Knowledge in Nutrition, 5th ed. The Nutrition Foundation. Washington, D.C.

Gothberg, G., S. Lundin, M. Aurell, and B. Folkow. 1983. Responses to slow graded bleeding in salt-depleted rats. J. Hypertens. Suppl. 2:24–26.

Greathouse, D.G., and G.F. Crown. 1979. Cardiovascular disease study—occurrence of inorganics in household tap water and relationships to cardiovascular mortality rates. Pp. 31–39 in D.D. Hemphill, ed. Trace Substances in Environmental Health-XII. Proceedings of the 12th Annual Conference, 1978, University of Missouri-Columbia, Columbia, Mo.

Grim, C.E., F.C. Luft, J.Z. Miller, G.R. Meneely, H.D. Battarbee, C.G. Hames, and L.K. Dahl. 1980. Racial differences in blood pressure in Evans County, Georgia:

relationship to sodium and potassium intake and plasma renin activity. J. Chronic Dis. 33:87–94.

Gross, S.J. 1983. Growth and biochemical response of preterm infants fed milk or modified infant formula. N. Engl. J. Med. 308:237.

Grossman, H., E. Duggan, S. McCamman, E. Welchert, and S. Hellerstein. 1980. The dietary chloride deficiency syndrome. Pediatrics 66:366–374.

Hamill, P.V.V., T.A. Drizd, C.L. Johnson, R.B. Reed, A.F. Roche, and W.M. Moore. 1979. Physical growth. National Center for Health Statistics Percentiles. Am. J. Clin. Nutr. 32:607–629.

Holliday, M.A., and W.E. Segar. 1957. The maintenance need for water in parental fluid therapy. Pediatrics 19:823.

Kempner, W. 1948. Treatment of hypertension vascular disease with rice diet. Am. J. Med. 4:545.

Khaw, K.T., and E. Barrett-Connor. 1987. Dietary potassium and stroke-associated mortality. A 12-year prospective population study. N. Engl. J. Med. 316:235–240.

Kurtz, T.W., H.A. Al-Bander, and R.C. Morris. 1987. 'Salt sensitive' essential hypertension in men. N. Engl. J. Med. 317:1043–1048.

Langford, H.G. 1985. Dietary potassium and hypertension. Pp. 147–153 in M.J. Horan, M. Blaustein, J.B. Dunbar, W. Kachadorian, N.M. Kaplan, and A.P. Simopoulos, eds. NIH Workshop on Nutrition and Hypertension: Proceedings from a Symposium. Biomedical Information Corp., New York.

Macy, I.C. 1949. Compositon of human colostrum and milk. Am. J. Dis. Child. 78:589.

Mickelson, O., D. Makdani, J.L. Gill, and R.L. Frank. 1977. Sodium and potassium intakes and excretions of normal men consuming sodium chloride or a 1:1 mixture of sodium and potassium chloride. Am. J. Clin. Nutr. 30:2033.

NRC (National Research Council). 1977. Drinking Water and Health. Report of the Safe Drinking Water Committee, Advisory Center on Toxicology, Assembly of Life Sciences. National Academy of Sciences, Washington, D.C. 939 pp.

NRC (National Research Council). 1980a. Drinking Water and Health, Vol. 3. Report of the Safe Drinking Water Committee, Board on Toxicology and Environmental Health Hazards, Assembly of Life Sciences. National Academy Press, Washington, D.C. 415 pp.

NRC (National Research Council). 1980b. Recommended Dietary Allowances, 9th Revised Ed. Committeee on Dietary Allowances, Food and Nutrition Board, Division of Biological Sciences, Assembly of Life Sciences. National Academy of Sciences, Washington, D.C. 185 pp.

NRC (National Research Council), 1989. Diet and Health: Implications for Reducing Chronic Disease Risk. Report of the Committee on Diet and Health, Food and Nutrition Board. National Academy Press, Washington, D.C. 750 pp.

Page, L.B. 1976. Epidemiologic evidence on the etiology of human hypertension and its possible prevention. Am. Heart J. 91:527–534.

Page, L.B. 1979. Hypertension and atherosclerosis in primitive and acculturating societies. Pp. 1–12 in J.C. Hunt, ed. Hypertension Update, Vol. 1. Health Learning Systems, Lyndhurst, N.J.

Pennington, J.A.T., D.B. Wilson, R.F. Newell, B.F. Harland, R.D. Johnson, and J.E. Vanderveen. 1984. Selected minerals in food surveys, 1974 to 1981/82. J. Am. Diet. Assoc. 84:771–780.

Pike, R.L., and H.A. Smiciklas. 1972. A reappraisal of sodium restriction during pregnancy. Int. J. Gynecol. Obstet. 10:1–8.

Rodriguez-Soriano, J., A. Vallo, G. Castillo, R. Oiveros, J.M. Cea, and M.J. Balzategui. 1983. Biochemical features of dietary chloride deficiency syndrome: a comparative study of 30 cases. J. Pediatr. 103:209–214.

Roy, S., and B.S. Arant. 1981. Hypokalemic metabolic alkalosis in normotensive infants with elevated plasma renin activity and hyperaldosteronism: role of dietary chloride deficiency. Pediatrics 67:423–429.

Roy, R.N., G.W. Chance, I.C. Radde, D.E. Hill, D.M. Willis, and J. Sheepers. 1976. Late hyponatremia in very low birthweight infants less than 1.3 kilograms. Pediatr. Res. 10:526–531.

Sanchez-Castillo, C.P., S. Warrender, T.P. Whitehead, and W.P. James. 1987a. An assessment of the sources of dietary salt in a British population. Clin. Sci. 72:95–102.

Sanchez-Castillo, C.P., W.J. Branch, and W.P. James. 1987b. A test of the validity of the lithium-marker technique for monitoring dietary sources of salt in men. Clin. Sci. 72:87–94.

Sebastian, A., E. McSherry, and R.C. Morris, Jr. 1971. Renal potassium wasting in renal tubular acidosis (RTA): its occurrence in Types 1 and 2 RTA despite sustained correction of systemic acidosis. J. Clin. Invest. 50:667–678.

Squires, R.D., and E.J. Huth. 1959. Experimental potassium depletion in normal human subjects. I. Relation of ionic intakes to the renal conservation of potassium. J. Clin. Invest. 38:1134–1148.

Tobian, L., Jr. 1979. The relationship of salt to hypertension. Am. J. Clin. Nutr. 32:2739–2748.

USDA (U.S. Department of Agriculture). 1984. Nationwide Food Consumption Survey. Nutrient Intakes: Individuals in 48 States, Year 1977–78. Report No. I-2. Consumer Nutrition Division, Human Nutrition Information Service, U.S. Department of Agriculture, Hyattsville, Md. 439 pp.

Whitescarver, S.A., B.J. Holtzclaw, J.H. Downs, O.H. Co, J.R. Sowers, and T.A. Kotchen. 1986. Effect of dietary chloride on salt-sensitive and renin-dependent hypertension. Hypertension 8:56–61.

12

Other Substances in Food

Several substances naturally present in foods are known to be required in the diets of various animal or microbial species, but there is little or no evidence of their dietary essentiality for humans. Because it is possible that some of the compounds within these classes of substances may eventually be shown to be needed in the diets of humans, and thus may one day be candidates for RDAs, they are included in this chapter.

Foods contain literally thousands of organic substances presumed to have a biological function in the plant or animal from which the food is derived or which are by-products of the plant's or animal's metabolism. Most of these substances can be synthesized in the human body in adequate amounts to meet biological needs and, thus, are not essential dietary nutrients. Examples include fatty acids, such as oleic, stearic, and palmitic acids; glycerol; free nonessential amino acids, such as glycine, alanine, aspartic acid, and glutamic acid; glucose and various less common sugars, such as pentoses and galactose; and derivatives and polymers of sugars.

Many inorganic elements that are not essential for humans enter the diet through foods of vegetable origin, either because they are essential for the plants or through nonspecific absorption from the soil. Indeed, most of the inorganic elements of the periodic table are present in foods and drinking water, usually in trace amounts. Some elements may occur in amounts that may be toxic under certain conditions. Inorganic elements in food that have no accepted biological function in animals or humans are aluminum, antimony, barium, beryllium, gallium, germanium, gold, mercury, rare earth minerals, silver, strontium, thallium, and titanium.

262

Natural foods contain many compounds that have no known nutritional effects. These include the flavonoids, rutin, quercetin, and hesperidin—the so-called vitamin P factors (Herbert, 1988)—and the proposed vitamin Q (Quick, 1975). Some of these naturally occurring compounds (e.g., caffeine in coffee and chocolate) have pharmacological effects.

NUTRIENTS ESSENTIAL FOR SOME HIGHER ANIMALS BUT NOT PROVED TO BE REQUIRED BY NORMAL HUMANS

Choline

Choline has been known to be present in mammalian tissues since it was first discovered and isolated from hog bile in 1862 (Strecker, 1862). It can be biosynthesized from ethanolamine and methyl groups derived from methionine, but it is likely that most tissue choline is derived from dietary phosphatides. Although choline is found in nature as the free compound, it has no known functions, except as a constituent of larger molecules (Kuksis and Mookerjea, 1984). As a component of phosphatidylcholine (lecithin), it is important to the structure of all cell membranes, plasma lipoproteins, and pulmonary surfactant (Kuksis and Mookerjea, 1984; Zeisel, 1981). In the central nervous system, it functions as a structural constituent of sphingomyelin and as a component of the neurotransmitter acetylcholine (Zeisel, 1981).

Choline is a dietary requirement of several animal species, including the dog, cat, rat, and guinea pig; however, it has not been shown to be essential for humans. Choline is found in a wide range of plant and animal foods. For example, eggs, liver, and soybeans are rich in lecithin, whereas free choline is found in such vegetables as cauliflower and lettuce (Wurtman, 1979). Lecithins are used as an emulsifying agent in foods such as chocolate or margarine. An average daily intake of choline is about 400 to 900 mg.

The oral administration of choline as choline chloride (2 to 5 g) or lecithin (10 to 15 g) will elevate plasma choline concentrations from 10 to 40 μmol (Jope et al., 1982; Zeisel, 1981). Large doses of dietary choline increase the level of the neurotransmitter acetylcholine, which may be deficient in certain neurological diseases, especially in the elderly (Zeisel, 1988).

The possibility that alcoholic cirrhosis results in part from inadequate dietary choline has been investigated (Baraona and Lieber, 1979). However, it is uncertain whether the liver damage is due to the toxic effect of the alcohol itself or to the alcohol in combination with deficiency of several nutritional factors (Kuksis and Mookerjea, 1984).

Both *de novo* synthesis and active transport of choline have been demonstrated in the placenta (Welsch, 1978). The demand for choline-containing compounds is high during growth and development, and may exceed synthetic capacity in the human newborn (Zeisel, 1981). It is likely that the neonate needs a dietary supply of choline, but the point is not yet firmly established. The American Academy of Pediatrics (AAP, 1985) has, however, recommended that infant formula contain 7 mg of choline per 100 kcal. This is based on the amount of choline in human milk, which also provides choline as phosphatidylcholine and sphingomyelin.

Taurine

Taurine (β-aminoethanesulfonic acid) is an important component of a wide range of metabolic activities in many tissues and is essential to the formation of conjugated forms of taurine (bile salts) present in bile. Deficiencies have been produced in young monkeys, felines, and other laboratory animals. It is not generally considered an essential nutrient for humans under normal physiological conditions, since it can be synthesized from dietary cysteine or methionine (Hayes, 1985). There is concern, however, that formula-fed infants may be at greater risk of taurine insufficiency than breastfed infants, because formulas based on cow's milk contain much lower levels of taurine than does human milk, i.e., 1 to 3 μmol/100 ml compared with 26 to 35 μmol/100 ml. Indeed, lower urine and plasma levels of taurine have been observed in premature infants fed formulas based on cow's milk than in breastfed infants (Sturman, 1988).

For full-term infants, differences in plasma and urine levels were also observed between those fed human milk and those fed taurine-deficient formulas (Gaull, 1982; Järvenpää et al., 1982). Yet, whether taurine is a dietary essential nutrient remains equivocal, since even in the premature infant, taurine supplementation did not produce changes in growth, nitrogen retention, or general metabolism (Järvenpää et al., 1983; Okamoto et al., 1984).

Because the essentiality of dietary taurine for infants has not been fully established, no RDA can be established at this time. For recent general reviews on taurine, see Chapman and Greenwood (1988), Chesney (1987), Sturman (1988), and Wright et al. (1986).

Carnitine

Carnitine is required metabolically for the transport of long-chain fatty acids into the matrix of the mitochondria—the site of β-oxidation. It therefore plays a critical rôle in energy metabolism. Carnitine is synthesized in the liver and kidney of the adult from the essential amino acids lysine and methionine (Broquist and Borum, 1982). Although the well-nourished adult can probably synthesize adequate amounts of carnitine, the newborn infant appears to have reduced stores of carnitine as well as a low capacity for synthesizing it. Human milk contains approximately 50 to 100 nmol/ml of carnitine. However, infants fed soy formulas or maintained on total parenteral nutrition receive no exogenous carnitine and have been shown to have plasma carnitine concentrations lower than those of infants fed human milk (Borum, 1983; Olson et al., 1989). A critical question that must be answered is whether these decreased carnitine concentrations have demonstrable functional consequences. Several laboratories are investigating the possibility that carnitine may be an essential nutrient for the newborn, especially for those born prematurely.

Animal products are the best dietary sources of carnitine. As a general rule, the redder the meat, the higher the carnitine concentration. Dairy products contain carnitine predominantly in the whey fraction (Borum, 1983, 1986).

Human carnitine deficiency was first described in 1973 (Engel and Angelini, 1973). Since then, more than a hundred people have been diagnosed as having genetic carnitine deficiency. The biochemical mechanism causing the carnitine deficiency has not been adequately identified in any patient. Deficiency of this substance appears to be characterized by a family of syndromes with a broad range of signs and symptoms that include progressive muscle weakness with lipid infiltration of the skeletal muscle and reduced muscle carnitine concentration, cardiomyopathy, severe hypoglycemia, elevated blood ammonia concentrations, and reduced ability to increase ketogenesis on fasting. Carnitine deficiency can also occur in conjunction with a variety of other conditions, such as organic aciduria, or with chronic hemodialysis of renal patients, long-term total parenteral nutrition, and treatment with valproic acid. Supplementation of carnitine-deficient patients with L-carnitine reduces symptoms in some but not all of the subjects (Borum, 1983, 1986; Bowyer et al., 1989). For representative recent reviews on carnitine, see Borum (1986), Carroll et al. (1987), Feller and Rudman (1988), and Rebouche (1986).

Carnitine was originally referred to as vitamin B_T because of its essentiality for the mealworm *Tenebrio molitor*. However, it has not been demonstrated to be a vitamin for the healthy adult human (Borum, 1983, 1986), and no RDA can be established at this time.

Myo-inositol

Myo-inositol is a cyclic alcohol (cyclohexanehexol) closely related chemically to glucose. Of the nine inositol isomers, only *myo*-inositol is of importance in plant and animal metabolism. It is found in plants, usually as phytic acid, and in animal tissues, primarily as a constituent of phospholipids in biomembranes (Holub, 1982). Consideration of *myo*-inositol as an essential nutrient is increasing because of the recent discovery that *myo*-inositol trisphosphate is a second messenger for receptor-mediated hormonal stimuli for mobilizing intracellular calcium (Berridge and Irvine, 1984). In addition, *myo*-inositol appears to have a lipotropic action that may originate from its vital role as a substrate for the biosynthesis of phosphatidyl inositol and polyphosphoinositides, which are essential components of biomembranes (Holub, 1982). The *myo*-inositol content of tissues is provided by the diet and through biosynthesis (Lewin and Beer, 1973; Middleton and Setchell, 1972). Dietary *myo*-inositol has not been shown to produce any known deleterious effect to any organ system when given in generous amounts (larger than present in normal diets). For a comprehensive account of the biological importance of *myo*-inositol, the reader is referred to see Agranoff (1986) and Prentki and Matschinsky (1987).

Although dietary essentiality has not been shown for humans, female gerbils have been shown to require *myo*-inositol in their diets (Hegsted et al., 1973, 1974). Deficiency is characterized by intestinal lipodystrophy (Chu and Geyer, 1983). In rats, *myo*-inositol deficiency has been reported to produce triglyceride accumulation and abnormal fatty acid metabolism. These studies have been summarized by Holub (1982). Altered *myo*-inositol levels have been found in rats, rabbits, and other animals with diabetes mellitus, chronic renal failure, or galactosemia, and a possible therapeutic role for *myo*-inositol has been suggested. In particular, restoration of nerve conduction velocity has been demonstrated in patients with diabetic neuropathy following the addition of *myo*-inositol to their diets (Greene et al., 1975; Mayer and Tomlinson, 1983; Winegrad and Greene, 1976). The importance of these studies for normal humans has not been established, so no RDA for *myo*-inositol can be established.

Trace Elements

Evidence for the essentiality of trace elements in humans is often difficult to obtain directly; it can be reliably predicted from proven essentiality in other mammalian species and from identification of certain elements as part of normal human enzyme systems. Evidence for a requirement in laboratory animals has been presented for many of the elements discussed below (especially arsenic, boron, nickel, and silicon), but in most cases the requirement has not been quantified. Deficiency in humans has not been established for any of these trace elements. Hence, there are no data from which a human requirement could be estimated and no provisional allowance can be given.

Arsenic, Nickel, Silicon, and Boron   There is substantial evidence to establish the essentiality of these trace elements in animals (Nielsen, 1988). Arsenic deficiency depresses growth and impairs reproduction in rats, minipigs, chickens, and goats. Nickel deficiency results in decreased growth in rats, sheep, cows, goats, and minipigs, and depressed hematopoiesis has been observed in rats, sheep, cows, and goats. Silicon deficiency leads to structural abnormalities of the long bones and skull in chickens (Carlisle, 1972; Schwarz and Milne, 1972). It apparently is involved in the normal growth of bone more through the mineralization process than through the formation of the organic matrix.

Boron deficiency has been reported in studies in rats, chickens, and humans (Nielsen, 1988; Nielsen et al., 1987). Boron appears to affect calcium and magnesium metabolism and may be needed for membrane function. Boron deficiency signs may be related to the level of vitamin D and possibly other nutrients in the diet. Boron has long been known to be essential for the growth of most plants.

Cadmium, Lead, Lithium, Tin, and Vanadium   Depressed growth, impaired reproductive performance, and other changes have been reported in laboratory animals fed diets extremely low in these elements and kept in an environment allowing the strictest control of contamination (Nielsen, 1988). Nutritional requirements, if they exist, are very low and easily met by the levels naturally occurring in foods, water, and air. The evidence for requirements and essentiality is weak.

Cobalt   The only known nutritional, but very vital, function of cobalt is as an integral part of vitamin B_{12}. Because all vitamin B_{12} is derived from bacterial synthesis, inorganic cobalt can be considered essential for animal species that depend totally on their bacterial flora for their vitamin B_{12}. This is the case for ruminant animal species in whom cobalt deficiency is well known; it might also have some relevance for strict vegetarians whose intake of the preformed vitamin is severely limited. However, there is no evidence that the intake of cobalt is ever limiting in the human diet, and no RDA is necessary.

GROWTH FACTORS AND COENZYMES

Various unidentified growth factors for several animal species, including infants, are known to exist in foods, but their role, if any, in normal nutrition is unknown (Berseth, 1987; Cheeke and Patton, 1978; Jaeger et al., 1987; Lofgren et al., 1974; Weaver et al., 1987).

Recently, there has been considerable interest in possible nutritional effects of compounds known to be important coenzymes, or related to them. Several polyamines, including spermine and spermidine, are required for the growth of normal and neoplastic cells (Celano et al., 1988) and for the induction of intestinal maturation in the rat (Dufour et al., 1988). Several recent studies have shown various immunologic suppression and metabolic effects of several dietary nucleotides in human infants and laboratory animals (DeLucchi et al., 1987; Kulkarni et al., 1987). Also, there are reports of deficiency signs in rats and mice fed highly purified diets in the absence of pyrroloquinoline quinone, a cofactor for oxidoreductases (Anonymous, 1988). Nutrition studies on such compounds will be watched with interest, but the data are far too few to establish even provisional requirements for humans.

Many other specific growth factors are known to be required in cell or tissue cultures and for bacteria, lower metazoa, or insects and other invertebrates. There is no evidence that such substances are required in the diets of humans or other higher animals, and since such substances can be synthesized in the tissues of higher animals, demonstration of need is highly unlikely. The substances in this category include asparagine, bifidus factor, biopterin, chelating agents, cholesterol, coenzyme Q (ubiquinones), hematin, lecithin, lipoic acid (thioctic acid), nerve-growth factors, p-aminobenzoic acid, various peptides and proteins, pimelic acid, and pteridines (Briggs and Calloway, 1984; Shils and Young, 1988).

SUBSTANCES WITH NO KNOWN ESSENTIALITY IN ANIMALS OR HUMANS

No essential nutrient function in animals or plants has ever been reported in reliable scientific literature for most other organic chemicals occurring naturally in foods or otherwise endogenously synthe-sized. Compounds in this category include amygdalin or laetrile (in-correctly referred to as vitamin B_{17}) (Herbert, 1988), chlorophyll, orotic acid, pangamic acid (an ill-defined mixture of dimethylglycine and sorbitol that is incorrectly called vitamin B_{15}), so-called vitamin U, and any other herbs, growth factors, enzymes, hormones, trace elements, or other compounds called vitamins or minerals not men-tioned elsewhere in this report (Briggs and Calloway, 1984; Shils and Young, 1988).

REFERENCES

AAP (American Academy of Pediatrics). 1985. Pediatric Nutrition Handbook, 2nd ed. Committee on Nutrition. American Academy of Pediatrics, Elk Grove Village, Ill.

Agranoff, B.W. 1986. Inositol trisphosphate and related metabolism. Fed. Proc. 45:2627–2652.

Anonymous. 1988. Is pyrroloquinoline quinone a cofactor derived from an undis-covered vitamin? Nutr. Rev. 46:139–142.

Baraona, E., and C.S. Lieber. 1979. Effects of ethanol on lipid metabolism. J. Lipid Res. 20:289–315.

Berridge, M.J., and R.F. Irvine. 1984. Inositol triphosphate, a novel second messenger in cellular signal transduction. Nature 312:315–321.

Berseth, C.L. 1987. Breast-milk-enhanced intestinal and somatic growth in neonatal rats. Biol. Neonate 51:53–59.

Borum, P.R. 1983. Carnitine. Annu. Rev. Nutr. 3:233–259.

Borum, P.R., ed. 1986. Clinical Aspects of Human Carnitine Deficiency. Pergamon Press, New York.

Bowyer, B.A., C.R. Fleming, M.W. Haymond, and J.M. Miles. 1989. L-carnitine: effect of intravenous administration on fuel homeostasis in normal subjects and home-parenteral-nutrition patients with low plasma carnitine concentrations. Am. J. Clin. Nutr. 49:618–623.

Briggs, G.M., and D.H. Calloway. 1984. Nutrition and Physical Fitness, 11th ed. Holt, Rinehart, and Winston, New York.

Broquist, H.P., and P.R. Borum. 1982. Carnitine biosynthesis: Nutritional implica-tions. Pp. 181–204 in H.H. Draper, ed. Advances in Nutritional Research. Plenum Press, New York.

Carlisle, E.M. 1972. Silicon: an essential element for the chick. Science 178:619–621.

Carroll, J.E., A.L. Carter, and S. Perlman. 1987. Carnitine deficiency revisited. J. Nutr. 117:1501–1503.

Celano, P., S.B. Baylin, F.M. Giardiello, B.D. Nelkin, and J.A. Casero, Jr. 1988. Effect of polyamine depletion on c-myc expression in human colon carcinoma cells. J. Biol. Chem. 263:5491–5494.

Chapman, G.E., and C.E. Greenwood. 1988. Taurine in nutrition and brain devel-opment. Nutr. Res. 8:955–968.

Cheeke, P.R., and N.M. Patton. 1978. Effect of alfalfa and dietary fiber on the growth performance of weanling rabbits. Lab. Anim. Sci. 28:167–172.

Chesney, R.W. 1987. New functions for an old molecule. Pediatric Res. 22:755–759.

Chu, S.-H.W., and R.P. Geyer. 1983. Tissue content and metabolism of myo-inositol in normal and lipodystrophic gerbils. J. Nutr. 113:293–303.

DeLucchi, C., M.L. Pita, M.J. Faus, J.A. Molina, R. Uauy, and A. Gil. 1987. Effects of dietary nucleotides on the fatty acid composition of erythrocyte membrane lipids in term infants. J. Pediatr. Gastro. Nutr. 6:568–574.

Dufour, C., G. Dandrifosse, P. Forget, F. Vermesse, N. Romain, and P. Lepoint. 1988. Spermine and spermidine induce intestinal maturation in the rat. Gastroenterology 95:112–116.

Engel, A.G., and C. Angelini. 1973. Carnitine deficiency of human skeletal muscle with associated lipid storage myopathy: a new syndrome. Science 179:899–902.

Feller, A.G., and D. Rudman. 1988. Role of carnitine in human nutrition. J. Nutr. 118:541–547.

Gaull, G.E. 1982. Taurine in the nutrition of the human infant. Acta Paediatr. Scand., Suppl. 296:38–40.

Greene, D.A., P.V. De Jesus, Jr., and A.I. Winegrad. 1975. Effects of insulin and dietary myoinositol on impaired peripheral motor nerve conduction velocity in acute streptozotocin diabetes. J. Clin. Invest. 55:1326–1336.

Hayes, K.C. 1985. Taurine requirements in primates. Nutr. Rev. 43:65–70.

Hegsted, D.M., K.C. Hayes, A. Gallagher, and H. Hanford. 1973. Inositol deficiency: an intestinal lipodystrophy in the gerbil. J. Nutr. 103:302–307.

Hegsted, D.M., A. Gallagher, and H. Hanford. 1974. Inositol requirement of the gerbil. J. Nutr. 104:588–592.

Herbert, V.D. 1988. Pseudovitamins. Pp. 471–477 in M.E. Shils and V.R. Young, eds. Modern Nutrition in Health and Disease, 7th ed. Lea & Febiger, Philadelphia.

Holub, B.J. 1982. The nutritional significance, metabolism and function of myo-inositol and phosphatidylinositol in health and disease. Pp. 107–141 in H.H. Draper, ed. Advances in Nutritional Research, Vol. 4. Plenum Press, New York.

Jaeger, L.A., C.H. Lamar, G.D. Bottoms, and T.R. Cline. 1987. Growth-stimulating substances in porcine milk. Am. J. Vet. Res. 48:1531–1533.

Järvenpää, A.-L., D.K. Rassin, N.C.R. Raiha, and G.E. Gaull. 1982. Milk protein quantity and quality in the term infant. II. Effects on acidic and neutral amino acids. Pediatrics 70:221–230.

Järvenpää, A.-L., N.C.R. Raiha, D.K. Rassin, and G.E. Gaull. 1983. Feeding the low-birth-weight infant: 1. Taurine and cholesterol supplementation of formula does not affect growth and metabolism. Pediatrics 71:171–178.

Jope, R.S., E.F. Domino, B.N. Mathews, N. Sitaram, D.J. Jenden, and A. Ortez. 1982. Free and bound choline blood levels after phosphatidylcholine. Clin. Pharmacol. Ther. 31:483–487.

Kuksis, A., and S. Mookerjea. 1984. Choline. Pp. 383–399 in R.E. Olson, ed. Present Knowledge in Nutrition, 5th ed. The Nutrition Foundation, Washington, D.C.

Kulkarni, A.D., W.C. Fanslow, F.B. Rudolph, and C.T. Van Buren. 1987. Modulation of delayed hypersensitivity in mice by dietary nucleotide restriction. Transplantation 44:847–849.

Lewin, L.M., and R. Beer. 1973. Prostatic secretion as the source of myo-inositol in human seminal fluid. Fertil. Steril. 24:666–670.

Lofgren, P.A., P.S. Reyes, K.W. McNutt, G.M. Briggs, and G.O. Kohler. 1974. Unidentified growth factor(s) present in alfalfa water-solubles for young guinea pigs. Proc. Soc. Exp. Biol. Med. 147:331–336.

Mayer, J.H., and D.R. Tomlinson. 1983. Prevention of defects of anoxal transport and nerve conduction velocity by oral administration of myo-inositol or an aldose reductase inhibitor in streptozotocin-diabetic rats. Diabetologia 25:433–438.

Middleton, A., and B.P. Setchell. 1972. The origin of inositol in the rete testis fluid of the ram. J. Reprod. Fertil. 30:473–475.

Nielsen, F.H. 1988. Possible future implications of ultratrace elements in human health and disease. Pp. 277–292 in A.S. Prasad, ed. Essential and Toxic Trace Elements in Human Health and Disease. Current Topics in Nutrition and Disease, Vol. 18. Alan R. Liss, New York.

Nielsen, F.H., C.D. Hunt, L.M. Mullen, and J.R. Hunt. 1987. Effect of boron on mineral, estrogen, and testosterone metabolism in postmenopausal women. FASEB J. 1:394.

Okamoto, E., D.K. Rassin, C.L. Zucker, G.S. Salen, and W.C. Heird. 1984. Role of taurine in feeding the low-birth-weight infant. J. Pediatr. 104:936–940.

Olson, A.L., S.E. Nelson, and C.J. Rebouche. 1989. Low carnitine intake and altered lipid metabolism in infants. Am. J. Clin. Nutr. 49:624–628.

Prentki, M., and F. M. Matschinsky. 1987. Ca^{2+}, cAMP, and phospholipid-derived messengers in coupling mechanisms of insulin secretion. Physiol. Rev. 67:1186–1235.

Quick, A.J. 1975. The correlated actions of vitamin C, K, and Q. Life Sci. 16:1017–1024.

Rebouche, C.J. 1986. Is carnitine an essential nutrient for humans? J. Nutr. 116:704–706.

Schwarz, K., and D.B. Milne. 1972. Growth-promoting effects of silicon in rats. Nature 239:333–334.

Shils, M.E., and V.R. Young, eds. 1988. Modern Nutrition in Health and Disease, 7th ed. Lea & Febiger, Philadelphia.

Strecker, A. 1862. Uber einige neue Bestandtheile der Schweingalle. Ann. Chem. Pharmacie. 123:353–360.

Sturman, J.A. 1988. Taurine in development. J. Nutr. 118:1169–1176.

Weaver, L.T., M.F. Laker, R. Nelson, and A. Lucas. 1987. Milk feeding and changes in intestinal permeability and morphology in the newborn. J. Pediat. Gastr. Nutr. 6:351–358.

Welsch, F. 1978. Choline metabolism in the human term placenta—studies on de novo synthesis and the effects of some drugs on the metabolic fate of [N-methyl-^{3}H] choline. Biochem. Pharmacol. 27:1231–1257.

Winegrad, A.I., and D.A. Greene. 1976. Diabetic polyneuropathy: the importance of insulin deficiency, hyperglycemia and alterations in myoinositol metabolism in its pathogenesis. N. Engl. J. Med. 295:1416–1421.

Wright, C.E., H. H. Tallan, Y.Y. Lin, and G.E. Gaull. 1986. Taurine: biological update. Ann. Rev. Biochem. 55:427–454.

Wurtman, R.J. 1979. Sources of choline and lecithin in the diet. Pp. 73–81 in A. Barbeau, J.H. Growdon, and R.J. Wurtman, eds. Nutrition and the Brain. Vol. 5. Choline and Lecithin in Brain Disorders. Raven Press, New York.

Zeisel, S.H. 1981. Dietary choline: biochemistry, physiology, and pharmacology. Annu. Rev. Nutr. 1:95–121.

Zeisel, S.H. 1988. "Vitamin-like" molecules. (A) Choline. Pp. 440–452 in M.E. Shils and V.R. Young, eds. Modern Nutrition in Health and Disease, 7th ed. Lea & Febiger, Philadelphia.

Index

SUMMARY TABLE   Estimated Safe and Adequate Daily Dietary Intakes of Selected Vitamins and Minerals[a]

Category	Age (years)	Vitamins	
		Biotin (μg)	Pantothenic Acid (mg)
Infants	0–0.5	10	2
	0.5–1	15	3
Children and	1–3	20	3
adolescents	4–6	25	3–4
	7–10	30	4–5
	11 +	30–100	4–7
Adults		30–100	4–7

Category	Age (years)	Trace Elements[b]				
		Copper (mg)	Man-ganese (mg)	Fluoride (mg)	Chromium (μg)	Molybdenum (μg)
Infants	0–0.5	0.4–0.6	0.3–0.6	0.1–0.5	10–40	15–30
	0.5–1	0.6–0.7	0.6–1.0	0.2–1.0	20–60	20–40
Children and	1–3	0.7–1.0	1.0–1.5	0.5–1.5	20–80	25–50
adolescents	4–6	1.0–1.5	1.5–2.0	1.0–2.5	30–120	30–75
	7–10	1.0–2.0	2.0–3.0	1.5–2.5	50–200	50–150
	11 +	1.5–2.5	2.0–5.0	1.5–2.5	50–200	75–250
Adults		1.5–3.0	2.0–5.0	1.5–4.0	50–200	75–250

[a] Because there is less information on which to base allowances, these figures are not given in the main table of RDA and are provided here in the form of ranges of recommended intakes.

[b] Since the toxic levels for many trace elements may be only several times usual intakes, the upper levels for the trace elements given in this table should not be habitually exceeded.